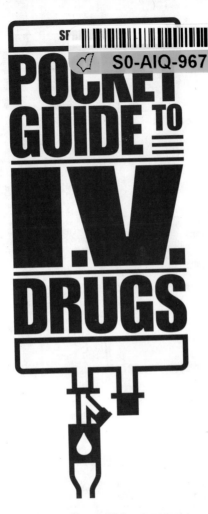

Dawn M. Philp, RN
Deborah L. Walz, RN

Springhouse Corporation
Springhouse, Pennsylvania

Staff

Publisher
Donna O. Carpenter, ELS

Editorial Director
William J. Kelly

Clinical Director
Ann M. Barrow, RN, MSN, CCRN

Creative Director
Jake Smith

Design Director
John Hubbard

Art Director
Elaine Kasmer Ezrow

Drug Information Editor
Lisa Truong, RPh, PharmD

Senior Associate Editor
Karen C. Comerford

Clinical Editor
Eileen Cassin Gallen, RN, BSN

Editors
Kevin D. Dodds, Catherine E. Harold

Copy Editors
Leslie Dworkin, Beth Pitcher

Designers
Arlene Putterman (Associate Design Director), Joseph John Clark, Jeff Sklarow, Donald G. Knauss

Typographers
Diane Paluba (manager), Joyce Rossi Biletz

Manufacturing
Deborah Meiris (director), Patricia K. Dorshaw (manager), Otto Mezei (book production manager)

Editorial Assistants
Arlene P. Claffee, Carol A. Caputo

Indexer
Barbara Hodgson

The clinical procedures described and recommended in this publication are based on research and consultation with nursing, medical, pharmaceutical, and legal authorities. To the best of our knowledge, these procedures reflect currently accepted practice; nevertheless, they can't be considered absolute and universal recommendations. For individual application, all recommendations must be considered in light of the patient's clinical condition and, before the administration of new or infrequently used drugs, in light of the latest package-insert information. The authors and publisher disclaim responsibility for adverse effects resulting directly or indirectly from the suggested procedures, from undetected errors, or from the reader's misunderstanding of the text.

A member of the Reed Elsevier plc group

Visit our Web site at www.eDrugInfo.com
ISBN 1-58255-044-1
PGIVD-D
02 01 00 99 10 9 8 7 6 5 4 3 2 1

Library of Congress Cataloging-in-Publication Data
Philp, Dawn N.
Pocket guide to I.V. drugs/Dawn M. Philp, Deborah L. Walz.
p. ; cm.
Includes index.
1. Intravenous therapy—Handbooks, manuals, etc. 2. Drugs—Handbooks, manuals, etc.
3. Nursing—Handbooks, manuals, etc. I. Walz, Deborah L. II. Title.
[DNLM: 1. Infusions, Intravenous—methods—Handbooks. WB 39 P571p2000]
RM170 .P487 2000
615'.6—dc21
ISBN 1-58255-044-1 (OTA binding : flexible cover : alk. paper)

99-052578

Contents

Consultants

Ruthie Bach, RN, MSN, CEN, CCRN
Emergency Staff Nurse
St. Elizabeth Hospital
Adjunct Faculty
Lamar University
Beaumont, Tex.

Shirley H. Brownell, RN,C, BSN
Clinical Team Coordinator
Bassett Health Care
Cooperstown, N.Y.

Karen T. Bruchak, RN, MSN
Director of Nursing, Medical Surgical & Specialty Unit
Mercy Fitzgerald Hospital
Darby, Pa.

Lawrence Carey, PharmD
Clinical Pharmacist Coordinator
Jefferson Home Infusion Service
Thomas Jefferson University Hospital
Philadelphia

Ellie Franges, RN, MSN, CNRN, CCRN
Director, Neuroscience Services
Sacred Heart Hospital
Allentown, Pa.

Anne Marie Frey, RN, BSN, CRNI
Clinical Nurse IV, I.V. Team
The Children's Hospital of Philadelphia

Colleen M. Fries, RN, BSN, CCRN
Clinical Leader
Abington (Pa.) Memorial Hospital

Bridget A. Haupt, PharmD
Director of Pharmacy
Children's Seashore House
Philadelphia

James A. Koestner, PharmD
Clinical Pharmacist, Trauma/Critical Care
Vanderbilt University Hospital
Nashville, Tenn.

Tamara Luedtke, RN, MSN, CCRN
Nurse Manager, Critical Care Unit
Hendrick Medical Center
Abilene, Tex.

Nancy F. Martin, RN
Independent Consultant
Wilmington, Del.

Kathleen A. McGrory, RN
Clinical Support Coordinator of Infusion Services
Jefferson Home Infusion Service
Bryn Mawr, Pa.

George Melko, PharmD
Clinical Pharmacist
Jefferson Home Infusion Service
Thomas Jefferson University Hospital
Philadelphia

Cathy Sellergren, RN, MSN, CCRN
Pulmonary Case Manager
Hinsdale (Ill.) Hospital

Kenneth K. Weiland, PharmD
Clinical Coordinator
Chestnut Hill Healthcare
Philadelphia

Preface

Today's health care professionals are awash in information. We have more data available to us from a wider range of sources than ever. What's more, our collective knowledge of health disorders and the drugs used to treat them continues to grow by leaps and bounds.

Bountiful information seems like a boon. But, in fact, it's a mixed blessing. The information in some sources may be less than reliable. The presentation isn't always convenient or practical. And few of us have the time to wade through all the facts to get to the pearls needed for daily practice.

That's why we created this book. Frankly, we set out to simplify our own lives as emergency department nurses by collecting the most pertinent information about I.V. drugs into a single, easy-to-use reference. The number of I.V. drugs currently available—and the rate by which this number grows each year—make it nearly impossible, and certainly dangerous, to rely on memory when preparing and administering these drugs.

Now, we don't have to—and neither do you. In this handy volume, truly a pocket-size book, you'll find up-to-date, practical, easy-to-use information about the most important and most common I.V. drugs available today. Designed for working professionals like us, it's organized alphabetically by generic drug name. For each drug, we've included what we consider to be the most essential information: trade names, therapeutic classes, pregnancy risk category, controlled substance schedule (when applicable), indications, dosages, storage and preparation tips, administration guidelines, and special considerations crucial for delivering safe, high quality patient care.

What started as a project to make our professional lives easier has become the book you now hold in your hands. It has indeed made our lives easier. We know it will do the same for you.

Dawn M. Philp, RN
Kaiser Permanente Emergency Department
San Diego, Calif.

Deborah L. Walz, RN
Kaiser Permanente Emergency Department
San Diego, Calif.

How to use this book

The *Pocket Guide to I.V. Drugs* brings you hands-on, need-to-know information about nearly 300 of the most important and commonly used I.V. drugs. Plus, the book is organized and designed to help you quickly find the most critical, practical information about each drug. For instance, the drugs are organized alphabetically by generic name. Next to each generic name, you'll find selected trade names. Just below that, you'll see the drug's therapeutic class, its pregnancy risk category and, where applicable, its controlled substance schedule.

Pregnancy risk categories: For each drug, you'll find the FDA's designated pregnancy risk category:

- A: Adequate studies in pregnant women have failed to show a risk to the fetus.
- B: Animal studies have not shown a risk to the fetus, but controlled studies have not been conducted in pregnant women; or animal studies have shown an adverse effect on the fetus, but adequate studies in pregnant women have not shown a fetal risk.
- C: Animal studies have shown an adverse effect on the fetus, but adequate studies have not been conducted in humans. The benefits may be acceptable despite potential risks.
- D: The drug may pose risks to the human fetus, but potential benefits may be acceptable despite the risks.
- X: Studies in animals or humans show fetal abnormalities, or reports of adverse reactions indicate evidence of fetal risk. The risks involved clearly outweigh the potential benefits.
- NR: Not rated.

Controlled substance schedules: When appropriate, you'll see the controlled substance schedule for a particular drug:

- I: High abuse potential, no accepted medical use.
- II: High abuse potential, severe dependence liability.
- III: Less abuse potential than schedule II drugs, moderate dependence liability.
- IV: Less abuse potential than schedule III drugs, limited dependence liability.
- V: Limited abuse potential.

Three-column format

The first column in each drug entry lists the drug's major indications and the most common dosages ordered for each indication.

The second column provides important instructions for storing the drug safely, reconstituting and diluting it before administration, and administering it by direct injection, intermittent infusion, and continuous infusion, as applicable.

The third column gives you key considerations to remember when administering the drug, including which adverse reactions to watch for, what to do if they arise, which tests and laboratory values to monitor during therapy, what to do in case of overdose or extravasation, and more.

Appendices and index

Finally, the appendices offer practical, helpful reference material for anyone who administers I.V. drugs. You'll find handy tables on infusion rates for dobutamine, dopamine, epinephrine, isoproterenol, nitroglycerin, and nitroprusside; the major electrolyte components of I.V. solutions; and antidotes for vesicant extravasation. The appendices also include nomograms for estimating surface area in adults and children.

If you're looking for a drug using its generic name, of course, you can find it quickly because of the book's A-to-Z organization. If you're looking up a drug by its trade name—or if you want to search for drugs by their indications—you can flip to the book's thorough index. Either way, you'll quickly and easily find the information you need to deliver the drug safely and correctly.

A guide to abbreviations

ABG	arterial blood gas
ACE	angiotensin-converting enzyme
AIDS	acquired immunodeficiency syndrome
ALT	alanine aminotransferase
APTT	activated partial thromboplastin time
AST	aspartate aminotransferase
AV	atrioventricular
b.i.d.	twice daily
BUN	blood urea nitrogen
C	Centigrade
CBC	complete blood count
CK	creatine kinase
CMV	cytomegalovirus
CNS	central nervous system
CO_2	carbon dioxide
COPD	chronic obstructive pulmonary disease
CSF	cerebrospinal fluid
CV	cardiovascular
CVA	cerebrovascular accident
D_5W	dextrose 5% in water
dl	deciliter
ECG	electrocardiogram
EEG	electroencephalogram
F	Fahrenheit
FDA	Food and Drug Administration
g	gram
G	gauge
GI	gastrointestinal
GU	genitourinary
H_1	histamine$_1$
H_2	histamine$_2$
HIV	human immunodeficiency virus
hr	hour
h.s.	at bedtime
ICU	intensive care unit
IgG	immunoglobulin G
I.M.	intramuscular
INR	international normalized ratio
IU	international unit
I.V.	intravenous
kg	kilogram
L	liter
lb	pound
M	molar
m^2	square meter
MAO	monoamine oxidase
mcg	microgram
mEq	milliequivalent
mg	milligram
MI	myocardial infarction
ml	milliliter
mm^3	cubic millimeter
mmol	millimole
NaCl	sodium chloride
ng	nanogram
NSAID	nonsteroidal anti-inflammatory drug
OTC	over the counter
oz	ounce
P.O.	by mouth
p.r.n.	as needed
PT	prothrombin time
PTT	partial thromboplastin time
PVC	premature ventricular contraction
q	every
q.d.	every day
q.i.d.	four times daily
RBC	red blood cell
RDA	recommended daily allowance
S.C.	subcutaneous
SIADH	syndrome of inappropriate antidiuretic hormone
T_3	triiodothyronine
T_4	thyroxine
t.i.d.	three times daily
U	units
USP	United States Pharmacopeia
UTI	urinary tract infection
WBC	white blood cell

COMMON INDICATIONS AND DOSAGES	ADMINISTRATION	SPECIAL CONSIDERATIONS

abciximab • ReoPro

Class: ***platelet aggregation inhibitor*** • *Pregnancy risk category C*

Adjunct to percutaneous transluminal coronary angioplasty or atherectomy for preventing acute ischemic complications in patients at high risk for abrupt closure of a treated coronary vessel.
Adults: 0.25 mg/kg as an I.V. bolus 10 to 60 minutes before the start of angioplasty or atherectomy, followed by a continuous I.V. infusion of 10 mcg/minute for 12 hr. The patient should also receive heparin and aspirin.

Available in 5-ml vials at a concentration of 2 mg/ml.
Incompatibilities: None reported, but don't add any drugs to the infusion solution.
Direct injection: Withdraw needed amount through a sterile, nonpyrogenic, low protein-binding 0.2- or 0.22-micron filter into syringe.
Continuous infusion: Withdraw 4.5 ml of drug through a sterile, nonpyrogenic, low protein-binding, 0.2- or 0.22-micron filter. Mix with 250 ml of sterile 0.9% NaCl or D_5W. Inspect for particulates before using and discard solution if they appear. Don't freeze or shake. Store at 36° to 46° F (2° to 8° C). Infuse at 10 mcg/minute for 12 hr in separate I.V. line with continuous infusion pump and in-line filter. Discard unused portion.

- Avoid noncompressible I.V. sites.
- Before infusion, check platelet count, PT, and APTT. Monitor platelet count, activated clotting time, and APTT during and after treatment.
- Institute bleeding precautions. Keep patient on bed rest for 6 to 8 hr after sheath is removed or infusion stopped, whichever is later. Minimize or avoid arterial and venous punctures, I.M. injections, urinary catheters, nasogastric tubes, automatic blood pressure cuffs, and nasotracheal intubation.
- Consider saline or heparin lock for drawing blood.
- Document and monitor vascular puncture sites.

acetazolamide sodium • Diamox◆

Classes: ***antiglaucoma agent, diuretic*** • *Pregnancy risk category C*

To rapidly lower intraocular pressure or when patient can't take drug orally.
Adults: 500 mg I.V., repeated in 2 to 4 hr if necessary. Therapy is usually continued with 125-250 mg P.O. q 4 to 6 hr, based on response.
Acute glaucoma. *Children:* 5 to 10 mg/kg I.V. q 6 hr.
As a diuretic. *Adults:* 5 mg/kg I.V. p.r.n.
Children: 5 mg/kg or 150 mg/m^2 I.V. once daily in morning for 1 or 2 days alternated with a drug-free day.

Available as powder in 500-mg vials. Reconstitute with 5 ml of sterile water for injection to provide a solution containing no more than 100 mg/ml. Use right away, if possible, or refrigerate and use within 24 hr.
Incompatibilities: Diltiazem and multivitamins.
Direct injection: Using a 21G or 23G needle, inject 100 to 500 mg/minute into a large vein.

- Give drug under continuous medical supervision. I.V. administration reduces intraocular pressure rapidly.
- Carefully monitor patient's intake, output, and serum electrolytes, especially potassium.
- Weigh patient daily. Elderly patients are especially susceptible to excessive diuresis.
- If patient has COPD, monitor arterial blood gases for respiratory acidosis.

acyclovir sodium (acycloguanosine) • Avirax◇, Zovirax◆

Class: ***antiviral*** • *Pregnancy risk category C*

Mucocutaneous herpes simplex virus (I and II) infections in immunocompromised patients with normal renal function. *Adults:* 5 mg/kg q 8 hr for 7 days. *Infants and children under age 12:* 250 mg/m^2 q 8 hr for 7 days.

Initial herpes genitalis in patients with normal renal function. *Adults:* 5 mg/kg q 8 hr for 5 days. *Children under age 12:* 250 mg/m^2 q 8 hr for 5 days.

Herpes simplex encephalitis. *Adults:* 10 mg/kg q 8 hr for 10 days. *Children ages 6 months to 12 years:* 500 mg/m^2 q 8 hr for 10 days.

Varicella zoster in immunocompromised patients. *Adults:* 10 mg/kg q 8 hr for 7 days (with normal renal function). *Children under age 12:* 500 mg/m^2 q 8 hr for 7 days.

Dosage adjustment. Dosage in renal failure is based on creatinine clearance. For adults, give 50% of dose q 24 hr if clearance is less than 10 ml/minute; 100% of dose q 24 hr if 10 to 25 ml/minute; 100% of dose q 12 hr if 25 to 50 ml/minute; and 100% of dose q 8 hr if clearance exceeds 50 ml/minute.

Available as powder in 10- and 20-ml sterile vials (equivalent to 500 and 1,000 mg of acyclovir, respectively). Store at 59° to 77° F (15° to 25° C). To reconstitute, add 10 ml of sterile water for injection to the 10-ml vial and 20 ml to the 20-ml vial to yield a concentration of 50 mg/ml. Precipitates may form if solution is refrigerated and will dissolve when returned to room temperature. Once reconstituted, drug should be used within 12 hr.

Incompatibilities: Biological solutions, colloidal solutions, and idarubicin. May precipitate when combined with parabens.

Intermittent infusion: Dilute reconstituted drug with at least 70 ml of commercially available electrolyte and glucose solution for a concentration of 7 mg/ml or less. Higher concentrations can cause phlebitis. Use within 24 hr. Administer over at least 1 hr using an intermittent infusion device or an I.V. line containing a free-flowing, compatible solution. Shorter infusion times risk nephrotoxicity.

- Use drug for infusion only. Avoid rapid infusion or bolus I.V. injection.
- Carefully monitor patient's intake and output. Because maximum drug concentration occurs in kidneys during first 2 hr of infusion, make sure that patient has adequate hydration and urine output during this period.
- Notify doctor if an increased serum creatinine level fails to return to normal within a few days. He may increase hydration, adjust dosage, or stop therapy.
- To treat overdose, make sure patient has enough urine output to prevent precipitation in renal tubules: 500 ml/g or more of drug infused. Drug also can be removed by hemodialysis.

◆ Also available in Canada. ◇ Available in Canada only.

COMMON INDICATIONS AND DOSAGES	ADMINISTRATION	SPECIAL CONSIDERATIONS
adenosine • Adenocard		
Class: ***antiarrhythmic*** • *Pregnancy risk category C*		
Conversion of paroxysmal supraventricular tachycardia to sinus rhythm. *Adults:* 6 mg I.V. by bolus injection over 1 to 2 seconds. If arrhythmia remains after 1 to 2 minutes, give 12 mg by rapid I.V. push. Repeat 12-mg dose once if necessary. Adenosine also can be used to treat Wolff-Parkinson-White syndrome (paroxysmal supraventricular tachycardia with accessory bypass tracts).	Available in vials containing 6 mg/2 ml. Store at controlled room temperature of 59° to 86° F (15° to 30° C). Inspect solution for crystals, which may appear if solution has been refrigerated. If crystals are visible, gently warm solution to room temperature. Don't use solutions that aren't clear. Discard unused drug because it lacks preservatives. ***Incompatibilities:*** Don't mix with other drugs. ***Direct injection:*** Administer rapidly over 1 to 2 seconds directly into a peripheral vein, if possible; if using an I.V. line, use the most proximal port and follow the injection with a rapid saline flush to hasten drug delivery to systemic circulation.	• Drug must reach systemic circulation in sufficient quantity to provide an adequate therapeutic effect. Therefore, rapid I.V. bolus injection is necessary. • Single doses over 12 mg aren't recommended. • Bolus dosages of 6 or 12 mg usually don't elicit systemic hemodynamic effects. • Adverse effects usually resolve quickly once injection is discontinued. • Give drug only under medical supervision with continuous ECG monitoring. Watch for arrhythmias.
alatrofloxacin mesylate • Trovan I.V.		
Class: ***antibiotic*** • *Pregnancy risk category C*		
Nosocomial pneumonia, gynecologic and pelvic infections, and complicated intra-abdominal infections, including postsurgical infections. *Adults:* 300 mg I.V. daily followed by 200 mg P.O. daily for 7 to 14 days (10 to 14 days for pneumonia). **Community-acquired pneumonia and complicated skin and skin-structure infections, including diabetic foot infections but not osteomyelitis.** *Adults:* 200 mg I.V. daily followed by 200 mg P.O. daily for 7 to 14 days (10 to 14 days for complicated skin and skin-structure infections).	Available as 40-ml and 60-ml vials that contain 5 mg/ml (200 and 300 mg, respectively). These single-use vials must be diluted with D_5W or 0.45% NaCl before administration. Don't dilute with 0.9% NaCl or lactated Ringer's solution. Follow package insert when preparing desired dosage. ***Incompatibilities:*** Don't mix with other drugs or infuse simultaneously through an I.V. line used for another drug, especially one that contains multivalent cations (such as magnesium). If the same I.V. line is used for sequential infusion of different drugs, flush the line before and after each infusion. ***Intermittent infusion:*** Administer diluted solution over 60 minutes by direct infusion or through a Y-type I.V. infusion set. Avoid rapid bolus administration or infusion.	• Check patient's liver function tests periodically, as ordered, to detect increases in ALT, AST, and alkaline phosphatase levels. • Moderate to severe phototoxicity reactions have occurred in patients exposed to direct sunlight. • No dosage adjustment is necessary when switching from I.V. to oral form. • If *Pseudomonas aeruginosa* is the known or presumed pathogen, the patient may receive combination therapy with an aminoglycoside or aztreonam.

Prophylaxis of infection after elective colorectal surgery or vaginal and abdominal hysterectomy. *Adults:* 200 mg I.V as a single dose 30 minutes to 4 hr before surgery.
Dosage adjustment. If patient has mild to moderate cirrhosis (Child-Pugh Class A or B), reduce 300-mg I.V. dose to 200 mg and 200-mg I.V. dose to 100 mg.

albumin (normal human serum albumin) • Albuminar-5, Albuminar-25, Albutein 5% and 25%, Buminate 5% and 25%, Plasbumin-5, Plasbumin-25◆

Class: ***plasma protein*** • *Pregnancy risk category C*

Shock. *Adults:* 25 g given over 15 to 30 minutes and repeated if no response. Thereafter, dosage reflects patient condition. Maximum of 125 g/day for up to 2 days (5 liters of 5% solution or 1 liter of 25% solution). *Children:* 25 g over 15 to 30 minutes. *Premature infants:* 1 g/kg. *Adults with nephrosis:* 25 to 50 g repeated q 1 to 2 days.
Hypoproteinemia. *Adults:* 50 to 75 g of 25% solution daily. *Children:* 25 g/day.
Burns. *Adults:* Amount sufficient to maintain serum albumin at 2 to 3 g/dl. Dosage varies with extent of burns, protein loss, denuded skin areas, and decreased albumin synthesis (which may persist for 60 days).
Preoperative adjunct in cardiopulmonary bypass. *Adults:* Amount sufficient to maintain serum albumin at 2 to 3 g/dl.

Available in sterile, nonpyrogenic vials packed with infusion kits; 5% solution supplied in 50-, 250-, 500-, and 1,000-ml vials and 25% solution in 20-, 50-, and 100-ml vials. Store below 99° F (37° C), but don't freeze. Discard unused portion after 4 hr.
Incompatibilities: Verapamil hydrochloride.
Intermittent infusion: Infuse at rate appropriate to patient's condition, usually over 15 to 30 minutes. For plasma volume expansion, don't exceed 2 to 4 ml/minute with 5% solution or 1 ml/minute with 25% solution. For hypoproteinemia, don't exceed 5 to 10 ml/minute with 5% solution or 2 to 3 ml/minute with 25% solution. For hypertension or mild to moderate cardiac failure, infuse 10% solution slowly.
Continuous infusion: Add 25% solution to 500 to 1,000 ml of D_5W or 0.9% NaCl. To obtain 10% solution, dilute 1 part 25% solution in 1.5 parts dextrose 10% in water. Infuse diluted solution slowly and adjust to patient response and blood pressure changes.

- Minimize allergic reactions by giving antihistamines, as ordered, before infusion and by slowing infusion rate.
- Albumin includes no clotting factors and may be administered regardless of patient's blood type or Rh factor.
- One volume of 25% albumin is equivalent to five volumes of 5% albumin in producing hemodilution and relative anemia.
- Sodium content (130 to 160 mEq/L) may require reduced dose if patient is on sodium-restricted diet.
- 5% albumin is isotonic and 25% albumin is hypertonic, equivalent to five times the normal oncotic pressure.
- Monitor vital signs before, during, and after infusion. Also monitor serum albumin, total protein, hemoglobin, electrolyte, and hematocrit levels.
- Watch closely for signs of circulatory overload.
- Check intake and output, and report changes in output. Increased colloid pressure mobilizes extracellular fluid, causing diuresis for 3 to 20 hr.

(continued)

◆ Also available in Canada. ◇ Available in Canada only.

COMMON INDICATIONS AND DOSAGES | **ADMINISTRATION** | **SPECIAL CONSIDERATIONS**

albumin *(continued)*

Hyperbilirubinemia. *Premature infants:* 4 ml (1 g)/kg or 120 ml (30 g)/m^2 of 25% solution given 1 to 2 hr before transfusion. *Premature infants with low serum protein levels:* 1.4 to 1.8 ml/kg of 25% solution.

aldesleukin (IL-2, interleukin-2) • Proleukin

Class: ***immunoregulator*** • *Pregnancy risk category C*

Metastatic renal cell carcinoma. *Adults ages 18 and over:* 600,000 IU/kg (0.037 mg/kg) infused over 15 minutes q 8 hr for 5 days (total of 14 doses). Repeat after a 9-day rest. Can repeat again at least 7 weeks after hospital discharge. Or give 18 million IU (1.1 mg)/m^2 of body surface area by 24-hr continuous infusion for 5 days. Repeat in 1 week.

Available as a powder for injection containing 22 million IU (1.3 mg) per vial. Reconstitute by adding 1.2 ml of sterile water for injection; resulting solution contains 18 million IU (1.1 mg)/ml. To avoid excessive foaming, direct water diluent toward side of vial and swirl gently; don't shake. The reconstituted drug should be particle-free and colorless to slightly yellow. Store powder for injection and reconstituted solutions in the refrigerator. To dilute, add the ordered dose of reconstituted drug to 50 ml of 5% dextrose injection, preferably in a plastic container for more consistent drug delivery. After reconstitution and dilution, drug must be administered within 48 hr. Discard unused drug. Return solution to room temperature before administration.

Incompatibilities: Albumin, bacteriostatic water for injection, and 0.9% NaCl. Avoid mixing with other drugs.

Intermittent infusion: Infuse diluted dose over 15 minutes without an in-line filter.

Continuous infusion: Give diluted solution over 24 hr.

- Be prepared to adjust dosages of patient's other drugs to compensate for aldesleukin-induced renal and hepatic impairment.
- Severe anemia or thrombocytopenia may occur. Administer packed RBCs or platelets as ordered.
- Withhold dose and notify doctor if patient develops moderate to severe lethargy or somnolence; continued administration can lead to coma.
- Drug has been linked to capillary leak syndrome (CLS), a condition in which loss of vascular tone allows plasma proteins and fluids into the extravascular space. Mean arterial blood pressure begins to drop within 2 to 12 hr of treatment; edema and effusions may be severe, and death can result from hypoperfusion of major organs.
- Treat CLS with careful monitoring of fluid status, pulse, mental status, urine output, central venous pressure, and organ perfusion.

alfentanil hydrochloride • Alfenta◆

Classes: ***analgesic, anesthetic*** • *Pregnancy risk category C* • *Controlled substance schedule II*

Adjunct to general anesthesia. *Adults:* Initially, 8 to 20 mcg/kg; then increments of 3 to 15 mcg/kg.
Primary anesthesia. *Adults:* Initially, 130 to 245 mcg/kg; then 0.5 to 1.5 mcg/kg/minute.
Monitored anesthesia care. *Adults:* Initially, 3 to 8 mcg/kg; then increments of 3 to 5 mcg/kg q 5 to 20 minutes to a total dose of 3 to 40 mcg/kg.
Dosage adjustment. Dose should be reduced in elderly or debilitated patients.

Only staff trained in administering I.V. anesthetics and managing their adverse effects should give this drug. It's available in ampules of 2, 5, 10, or 20 ml at a concentration of 500 mcg/ml. Drug may be injected full strength using a tuberculin or 1-ml syringe. Store undiluted drug between 59° and 86° F (15° and 30° C). Protect from light and don't freeze.
Incompatibilities: None reported.
Direct injection: Over 90 seconds to 3 minutes, inject undiluted drug into I.V. tubing of a free-flowing, compatible solution.
Continuous infusion: Dilute in 0.9% NaCl, D_5W, dextrose 5% in 0.9% NaCl, or lactated Ringer's solution. Using an I.V. piggyback, infuse at ordered rate through tubing containing a free-flowing, compatible solution.

- Closely monitor patient's respiratory, CV, and neurologic systems during and after surgery.
- Stop drug 10 to 15 minutes before end of surgery.
- Periodically monitor postoperative vital signs and bladder function.
- Patient may need analgesics shortly after surgery.
- For overdose, reverse effects with naloxone and then give symptomatic care. For apnea, administer oxygen and provide mechanical ventilation. Use positive-pressure ventilation via bag or mask. For hypotension, give I.V. fluids and vasopressors. For muscle rigidity, give a neuromuscular blocking drug.

alprostadil (prostaglandin E_1) • Prostin VR Pediatric◆

Class: ***prostaglandin derivative*** • *Pregnancy risk category NR*

Temporary maintenance of ductus arteriosus patency until surgery can be performed. *Neonates:* 0.05 to 0.1 mcg/kg/minute, not to exceed 0.4 mcg/kg/minute. When therapeutic response is achieved, reduce dosage to lowest level that maintains response.

Only staff trained in pediatric intensive care should give this drug. To prepare, dilute 1 ml (500 mcg/ml) in 25 to 250 ml of 0.9% NaCl or D_5W to yield a concentration of 20 to 2 mcg/ml. Don't use a diluent that contains benzyl alcohol because fatal toxic syndrome could result. Store solution at 36° to 46° F (2° to 8° C). Don't freeze. Use prepared solution within 24 hr.
Incompatibilities: None reported.
Continuous infusion: Using a continuous-rate pump, infuse drug through a large peripheral or central vein or through an umbilical artery catheter placed at the level of ductus arteriosus.

- Patients with low partial pressure of oxygen values respond best.
- Drug must be given before ductus closes to maintain patency.
- Infusion may continue during cardiac catheterization.
- Monitor respiratory status during treatment and keep resuscitation equipment readily available. Apnea usually occurs in first hr of infusion in 10% to 12% of neonates who weigh less than 2 kg at birth.
- Monitor arterial pressure by umbilical artery catheter, auscultation, or Doppler transducer.
- Expect to reduce the infusion rate if hypotension, bradycardia, apnea, or fever develops.
- In infants with restricted pulmonary blood flow,

(continued)

◆ Also available in Canada. ◇ Available in Canada only.

COMMON INDICATIONS AND DOSAGES	ADMINISTRATION	SPECIAL CONSIDERATIONS
alprostadil *(continued)*		measure drug's effectiveness by monitoring blood oxygenation. In infants with restricted systemic blood flow, measure drug's effectiveness by monitoring systemic blood pressure and blood pH. • If flushing occurs from peripheral vasodilation, catheter may require repositioning.

alteplase (recombinant alteplase, tissue plasminogen activator, t-PA) • Activase♦

Class: ***thrombolytic*** • *Pregnancy risk category C*

COMMON INDICATIONS AND DOSAGES	ADMINISTRATION	SPECIAL CONSIDERATIONS
Destruction of coronary artery thrombi in acute MI. *Adults who weigh 143 lb (65 kg) or more:* 100 mg over 3 hr, with 60 mg given in first hr (6 to 10 mg in first 1-2 minutes), 20 mg in second hr, and 20 mg in third hr. Doses above 100 mg have been linked with intracranial bleeding. *Adults who weigh less than 143 lb:* 1.25 mg/kg over 3 hr, with 60% of dose given in first hr (10% in first 1 to 2 minutes) and remainder over next 2 hr. **Accelerated dosing for acute MI.** *Adults who weigh more than 148 lb (67 kg):* 15 mg by rapid I.V. bolus over 1 to 2 minutes, then 50 mg I.V. over the next 30 minutes, followed by 35 mg I.V. over 1 hr for a total dosage of 100 mg. *Adults who weigh 148 lb or less:* 15 mg by rapid I.V. bolus over 1 to 2 minutes; followed by 0.75 mg/kg (not to exceed 50 mg) over the next 30 minutes; then 0.5 mg/kg (not to exceed 35 mg) over the next hr. **Acute ischemic stroke within 3 hr of**	Available as lyophilized powder in 20-, 50-, and 100-mg vials. Store at room temperature or refrigerate. Reconstitute just before injection. Using an 18G needle, reconstitute to 1 mg/ml by adding 50 ml (50-mg vial) or 100 ml (100-mg vial) of preservative-free, sterile water for injection, provided by manufacturer. (Do not use bacteriostatic water for injection.) Aim diluent at lyophilized cake and expect slight foaming. Let vial stand for several minutes. If necessary, dilute drug to 0.5 mg/ml in glass bottle or polyvinyl chloride bag. Avoid undue agitation. Diluted solution remains stable for 8 hr at room temperature. ***Incompatibilities:*** Don't mix with other drugs. ***Direct injection:*** Bolus doses can be administered over 1 to 2 minutes. ***Continuous infusion:*** Infuse diluted solution at recommended rate.	• Recanalization of occluded coronary arteries and improvement of heart function require that treatment start within 6 to 12 hr after onset of symptoms. Treatment of acute ischemic stroke must begin within 3 hr after onset. • If possible, obtain coagulation studies (PT, PTT, INR, fibrin split products) before starting therapy. • Have antiarrhythmic drugs readily available, and carefully monitor ECG. • To prevent new clot formation (except in ischemic stroke), give heparin during or after alteplase infusion, if ordered. • Avoid venipuncture and arterial puncture during therapy because of increased risk of bleeding. If arterial puncture is necessary, select a site on an arm and apply pressure for 30 minutes afterward. Also, use pressure dressings, sandbags, or ice packs on recent puncture sites to prevent bleeding. • Avoid I.M. injections because of high risk of bleeding into muscle. Also, avoid turning and moving the patient excessively during infusion. • If unable to stop severe bleeding with local pressure, discontinue alteplase and heparin infusions.

symptom onset. *Adults:* 0.9 mg/kg (maximum, 90 mg) I.V. infusion over 1 hr, with 10% of the dose given as an I.V. bolus during the first minute.
Lysis of acute pulmonary emboli. *Adults:* 100 mg over 2 hr.

amifostine • Ethyol

Class: ***cytoprotective agent*** • *Pregnancy risk category C*

Reduction of cumulative renal toxicity from repeated administration of cisplatin in patients with advanced ovarian cancer or non-small-cell lung cancer. *Adults:* 910 mg/m^2/day as a 15-minute I.V. infusion starting 30 minutes before chemotherapy. If hypotension develops and blood pressure fails to return to normal within 5 minutes after treatment stops, give 740 mg/m^2 during later cycles.

Supplied as a sterile lyophilized powder in 10-ml, single-use vials. Each vial contains 500 mg of amifostine (anhydrous basis) and 500 mg of mannitol. Reconstitute with 9.7 ml of normal saline solution. Resulting solution is stable for up to 5 hr at room temperature (about 77° F [25° C]) or up to 24 hr if refrigerated at 35° to 46° F (1.7° to 8° C). Don't use if solution becomes cloudy or you see precipitates.
Incompatibilities: Unknown, but don't mix with other solutions.
Intermittent infusion: Infuse over 15 minutes. Longer infusion can lead to increased adverse reactions.

- Patient should be adequately hydrated before administration.
- Administer antiemetic drug before and with amifostine.
- Keep patient in a supine position during infusion.
- Monitor blood pressure every 5 minutes during infusion.
- Monitor serum calcium levels in patients at risk for hypocalcemia such as those with nephrotic syndrome.
- The most common symptom of overdose is hypotension, which should be treated with supportive measures.

amikacin sulfate • Amikin◆

Class: ***antibiotic*** • *Pregnancy risk category D*

Septicemia, peritonitis, and severe infections of burns, bones, joints, respiratory tract, skin, or soft tissue caused by susceptible organisms. *Adults and children with normal renal function:* 15 mg/kg/day in equally divided doses at 8- or 12-hr intervals for 7 to 10 days, not to exceed 1.5 g/day.

Available as a 50 mg/ml concentration in 2-ml vials or as a 250 mg/ml concentration in 2- and 4-ml vials. Diluted solutions remain stable for 24 hr at room temperature. Yellowing of solution doesn't indicate loss of potency.
Incompatibilities: Amphotericin B, bacitracin, cephalothin, cephapirin, cisplatin, heparin, phenytoin, thiopental, vancomycin, and vitamin B complex with C. Manufacturer recommends not mixing with other drugs.

- Drug may contain sulfites.
- Evaluate patient's hearing before and during treatment.
- Obtain periodic peak and trough levels, and adjust dosage as ordered.
- Keep patient well hydrated to reduce risk of nephrotoxicity. Measure intake and output and monitor

(continued)

◆ Also available in Canada. ◇ Available in Canada only.

COMMON INDICATIONS AND DOSAGES	ADMINISTRATION	SPECIAL CONSIDERATIONS
amikacin sulfate *(continued)* **Dosage adjustment.** *Adults and children with renal impairment:* Loading dose of 7.5 mg/kg, adjusted based on serum levels and degree of impairment. *Neonates with normal renal function:* Initially 10 mg/kg, then 7.5 mg/kg q 12 hr.	***Intermittent infusion:*** Add 500 mg of amikacin to 100 to 200 ml of 0.9% NaCl or D_5W. Infuse diluted drug over 30 to 60 minutes in adults and children, over 1 to 2 hr in infants.	urine for decreased specific gravity. • Be alert to loss of balance in ambulatory patients who receive drug for more than 2 weeks. • For overdose, patient may receive hemodialysis, peritoneal dialysis, or (for a neonate) exchange transfusions.

amino acid injection • Aminosyn◆, BranchAmin, FreAmine◆, HepatAmine, NephrAmine, Novamine, ProcalAmine, RenAmin, Travasol◆, TrophAmine

Classes: ***parenteral nutritional therapy, caloric agent*** • *Pregnancy risk category C*

COMMON INDICATIONS AND DOSAGES	ADMINISTRATION	SPECIAL CONSIDERATIONS
Total parenteral nutrition for patients who can't or won't eat. *Adults:* 1 to 1.5 g/kg daily. *Children over 22 lb (10 kg):* 20 to 25 g daily for the first 10 kg, plus 1 to 1.25 g/kg daily for each kilogram over 10 kg. *Children under 22 lb:* 2 to 4 g/kg daily. **Nutritional support for patients with cirrhosis, hepatitis, or hepatic encephalopathy.** *Adults:* 80 to 120 g of amino acids (12 to 18 g of nitrogen) daily of the formulation for hepatic failure. **Nutritional support for patients with high metabolic stress.** *Adults:* 1.5 g/kg daily of the formulation for high metabolic stress. **Nutritional support for patients with renal failure.** *Adults:* 0.3 to 0.5 g/kg daily (to 26 g daily). Patients on dialysis may require 1 to 1.2 g/kg daily. **Dosage adjustment.** Adjust dosage as needed based on nitrogen balance and body weight corrected for fluid balance.	Available in bottles containing 250 to 1,000 ml. Dextrose 5% to 70% in water, electrolytes, trace elements, and vitamins, may be added as needed. When modifying solutions, use strict aseptic technique, follow manufacturer's instructions, and administer within 24 hr. Discard remaining solution. Use only clear solution; hold up to light to find precipitate or evidence of damaged container. ***Incompatibilities:*** Bleomycin, ganciclovir, and indomethacin sodium trihydrate. Because of the high risk of incompatibility with other substances, add only required nutritional products. ***Continuous infusion:*** Infuse over 8 hr based on patient tolerance. For severely debilitated patients or those who need long-term parenteral nutrition, give hypertonic solutions (more than 12.5% dextrose) via subclavian catheter into the superior vena cava. For moderately debilitated patients, administer solutions mixed with D_5W or dextrose 10% in water via peripheral route.	• Begin with a 5% to 10% dextrose concentration and gradually increase to hypertonicity if needed. • Special solutions can be prepared by the pharmacy for patients with specific nutrient requirements or intolerance to the components of conventional solutions. For example, solutions are available for patients with renal or hepatic failure. • Monitor serum electrolytes, BUN, and renal and liver function studies. Check serum calcium frequently. Check blood glucose every 6 hr to guide dosage of dextrose and insulin (if required). • If flow rate lags behind ordered rate, don't try to catch up by increasing beyond original order. • Monitor patient for signs of fluid overload. • Check infusion site frequently. Change peripheral I.V. site every 48 hr or according to facility policy to prevent irritation and infection.

aminocaproic acid • Amicar◆

Class: ***fibrinolysis inhibitor*** • *Pregnancy risk category C*

Life-threatening hemorrhage caused by systemic hyperfibrinolysis from complications of cardiac surgery and portacaval shunt; cancer of the lung, prostate, cervix, or stomach; abruptio placentae; hematologic disorders, such as aplastic anemia; and urinary fibrinolysis from severe trauma, shock, and anoxia. *Adults:* 4 to 5 g over 1 hr, then either 1 to 1.25 g hourly, or a continuous infusion of 1 g/hr for about 8 hr to maintain plasma level of 130 mcg/ml. Maximum 30 g/day. *Children:* 100 mg/kg or 3 g/m^2 of body surface area during first hr, then continuous infusion of 33 mg/kg/hr or 1 g/m^2/hr. Maximum 18 g/m^2/day.

Available in 250 mg/ml solutions containing 5 g (20 ml) or 24 g (96 ml) with benzyl alcohol. Dilute with 0.9% NaCl, D_5W, lactated Ringer's solution, or sterile water for injection. (Don't use sterile water for injection if patient has subarachnoid hemorrhage.) Store at 59° to 86° F (15° to 30° C) and protect from freezing.
Incompatibilities: Fructose solution.
Continuous infusion: Slowly infuse 4 to 5 g of diluted drug during first hr. Then infuse 1 g/hr to maintain serum level of 130 mcg/ml.

- Monitor patient for changes in coagulation studies, heart rhythm, and blood pressure.
- Guard against thrombophlebitis by using proper technique for needle insertion and positioning.
- Rapid infusion may cause hypotension and bradycardia.
- Drug has been used as antidote for alteplase, anistreplase, streptokinase, and urokinase. It isn't beneficial in treating thrombocytopenia.

aminophylline

Class: ***bronchodilator*** • *Pregnancy risk category C*

Acute bronchial asthma and reversible bronchospasm caused by chronic bronchitis and emphysema. *Adults not currently receiving theophylline:* Initially 6 mg/kg, then maintenance doses. For nonsmoking adults, 0.7 mg/kg/hr for first 12 hr, then 0.5 mg/kg/hr for next 12 hr. For elderly patients and those with cor pulmonale, 0.6 mg/kg/hr for first 12 hr, then 0.3 mg/kg/hr for next 12 hr. For patients with heart failure or liver failure, 0.5 mg/kg/hr for first 12 hr, then 0.1 to

Available as a 25 mg/ml solution in 10-ml (250 mg) and 20-ml (500 mg) ampules. Store at room temperature and protect from freezing and light. Inspect for precipitate and discoloration before use.
Incompatibilities: Amikacin, amiodarone, ascorbic acid, bleomycin, cephalothin, cephapirin, chlorpromazine, ciprofloxacin, clindamycin phosphate, codeine phosphate, corticotropin, dimenhydrinate, dobutamine, doxapram, doxorubicin, epinephrine hydrochloride, erythromycin gluceptate, fat emulsion 10%, fructose 10% in 0.9% NaCl, hydralazine, hydroxyzine hydrochloride, insulin (regular), invert sugar 10% in 0.9% NaCl injection, invert sugar 10% in water, levor-

- Base dosage on lean body weight and serum theophylline level. Monitor serum trough levels to manage regimen; monitor serum peak levels to assess for toxicity. Optimum therapeutic levels, 10 to 20 mcg/ml.
- I.V. administration can cause vein irritation and burning. Dilute with compatible solution if necessary.
- Warn elderly patient that dizziness, a common adverse reaction, may occur at the start of therapy.
- For overdose, stop drug immediately and provide

(continued)

◆ Also available in Canada. ◇ Available in Canada only.

COMMON INDICATIONS AND DOSAGES	ADMINISTRATION	SPECIAL CONSIDERATIONS
aminophylline *(continued)* 0.2 mg/kg/hr for next 12 hr. *Children not currently receiving theophylline:* Initially 6 mg/kg, then maintenance doses. For children ages 6 months to 9 years, 1.2 mg/kg/hr for first 12 hr, then 1 mg/kg/hr for next 12 hr. For children ages 9 to 16, 1 mg/kg/hr for first 12 hr, then 0.8 mg/kg/hr for next 12 hr. *Adults and children currently receiving theophylline:* dosage form, amount, time, and administration rate of last theophylline dose determine initial aminophylline dose. Ideally, initial dose should be deferred until serum theophylline level can be obtained. If the patient is in respiratory distress, a loading dose of 2.5 mg/kg may be given.	phanol, meperidine, methadone, methylprednisolone sodium succinate, morphine sulfate, nafcillin, norepinephrine, ondansetron, papaverine, penicillin G potassium, pentazocine lactate, phenobarbital sodium, phenytoin sodium, procaine, prochlorperazine edisylate, promazine, promethazine hydrochloride, vancomycin, verapamil, and vitamin B complex with C. ***Direct injection:*** Give undiluted loading dose (25 mg/ml) slowly, not exceeding 25 mg/minute. Don't use a central venous catheter because rapid injection can be fatal. ***Continuous infusion:*** For maintenance therapy, give desired dose in a large volume (500 to 1,000 ml) of compatible solution. Adjust infusion rate to deliver prescribed amount each hr.	supportive and symptomatic treatment. Avoid giving sympathomimetic drugs.

amiodarone hydrochloride • Cordarone◆

Class: ***ventricular and supraventricular antiarrhythmic*** • *Pregnancy risk category C*

COMMON INDICATIONS AND DOSAGES	ADMINISTRATION	SPECIAL CONSIDERATIONS
Prevention and treatment of frequently recurring ventricular fibrillation and hemodynamically unstable ventricular tachycardia in patients unresponsive to other therapy or who can't take the oral form. *Adults:* Rapid loading infusion of 150 mg over 10 minutes (15 mg/minute), then a slow loading phase of 1 mg/minute over 6 hr (total of 360 mg), followed by a maintenance phase of 0.5 mg/minute for 18 hr (total of 540 mg). After the first 24 hr, continue	Available in 3-ml ampules at a concentration of 50 mg/ml. Store at room temperature and protect from light. Dilute before use. ***Incompatibilities:*** Aminophylline, cefamandole, cefazolin, heparin sodium, mezlocillin, quinidine gluconate, and sodium bicarbonate. ***Direct injection:*** For rapid loading dose, dilute 150 mg of drug in 100 ml D_5W and give initial bolus over 10 minutes. ***Continuous infusion:*** For maintenance infusion, final concentrations can range from 1 to 6 mg/ml. Administer with a volumetric infusion pump and an in-line filter. Use a central venous catheter when possible.	• Little is known about effects of using I.V. amiodarone for more than 3 weeks. • Monitor ECG continuously for AV block, bradycardia, paradoxical arrhythmias, and prolonged QT segments. • Assess respiratory system for pulmonary toxicity. • Monitor for dry eyes, halo vision, and photophobia. • For overdose, give symptomatic and supportive care. Monitor ECG and blood pressure. If needed, give an I.V. beta-adrenergic antagonist (such as isoproterenol) or assist with transvenous pacemaker insertion to treat bradycardia. Infuse I.V. fluids and use the

the maintenance infusion of 0.5 mg/minute or increase it to control arrhythmia.

Trendelenburg position to correct hypotension. Give an I.V. vasopressor or inotropic drug (such as norepinephrine or dopamine) to improve tissue perfusion.

ammonium chloride

Class: ***acidifying agent*** *• Pregnancy risk category B*

Metabolic alkalosis caused by chloride loss from vomiting, gastric suctioning, pyloric stenosis, gastric fistula drainage, or diuretic use. *Adults:* Dosage is calculated by the amount of chloride deficit and estimated in milliequivalents. First, estimate patient's fluid volume by multiplying 20% of body weight in kilograms by serum chloride level. For example, in a patient weighing 154 lb (70 kg) with a chloride level of 94 mEq/ml, multiply 14 by 94 for a dosage of 1,316 mEq. One liter of 2.14% solution provides 400 mEq of ammonium and chloride ions.

Prepare diluted solution by adding one or two vials (100 or 200 mEq) of aqueous ammonium chloride to 500 or 1,000 ml of 0.9% NaCl for injection. Also available as prepared solution in a 500-ml bottle containing 2.14 g/dl (0.4 mEq/ml). Solution may crystallize if stored at low temperature. Crystals will dissolve when solution is placed in warm water.

Incompatibilities: Alkalis and their carbonates, dimenhydrinate, levorphanol, methadone, and strong oxidizing agents such as potassium chloride.

Continuous infusion: Infuse diluted solution at no more than 5 ml/minute to avoid pain, toxic effects, and local irritation. Infuse the 2.14% solution at 0.9 to 1.3 ml/minute (but always under 2 ml/minute). Start infusion at half the calculated rate to determine patient tolerance.

- Assess for pain at infusion site and adjust rate if necessary.
- Assess respiratory pattern frequently.
- To prevent acidosis, determine serum electrolyte levels during therapy.
- Monitor input and output, edema, weight, and urine pH during therapy. Expect diuresis for the first 2 days.
- For overdose, stop drug and give potassium chloride or sodium bicarbonate I.V. for acidosis. Signs of overdose include arrhythmias, asterixis, bradycardia, coma, Kussmaul's respirations, pallor, local or generalized twitching, sweating, tonic seizures, and vomiting.

amobarbital sodium • Amytal Sodium◆

Classes: ***anticonvulsant, sedative-hypnotic*** *• Pregnancy risk category D • Controlled substance schedule II*

Agitation in psychoses, insomnia, seizures, and status epilepticus. *Adults and children over age 6 when used as a hypnotic or anticonvulsant:* Dosage varies by patient from 65 to 500 mg, not to exceed 1 g.

To prepare the standard 100-mg/ml (10%) injection, dissolve 250 or 500 mg of sterile powder in 2.5 or 5 ml of sterile water, respectively, for injection. Rotate the ampule to mix; don't shake it. If the solution becomes cloudy after 5 minutes, discard it. Drug breaks down in solution or on exposure to air. Drug also precipitates if diluent pH is 9.2 or less. Give within 30 minutes of reconstitution.

Incompatibilities: Cefazolin, cephalothin, chlorpromazine, cimetidine, clindamycin, droperidol, isoproterenol, metaraminol, methyldopate, norepinephrine, penicillin G, pen-

- I.V. route typically used only in emergencies. Give drug only to hospitalized patients under close observation and respiratory monitoring. Keep resuscitation equipment available.
- Barbiturates potentiate narcotic effect. If given during labor, reduce narcotic dose to lessen risk of neonatal respiratory depression.
- Don't give drug within 24 hr of liver function test.
- Monitor PT carefully when patient starts or ends an-

(continued)

◆ Also available in Canada. ◇ Available in Canada only.

COMMON INDICATIONS AND DOSAGES	ADMINISTRATION	SPECIAL CONSIDERATIONS
amobarbital sodium *(continued)*	tazocine lactate, propiomazine, succinylcholine, and thiamine. ***Direct injection:*** Don't exceed 100 mg/minute for adults or 60 mg/m²/minute for children. Avoid extravasation, which can cause necrosis.	ticoagulant therapy. Anticoagulant dose may need adjustment. • Signs of overdose include clammy skin, cyanosis, hypotension, constricted pupils, and coma. If they occur, maintain airway and, if needed, provide ventilatory support. Monitor vital signs and fluid balance. Forced diuresis may help remove drug if patient has normal renal function; hemodialysis or hemoperfusion may help as well.

amphotericin B • Fungizone◆

Class: ***antifungal*** • *Pregnancy risk category B*

COMMON INDICATIONS AND DOSAGES	ADMINISTRATION	SPECIAL CONSIDERATIONS
Systemic fungal infection (aspergillosis, blastomycosis, candidiasis, coccidioidomycosis, cryptococcosis, histoplasmosis, and phycomycosis). *Adults and children:* Test dose of 1 mg in 20 ml of D_5W given over 20 to 30 minutes, followed by 0.25 mg/kg over 6 hr (3 to 4 hr if tolerated). Dosage increased gradually based on patient tolerance and severity of infection to a maximum of 1 mg/kg/day. Dosage must never exceed 1.5 mg/kg/day. If discontinued for 1 week or more, therapy resumes with initial dose and gradually increases again. Therapy may last for months.	For 50-mg vial, reconstitute with 10 ml of sterile (not bacteriostatic) water for injection. Shake until solution clears. Dilute in 500 ml of D_5W with a pH above 4.2. Final concentration will be 0.1 mg/ml. Store concentrate at room temperature for 24 hr or refrigerate for 1 week. When diluted, use drug promptly. Protect from light until ready to hang. ***Incompatibilities:*** 0.9% NaCl, amikacin, calcium chloride, calcium gluceptate, chlorpromazine, cimetidine, diphenhydramine, edetate calcium disodium, gentamicin, kanamycin, lactated Ringer's solution, melphalan, metaraminol, methyldopate, paclitaxel, penicillin G potassium, penicillin G sodium, polymyxin B, potassium chloride, prochlorperazine mesylate, streptomycin, and verapamil. ***Continuous infusion:*** Administer 500 ml of diluted solution over 3 to 6 hr. In-line filter should have a pore diameter exceeding 1 micron. Because severe adverse reactions can occur, stay with home care patient throughout infusion.	• Monitor patient's vital signs q 30 minutes for 4 hr at start of therapy. Fever may arise 1 to 2 hr after start of infusion; it should subside within 4 hr after stopping drug. • Adding a small amount of heparin (1,200 to 1,600 U) to solution may lessen risk of thrombophlebitis. • Antihistamines, antipyretics, corticosteroids, and antiemetics may be ordered to prevent adverse reactions. • Monitor intake and output, serum potassium and magnesium levels, and hemoglobin and hematocrit. • For overdose, stop therapy, monitor patient's clinical status, and give supportive therapy. Drug can't be removed by dialysis.

amphotericin B cholesteryl sulfate complex • Amphotec

Class: ***antifungal*** • *Pregnancy risk category B*

Invasive aspergillosis in patients not eligible for amphotericin B deoxycholate because of failed previous therapy, renal impairment, or unacceptable toxicity. *Adults and children:* For new courses of treatment, test dose of 10 ml of final drug preparation (1.6 to 8.3 mg of drug) over 15 to 30 minutes. If no adverse reaction after 30 minutes, 3 to 4 mg/kg/day. Can increase to 6 mg/kg/day if no improvement or if infection progresses.

Available in preservative-free, 50- and 100-mg lyophilized powder vials. Store at room temperature. Reconstitute by rapidly adding 10 ml of sterile water for injection to 50-mg vial or 20 ml to 100-mg vial with a sterile syringe and 20G needle. Shake vial gently. Don't use any other diluent. Reconstituted drug is clear or opalescent and stable for 24 hr when refrigerated. Discard partially used vials. Dilute to final concentration of about 0.6 mg/ml (0.16 to 0.83 mg/ml) with D_5W. Final product is stable for 24 hr when refrigerated. Don't freeze. Don't filter or use an in-line filter.
Incompatibilities: Bacteriostatic agents, electrolyte solutions, and saline solution.
Intermittent infusion: Infuse over at least 2 hr. Don't mix with other drugs. If given through an existing I.V. line, flush with D_5W before infusion or use a separate line.
Continuous infusion: Administer by continuous infusion at rate of 1 mg/kg/hr. Infusion time can be lengthened based on tolerance.

- To help reduce acute infusion-related reactions, pretreat or promptly treat with antihistamines and corticosteroids, reduce the rate of infusion, or both.
- Monitor patient's vital signs every 30 minutes during initial therapy.
- Monitor intake and output, renal and hepatic function tests, CBC, PT, and serum electrolytes, especially potassium, magnesium, and calcium.
- For overdose, stop therapy, monitor clinical status, and give supportive therapy. Drug can't be removed by dialysis.

ampicillin sodium • Ampicin◇, Omnipen-N

Class: ***antibiotic*** • *Pregnancy risk category B*

Systemic, respiratory tract, skin, GI, and acute urinary tract infections.
Adults: 250 to 500 mg q 6 hr. In more severe infections, 500 mg q 6 hr. *Children:* 25 to 50 mg/kg q 6 hr.
Bacterial meningitis. *Adults:* 1 to 2.5 g q 3 to 4 hr for 3 days, then give I.M. *Children:* 12.5 to 50 mg/kg q 3 to 4 hr for 3 days, then give I.M.

Supplied in vials containing 125 mg, 250 mg, 500 mg, 1 g, and 2 g. Reconstitute by adding 5 ml of sterile water for injection to the 125-, 250-, or 500-mg vial; 7.5 ml to the 1-g vial; or 10 ml to the 2-g vial. Dilute for infusion with 50 or 100 ml 0.9% NaCl, D_5W, dextrose 5% and 0.45% NaCl, invert sugar 10% and water, 1/6 M sodium lactate, lactated Ringer's solution, or sterile water for injection. Concentration of the drug should not exceed 30 mg/ml. Solution remains stable for 2 to 4 hr in dextrose solutions and for up to 8 hr in other solutions

- Obtain specimens for culture and sensitivity testing before giving first dose. Therapy may start before results are available.
- Intermittent infusion reduces risk of vein irritation.
- Monitor hematologic and renal function studies during therapy.
- Monitor for signs of bacterial or fungal superinfection.

(continued)

◆ Also available in Canada. ◇ Available in Canada only.

COMMON INDICATIONS AND DOSAGES	ADMINISTRATION	SPECIAL CONSIDERATIONS
ampicillin sodium *(continued)* **Dosage adjustment.** In adult patients with creatinine clearance of 10 ml/minute or less, increase dosage interval to q 12 hr.	when refrigerated. When frozen, drug is stable for 30 days. Allow solution to thaw for 8 hr before administration. ***Incompatibilities:*** Amikacin, amino acid solutions, chlorpromazine, dextran solutions, dopamine, erythromycin lactobionate, 10% fat emulsions, fructose, gentamicin, heparin sodium, hetastarch, hydrocortisone sodium succinate, hydromorphone, kanamycin, lidocaine, lincomycin, polymyxin B, prochlorperazine edisylate, sodium bicarbonate, and streptomycin. ***Direct injection:*** Inject reconstituted drug into a large vein or cannula over 10 to 15 minutes. After injection, flush cannula with 0.9% NaCl. ***Intermittent infusion:*** Give diluted solution through I.V. piggyback or cannula over 30 to 60 minutes.	• Discontinue drug if patient develops acute interstitial nephritis, bone marrow depression, or pseudomembranous colitis.

ampicillin sodium/sulbactam sodium • Unasyn

Class: ***antibiotic*** *• Pregnancy risk category B*

COMMON INDICATIONS AND DOSAGES	ADMINISTRATION	SPECIAL CONSIDERATIONS
Peritonitis and gynecologic, skin, and skin-structure infections caused by susceptible organisms. *Adults:* 1.5 g (1 g ampicillin, 0.5 g sulbactam) to 3 g (2 g ampicillin, 1 g sulbactam) q 6 hr, not to exceed 4 g/day of sulbactam. **Dosage adjustment.** Dosage in renal failure is based on creatinine clearance. In adults, give 1.5 to 3 g q 6 to 8 hr if creatinine clearance exceeds 29 ml/minute; 1.5 to 3 g q 12 hr if 15 to 29 ml/minute; or 1.5 to 3 g q 24 hr if 5 to 14 ml/minute.	Available in 1.5- and 3-g vials and in piggyback vials. Reconstitute with sterile water for injection to yield a concentration of 375 mg/ml. For infusion, immediately dilute reconstituted solution with compatible diluent to yield 3 to 45 mg/ml. Storage times reflect diluent and concentration. Using sterile water for injection or 0.9% NaCl injection, a 45-mg/ml solution remains stable for 8 hr at 77° F (25° C) and 48 hr at 39° F (4° C); a 30-mg/ml solution remains stable for 72 hr at 39° F. Using D_5W, a 30-mg/ml solution is stable for 2 hr at 77° F and 24 hr at 39° F. Using lactated Ringer's solution, a 45-mg/ml solution remains stable for 8 hr at 77° F and 24 hr at 39° F. Other compatible diluents include dextrose 5% and 0.45% NaCl or 10% invert sugar. ***Incompatibilities:*** Amikacin, amino acid solutions, chlorpromazine, dextran solutions, dopamine, erythromycin lactobionate, 10% fat emulsions, fructose, gentamicin, heparin	• Obtain specimens for culture and sensitivity testing before administering first dose. Therapy may start before results of tests are known. • Give ampicillin sulbactam at least 1 hr before bacteriostatic antibiotics. • If patient has renal impairment, monitor for signs of toxicity. • Discontinue drug if patient develops acute interstitial nephritis, bone marrow depression, or pseudomembranous colitis. • Observe patient for fungal and bacterial superinfection with large doses or prolonged use. • For overdose, patient may undergo hemodialysis.

sodium, hetastarch, hydrocortisone sodium succinate, kanamycin, lidocaine, lincomycin, netilmicin, polymyxin B, prochlorperazine edisylate, sodium bicarbonate, streptomycin, and tobramycin.

Direct injection: Inject reconstituted drug into large vein or cannula over at least 10 to 15 minutes. Then flush with 0.9% NaCl.

Intermittent infusion: After diluting reconstituted drug (usually in 100 ml of solution), infuse over 15 to 30 minutes.

amrinone lactate • Inocor◆

Classes: ***inotropic, vasodilator*** • *Pregnancy risk category C*

Short-term management of heart failure, primarily in patients unresponsive to cardiac glycosides, diuretics, and vasodilators. *Adults:* initially, 0.75 mg/kg given over 2 to 3 minutes, followed by 200 mg in 100 ml of 0.9% NaCl given at 5 to 10 mcg/kg/minute. If needed, additional bolus of 0.75 mg/kg can be given 30 minutes after therapy starts. Dosages should be individualized based on patient response. Maximum daily dosage is 10 mg/kg. Steady-state plasma level should be maintained at 3 mcg/ml.

Available in 20-ml ampules of clear yellow solution containing 5 mg/ml. Protect ampules from light and store at room temperature. Don't use if solution is discolored or has precipitates. Administer undiluted or dilute in 0.45% or 0.9% NaCl. Concentrations of 1 to 3 mg/ml remain stable for 24 hr.

Incompatibilities: Bicarbonate, dextrose-containing solutions, furosemide, and glucose.

Direct injection: Inject diluted or undiluted drug into vein or I.V. tubing containing a free-flowing, compatible solution. Avoid extravasation. After injection, flush with 0.9% NaCl.

Continuous infusion: Dilute with NaCl to 1 to 3 mg/ml. May be piggybacked into line close to insertion site containing D_5W. Infusion rate should be controlled by pump.

- Don't use drug in patients hypersensitive to bisulfites.
- Because amrinone may increase ventricular response rate, patients with atrial fibrillation or flutter may require concomitant therapy with cardiac glycosides.
- During infusion, check vital signs every 5 to 15 minutes. If blood pressure drops, slow or stop infusion and notify doctor.
- Carefully monitor fluid and electrolyte levels, hepatic and renal function, and platelet count. Expect to decrease dosage if platelet count drops below 150,000/mm^3.
- For overdose, reduce infusion rate and treat hypotension symptomatically.

anistreplase (anisoylated plasminogen-streptokinase activator complex, APSAC) • Eminase◆

Class: ***thrombolytic enzyme*** • *Pregnancy risk category C*

Lysis of coronary artery thrombi following acute MI. *Adults:* 30 U I.V. injection.

Available in vials containing 30 U. Refrigerate at 36° to 46° F (2° to 8° C). Reconstitute by slowly directing 5 ml of sterile water for injection at the side of the vial, not at the drug itself. Gently roll the vial to mix, don't shake to avoid foaming.

- Give drug within 6 hr after onset of symptoms.
- Monitor for reperfusion arrhythmias, such as sinus bradycardia, accelerated idioventricular rhythm,

(continued)

◆ Also available in Canada. ◇ Available in Canada only.

COMMON INDICATIONS AND DOSAGES	ADMINISTRATION	SPECIAL CONSIDERATIONS
anistreplase *(continued)*	Solution should be colorless to pale yellow. Inspect for precipitate. Discard drug if not administered within 30 minutes of reconstituting. Don't dilute it. ***Incompatibilities:*** Don't mix with other drugs. ***Direct injection:*** Inject drug over 2 to 5 minutes into an I.V. line or vein.	ventricular tachycardia, and PVCs. Have emergency treatment readily available. • If arterial puncture is necessary, select a compressible site and apply pressure for 30 minutes afterward. Use pressure dressings, sandbags, or ice packs on recent punctures to prevent bleeding. • Avoid I.M. injections because of the risk of bleeding into muscle. Also, avoid turning and moving the patient excessively.

antihemophilic factor (AHF, factor VIII) • Hemofil M, Humate-P, Koate HP♦, Monoclate-P

Class: ***antihemophilic*** • *Pregnancy risk category C*

COMMON INDICATIONS AND DOSAGES	ADMINISTRATION	SPECIAL CONSIDERATIONS
The following dosages provide guidelines. Refer to specific brand for actual dosing. **Mild bleeding.** *Adults and children:* 8 to 15 IU/kg daily for 2 to 3 days. **Moderate bleeding and minor surgery.** *Adults and children:* Initially, 15 to 25 IU/kg, then 10 to 15 IU/kg q 8 to 12 hr p.r.n. **Severe bleeding and bleeding near vital organs.** *Adults and children:* Initially, 40 to 50 IU/kg, then 20 to 25 IU/kg q 8 to 12 hr p.r.n. **Major surgery.** *Adults and children:* 40 to 50 IU/kg 1 hr before surgery, then 20 to 25 IU/kg 5 hr after first dose.	Available in a kit that includes a single-dose vial with diluent, sterile needles for reconstitution and withdrawal, a winged infusion set with microbore tubing, and alcohol swabs. Refrigerate unreconstituted drug, but avoid freezing. Reconstitute by using the double-ended needle to transfer diluent into vial (drawn in by vacuum). Gently swirl vial until contents dissolve. Use within 3 hr. ***Incompatibilities:*** None reported. ***Direct injection:*** Using a plastic syringe (concentrate may adhere to glass) and the winged infusion set, inject into vein at 2 ml/minute. Consult specific product information; some can be given at a rate of 10 ml/minute.	• Product is a sterile, lyophilized concentrate of factor VIII:C (coagulant portion of factor VIII complex) and small amounts of factor VIII:R (responsible for von Willebrand's factor activity). • Drug provides hemostasis in factor VIII deficiency (hemophilia A). Dosage based on patient's weight, severity of hemorrhage, and presence of inhibitors. Mild bleeding episodes require a circulating factor VIII:C level of 30% or more of normal. Moderate bleeding episodes and minor surgery require 30% to 50% of normal. Severe bleeding or major surgery require 80% to 100% of normal. • I.V. administration of 1 IU/kg increases circulating antihemophilic activity by about 2%. • Tell patient to notify doctor if drug seems less effective. It could signal formation of antibodies.

anti-inhibitor coagulant complex • Autoplex T, Feiba VH Immuno

Class: ***hemostatic*** • *Pregnancy risk category C*

Prevention and control of hemorrhage in some patients with hemophilia A in whom inhibitor antibodies to antihemophilic factor have developed; management of bleeding in patients with acquired hemophilia who have spontaneously acquired inhibitors to factor VII. *Adults and children:* Dosage is highly individualized and varies among manufacturers. For Autoplex T, 25 to 100 U/kg I.V.; if no hemostatic improvement within 6 hr after initial dose, repeat. For Feiba VH Immuno, 50 to 100 U/kg I.V. q 6 or 12 hr until patient shows signs of improvement. Maximum daily dosage of Feiba VH Immuno is 200 U/kg.

Available in a package containing a vial of dry concentrate, a vial of sterile water for injection, a double-ended transfer needle, and a filter needle. Refrigerate vials before use. To reconstitute, bring vials to room temperature and follow manufacturer's instructions. If drawing more than 1 vial into a syringe, use a new filter needle for each vial. Don't refrigerate after reconstitution. Use Autoplex T within 1 hr and Feiba VH Immuno within 3 hr. Otherwise, patient will become hypotensive from increased prekallikrein activator.

Incompatibilities: None reported, but don't mix with any other drugs or solutions.

Direct injection: Inject Autoplex T directly into vein at 2 ml/minute, increasing to 10 ml/minute based on patient tolerance. Stop if patient develops a headache, flushing, or change in pulse or blood pressure. Resume at slower rate when symptoms disappear. Inject Feiba VH Immuno no faster than 2 U/kg/minute.

Intermittent infusion: Not recommended for Autoplex T. For Feiba VH Immuno, follow manufacturer's instructions for using the administration set. Use a standard blood filter and infuse at no faster than 2 U/kg/minute.

- Although treated to minimize viral transmission, anti-inhibitor coagulant complex has a small risk of transmitting severe infection, such as hepatitis and HIV. If patient is negative for hepatitis B surface antigen, encourage hepatitis B vaccination.
- Before therapy, verify that patient has a diagnosed clotting deficiency caused by factor VIII inhibitors.
- Keep epinephrine available to treat anaphylaxis.
- Watch for signs of intravascular coagulation, such as dyspnea, chest pain, cough, and changes in pulse and blood pressure. If they appear, stop and check lab indicators, such as prolonged thrombin, PT, and APTT; reduced fibrinogen levels and platelet count; and the presence of fibrin split products.

antithrombin III, human • ATnativ, Thrombate III

Classes: ***anticoagulant, antithrombotic*** • *Pregnancy risk category C*

Hereditary antithrombin III deficiency, surgery, obstetric procedures, or thromboembolism. *Adults and children:* Initial dose is calculated based on amount needed to increase antithrombin III activity to 120% of normal at 30 minutes after

Available as a lyophilized powder in 50-ml infusion bottles containing 500 or 1,000 IU of antithrombin III. Store at 36° to 46° F (2° to 8° C). Reconstitute using 10 to 20 ml sterile water for injection (provided), 0.9% NaCl, or D_5W. Gently swirl vial to dissolve powder. Do not shake. Bring solution to room temperature and administer within 3 hr of reconstitution. Use

- One IU is equivalent to the amount of endogenous antithrombin-III in 1 ml of normal human plasma.
- Treatment usually lasts 2 to 8 days, maybe longer if patient is pregnant, immobile, or having surgery.
- Measure plasma antithrombin-III levels before and

(continued)

◆ Also available in Canada. ◇ Available in Canada only.

COMMON INDICATIONS AND DOSAGES	ADMINISTRATION	SPECIAL CONSIDERATIONS
antithrombin III, human *(continued)* administration. Usual dose is 50 to 100 IU/minute I.V., not to exceed 100 IU/minute. Maintenance dose is calculated based on amount needed to increase antithrombin III activity to 80% of previous normal and is administered at 24-hr intervals.	same diluent to dilute further if needed. Inspect for precipitate and discoloration before use. ***Incompatibilities:*** None reported. ***Intermittent infusion:*** Infuse over 10 to 20 minutes at 50 IU/minute (1 ml/minute). Don't exceed 100 IU/minute (2 ml/minute).	20 minutes after treatment, and calculate patient's expected recovery. If it differs from expected rise of 1.4% for each IU/kg given, modify formula. • An infant born to parents with hereditary antithrombin-III deficiency has an increased risk of possibly fatal neonatal thromboembolism. Measure the infant's antithrombin-III levels immediately. • Dyspnea and increased blood pressure may occur at increased rates (1,500 IU in 5 minutes). • Heparin binds to antithrombin-III lysine binding sites at 1:1 M ratio, making heparin more effective. • Drug isn't recommended for long-term prevention of thrombosis.

aprotinin • Trasylol ♦

Class: ***systemic hemostatic*** • *Pregnancy risk category B*

COMMON INDICATIONS AND DOSAGES	ADMINISTRATION	SPECIAL CONSIDERATIONS
Reduction of blood loss and transfusions during cardiopulmonary bypass. *Adults:* 1-ml (1.4 mg or 10,000 U) test dose 10 minutes before scheduled administration, followed by loading dose of 200 ml (280 mg or 2 million U) given over 20 to 30 minutes after induction of anesthesia. Patient should be supine. A 200-ml pump-priming dose is delivered to the machine before bypass begins. During surgery, patient receives constant infusion of 50 ml/hr (70 mg/hr or 500,000 U/hr) until incision closed. Then infusion stops. *Children:* Dosage hasn't been established.	Available as 100- and 200-ml vials containing 1.4 mg/ml (10,000 U) aprotinin. Store at room temperature. May dilute with D_5W or 0.9% NaCl before infusion. ***Incompatibilities:*** Corticosteroids, heparin, tetracycline, and nutrient solutions containing amino acids or fat emulsions. If aprotinin given with other drugs, each drug should be given separately through different I.V. lines or catheters. ***Direct injection:*** By slow I.V. injection over at least 4 minutes. ***Intermittent infusion:*** By slow I.V. infusion at 200 ml over 20 to 30 minutes. ***Continuous infusion:*** During surgery at 50 ml/hr until incision is closed.	• A test dose is recommended before infusion because allergic reactions, including anaphylaxis, have occurred. • Administer drug through a central line. • Make sure patient is supine when giving test dose to avoid hypotension. • Watch for increased serum creatinine, which signals nephrotoxicity.

arbutamine hydrochloride • GenESA

Class: ***sympathomimetic diagnostic aid*** *• Pregnancy risk category B*

Single-dose diagnostic aid in patients with suspected coronary artery disease who can't exercise adequately. *Adults:* 0.1 mcg/kg/minute for 1 minute via GenESA I.V. infusion system. The device adjusts dose until it reaches either maximum heart rate (set by user) or maximum infusion rate of 0.8 mcg/kg/minute (maximum total dosage, 10 mcg/kg).

Available as 20-ml prefilled glass syringe containing 1 mg (0.05 mg/ml). Inspect syringe for particulates or discoloration before use.

Intermittent infusion: Don't dilute before administration. Administer only with prefilled syringe and GenESA system (a closed-loop, computer-controlled I.V. infusion device).

- Before using the GenESA system, you must read and understand manufacturer's directions for use.
- Tell patient to stop beta-blockers at least 48 hr before having cardiac stress testing with arbutamine, as ordered.
- Keep crash cart at bedside during administration.
- Monitor blood pressure, heart rate, and a diagnostic quality ECG continuously throughout infusion. Corrected QT interval, as measured from surface ECG, will be prolonged during administration.
- Serum potassium levels may decrease transiently but rarely to hypokalemic levels.
- Don't give atropine to enhance drug-induced chronotropic response; it could lead to tachyarrhythmias.

ascorbic acid (vitamin C) • Cenolate

Class: ***vitamin*** *• Pregnancy risk category A (C above recommended dosage)*

Vitamin C deficiency (scurvy). *Adults:* 100 to 250 mg once or twice daily. *Pregnant or breast-feeding women:* 60 to 80 mg daily, not to exceed 1 g/day. *Children:* 100 to 300 mg daily in divided doses. *Infants:* 50 to 100 mg daily.

Prevention of vitamin C deficiency during hemodialysis. *Adults:* 100 to 200 mg daily.

Severe burns. *Adults and children:* Usually 1 to 2 g daily.

Available in 100-, 250-, and 500-mg/ml parenteral formulations. Refrigerate if required by manufacturer. Solution stable at room temperature for 96 hr. Light darkens drug but doesn't reduce its effectiveness. If required, dilute drug in 50 to 100 ml of compatible solution.

Incompatibilities: Aminophylline, bleomycin, cefazolin, cephapirin, chlorothiazide, conjugated estrogens, erythromycin lactobionate, nafcillin, and sodium bicarbonate. May be incompatible with chloramphenicol and hydrocortisone.

Direct injection: Slowly inject into vein over 2 to 3 minutes. Alternatively, inject into I.V. tubing containing a compatible solution. Avoid rapid injection, which may cause transient dizziness or faintness.

- Drug may contain sulfites.
- Infiltration may cause local tissue irritation and damage. Assess I.V. site frequently.
- Stress proper nutritional habits to prevent recurrence of deficiency.
- Prolonged use of high doses may increase metabolism.
- Therapeutic value of ascorbic acid is controversial when used for acne, anemia, burns, cancer, common cold, depression, fractures, hemorrhage, infections, infertility, and pressure sores.
- Hemodialysis can remove vitamin.

(continued)

COMMON INDICATIONS AND DOSAGES	ADMINISTRATION	SPECIAL CONSIDERATIONS
ascorbic acid *(continued)*	***Intermittent infusion:*** Infuse diluted drug over 20 to 30 minutes. ***Continuous infusion:*** Add drug to compatible I.V. solution.	

asparaginase (colaspase, L-asparaginase) • Elspar, Kidrolase◇

Class: ***antineoplastic*** • *Pregnancy risk category C*

COMMON INDICATIONS AND DOSAGES	ADMINISTRATION	SPECIAL CONSIDERATIONS
Asparaginase may be used in combination regimens. Dosage varies with protocol; consult current medical literature determine most appropriate dosage. **Induction phase of acute lymphocytic leukemia (in combination therapy).** *Adults and children:* 1,000 IU/kg/day for 10 days. **Induction phase of acute lymphocytic leukemia (as sole agent).** *Adults and children:* 200 IU/kg/day for 28 days.	Use extreme caution when preparing or giving drug to avoid mutagenic, teratogenic, and carcinogenic risks. Use biological containment cabinet, wear mask and gloves, and avoid skin contact. If drug contacts skin or mucosa, immediately wash thoroughly with soap and water. Correctly dispose of needles, syringes, vials, and unused drug. Drug is available in 10,000-IU vials stable for 2 years at room temperature or 4 years if refrigerated. Reconstitute with 2 to 5 ml of preservative-free 0.9% NaCl or sterile water for injection. Drug may be clear or slightly cloudy. Dilute in D_5W or 0.9% NaCl within 8 hr after reconstitution. ***Incompatibilities:*** None reported. ***Intermittent infusion:*** Start new I.V. site in distal vein to allow several venipunctures, if necessary, using a 23G or 25G butterfly needle. Give drug through side port of rapidly infusing D_5W or 0.9% NaCl over at least 30 minutes.	• Skin testing and desensitization are mandatory before first dose or if more than 1 week has elapsed between treatments. Life-threatening hypersensitivity occurs in 20% to 35% of patients. Keep emergency equipment nearby during therapy. • Adequate hydration, alkalinization of urine, and possibly allopurinol administration reduce risk of uric acid nephropathy. • Loss of potency has been observed with use of 0.2-micron filter. • Observe patient for signs of CNS toxicity or thromboembolism. Be especially alert for dyspnea and chest pain, which may indicate pulmonary embolism. • Teach patient to recognize signs of hepatic impairment (jaundice, dark orange urine, and clay-colored stools).

atenolol • Tenormin

Classes: ***antianginal, antihypertensive*** • *Pregnancy risk category D*

COMMON INDICATIONS AND DOSAGES	ADMINISTRATION	SPECIAL CONSIDERATIONS
To reduce CV mortality and risk of reinfarction in hemodynamically stable patient who has survived acute phase of MI. *Adults:* 5 mg I.V., followed by anoth-	Available in 10-ml ampules containing 5 mg atenolol. Store at room temperature of 59° to 86° F (15° to 30° C) and protect from light. Dilute with 0.9% NaCl, D_5W, or NaCl and dextrose injection. Dilutions are stable for 48 hr.	• Administration of I.V. atenolol should be restricted to critical care areas, such as cardiac care unit. • During administration, monitor blood pressure, heart rate, and ECG. Stop drug if significant hy-

of 5 mg I.V. 10 minutes later. Initiate oral therapy 10 minutes after final I.V. dose in patient who can tolerate full I.V. dose. Give 50 mg P.O., followed by another 50 mg P.O. q 12 hr later. Then give 50 mg P.O. b.i.d. or 100 mg P.O. once daily for at least 6 to 9 days, or until patient is discharged from the hospital. If not contraindicated, therapy may sometimes be continued for 1 to 3 years.
Dosage adjustment. Adjustment may be required if patient has renal failure.

Incompatibilities: Don't mix with other drugs.
Direct injection: Administer over at least 5 minutes into a large vein.

potension or bradycardia occurs.
- Administer drug as soon as patient's eligibility is established and hemodynamic condition has stabilized. Results are best during first 24 hr after MI.
- During the acute phase of MI, beta-adrenergic blocker therapy should supplement standard treatment.

atracurium besylate • Tracrium ◆

Class: ***skeletal muscle relaxant*** • *Pregnancy risk category C*

Facilitation of endotracheal intubation and muscle relaxation during surgery or mechanical ventilation. *Adults:* Initially, 0.4 to 0.5 mg/kg (double the dose needed for nearly complete neuromuscular blockade). Maintenance dose of 0.08 to 0.10 mg/kg p.r.n. depends on response to peripheral nerve stimulation or observation of muscle tone recovery, spontaneous breathing, coughing, or resistance to tube. *Children ages 1 month to 2 years:* Initially, 0.3 to 0.4 mg/kg. Frequent maintenance doses may be needed. Dosage must be individualized for adults and children.

Only staff trained in giving I.V. neuromuscular blockers and managing adverse reactions should give drug. Available in 5- and 10-ml ampules. Each ml contains 10 mg of drug. Dilute with D_5W or 0.9% NaCl for intermittent or continuous infusion. Refrigerate at 36° to 46° F (2° to 8° C). Don't freeze.
Incompatibilities: Alkaline solutions, because of drug's acid pH.
Direct injection: Inject rapidly into an I.V. line containing a free-flowing, compatible solution.
Intermittent infusion: Infuse diluted drug during procedure, as needed, into I.V. line containing compatible solution.
Continuous infusion: After direct injection, give a 0.02% to 0.05% solution at 7.5 mcg/kg/minute during procedure.

- Keep emergency resuscitation equipment readily available.
- Maintain a patent airway.
- Protect corneas because patient can't blink.
- Patient won't have usual reflexes (such as cough and gag reflexes) except for pupillary constriction to light while under effects of drug.
- Drug doesn't alter consciousness or relieve pain. Assess patient's need for sedation and analgesics.
- For overdose, maintain a patent airway and assist breathing, as needed. Give fluids and vasopressors for hypotension and edrophonium, neostigmine, or pyridostigmine for neuromuscular blockade. Effects usually reverse in 8 to 10 minutes.

COMMON INDICATIONS AND DOSAGES	ADMINISTRATION	SPECIAL CONSIDERATIONS

atropine sulfate

Classes: ***antiarrhythmic, vagolytic*** • *Pregnancy risk category C*

COMMON INDICATIONS AND DOSAGES

Symptomatic bradycardia. *Adults:* 0.5 to 1 mg q 5 minutes until reach desired heart rate (usually 60 beats/minute). Maximum total dose is 3 mg; minimum is 0.5 mg. Lower dose could cause paradoxical bradycardia by vagal stimulation.
Ventricular asystole in advanced life support. *Adults:* 1 mg q 5 minutes if asystole persists. *Adolescents and children:* 0.02 mg/kg (minimum 0.1 mg and maximum 1 mg in children) q 5 minutes, if needed. In adolescents, maximum total dose is 2 mg.
Blocked muscarinic effects of anticholinesterase agents. *Adults:* 0.6 to 1.2 mg for each 0.5 to 2.5 mg of neostigmine methylsulfate or each 10 to 20 mg of pyridostigmine bromide.
Antidote for anticholinesterase toxicity. *Adults:* Initially, 1 to 2 mg; then 2 mg q 5 to 60 minutes until symptoms subside. In severe cases, initial dose may be as much as 6 mg q 5 to 60 minutes p.r.n.

ADMINISTRATION

Available in single-dose ampules or vials of 0.1, 0.4, 0.5, 1, and 1.2 mg/ml; in multidose 20-ml vials of 0.4 mg/ml; and in prefilled syringes containing 0.5 and 1 mg of drug. Store at room temperature.
Incompatibilities: Alkalides, bromides, iodides, isoproterenol, metaraminol, methohexital, norepinephrine, pentobarbital sodium, and sodium bicarbonate.
Direct injection: Inject prescribed amount of undiluted drug into vein or I.V. tubing over 1 to 2 minutes.

SPECIAL CONSIDERATIONS

- Monitor blood pressure closely to evaluate drug tolerance.
- Monitor ECG if patient has bradycardia or heart block and notify doctor if heart rate exceeds 100 beats/minute, PVCs increase, or ventricular tachycardia develops.
- Initial drug bolus may cause bradycardia, which usually resolves in 1 to 2 minutes.
- Encourage fluids and provide mouth care when appropriate.
- For overdose, give fluids for shock, diazepam for CNS irritability, pilocarpine for mydriasis, and cooling blanket for hyperthermia. Provide respiratory support and possibly give physostigmine to treat delirium, hallucinations, coma, or supraventricular tachycardia.

aztreonam • Azactam

Class: ***antibiotic*** • *Pregnancy risk category B*

COMMON INDICATIONS AND DOSAGES

Infections of the respiratory tract, GU tract, bone, skin, or soft tissues caused

ADMINISTRATION

Available in 15-ml vials or 100-ml piggyback infusion bottles containing 500 mg, 1 g, or 2 g of drug. Before reconstitution,

SPECIAL CONSIDERATIONS

- Obtain specimens for culture and sensitivity testing before giving first dose. Therapy may start before

500 mg to 2 g q 8 to 12 hr. For severe systemic or life-threatening infections, 2 g may be given q 6 to 8 hr. Maximum daily dosage is 8 g.
Dosage adjustment. Dosage may need to be adjusted for renal impairment.

add 6 to 10 ml of sterile water for injection to vial and shake well. For infusion, add at least 3 ml sterile water for each gram of drug. Dilute with 50 to 100 ml of 0.9% NaCl, D_5W, dextrose 5% in 0.9% NaCl injection, or lactated Ringer's solution. Solutions reconstituted with 0.9% NaCl or sterile water retain potency for 48 hr at room temperature or 7 days if refrigerated. Promptly use any solution over 2% concentration and discard the unused amount. Slight pink tint does not affect potency.
Incompatibilities: Ampicillin, amsacrine, cephradine, metronidazole, nafcillin, and vancomycin. Don't mix with other drugs.
Direct injection: Using a 21G to 23G needle, inject reconstituted drug over 3 to 5 minutes into vein or I.V. line containing a free-flowing, compatible solution.
Intermittent infusion: Over 20 to 60 minutes, infuse into I.V. tubing of a free-flowing, compatible solution or use a volume-control device. In latter case, final dilution should not exceed 2% (20 mg/ml).

- Monitor for phlebitis at infusion site.
- Monitor BUN and creatinine levels during therapy.
- Assess patient for fungal and bacterial superinfection with prolonged use.
- For overdose, patient may receive hemodialysis, peritoneal dialysis, or both.

basiliximab • Simulect

Class: ***immunosuppressive*** • *Pregnancy risk category B*

Prevention of acute organ rejection in renal transplant patients receiving immunosuppression with cyclosporine and corticosteroids. *Adults:* 20 mg I.V. given within 2 hr before transplant surgery and 20 mg I.V. given 4 days after surgery. *Children 2 to 15 years:* 12 mg/m² (maximum 20 mg) I.V. given within 2 hr before transplant surgery and 12 mg/m² (maximum 20 mg) I.V. given 4 days after surgery.

Available as single use vials containing 20 mg of lyophilized powder. Reconstitute with 5 ml sterile water for injection. Shake vial gently to dissolve powder. Dilute reconstituted solution to 50 ml with normal saline or dextrose 5% for infusion. Gently invert bag to avoid foaming. Don't shake. Use reconstituted solution immediately. May be refrigerated at 36° to 46° F (2° to 8° C) for 24 hr or room temperature for 4 hr.
Incompatibilities: None reported, but don't add or infuse drugs simultaneously through same I.V. line.
Intermittent infusion: Infuse medication over 20 to 30 minutes via a central or peripheral vein.

- Anaphylactoid reactions may result from proteins. Keep drugs for treating severe hypersensitivity reactions readily available.
- Monitor for electrolyte imbalances and acidosis during drug therapy.
- Monitor patient's intake and output, vital signs, hemoglobin, and hematocrit during therapy.
- Tell women of child-bearing age to use birth control before starting therapy and until 2 months after.
- Tell patient that immunosuppressive therapy increases the risk of lymphoproliferative disorders and infections. Tell him to report infections promptly.

COMMON INDICATIONS AND DOSAGES	ADMINISTRATION	SPECIAL CONSIDERATIONS

benztropine mesylate • Cogentin◇

Class: ***antiparkinsonian*** • *Pregnancy risk category C*

COMMON INDICATIONS AND DOSAGES	ADMINISTRATION	SPECIAL CONSIDERATIONS
Arteriosclerotic, idiopathic, or postencephalitic parkinsonian syndrome. *Adults:* Usually 1 to 2 mg daily (range, 0.5 to 6 mg). Started at low dose and raised by 0.5-mg increments over 5 to 6 days until symptoms subside or dose reaches 6 mg daily. **Drug-induced extrapyramidal symptoms.** *Adults:* 1 to 4 mg once or twice daily, as needed and tolerated. **Drug-induced extrapyramidal symptoms that start shortly after antipsychotic therapy begins.** *Adults:* 1 to 2 mg b.i.d or t.i.d. Reevaluate after 1 to 2 weeks of therapy. **Acute dystonic reactions.** *Adults:* Initially, 1 to 2 mg I.V., then 1 to 2 mg P.O. b.i.d. to prevent recurrence, altered as needed and tolerated. *Children age 3 and older:* Individualized dosage.	Supplied in 1-mg/ml concentration. Store in light-resistant container at room temperature. ***Incompatibilities:*** None reported. ***Direct injection:*** Inject over 3 to 5 minutes into vein or I.V. tubing that contains a free-flowing, compatible solution. ***Intermittent infusion:*** Dilute in 50 to 100 ml of a compatible solution. Give diluted solution over 15 to 30 minutes.	• Use I.V. or I.M. route for patients who can't tolerate oral drug or who need rapid response. I.V. route rarely used because onset isn't much faster than I.M. • Individualize dosage according to age, weight, and type of parkinsonism being treated. • Monitor patient's temperature, heart rate and ECG for tachycardia, and input and output for anhidrosis and urine retention. • Monitor closely if patient has a history of mental illness because symptoms may intensify. • Full drug effects may not occur for 2 to 3 days. • Discontinue drug gradually, never abruptly. • For overdose, give physostigmine salicylate 1 to 2 mg S.C. or I.V., as ordered. Repeat in 2 hr, if necessary.

betamethasone sodium phosphate • Celestone Phosphate, Cel-U-Jec

Class: ***anti-inflammatory*** • *Pregnancy risk category C*

COMMON INDICATIONS AND DOSAGES	ADMINISTRATION	SPECIAL CONSIDERATIONS
Severe inflammation or immunosuppression. *Adults:* 0.5 to 9 mg daily. After achieving satisfactory response, reduce dosage gradually and maintain at lowest level that produces therapeutic response.	Available in 5-ml multidose vials containing 3 mg/ml. Dilute as needed with D_5W, 0.9% NaCl, lactated Ringer's, or dextrose 5% in Ringer's or lactated Ringer's. Store between 59° and 86° F (15° and 30° C). Don't freeze, and protect from light.	• Use I.V. route only in an emergency or when oral therapy isn't possible. • Patient may need a potassium supplement. • Because of drug's hyperglycemic effect, diabetic patient may need larger dosages of antidiabetic drug.

Incompatibilities: Parenteral local diluents or anesthetics containing preservatives, such as parabens or phenols, because betamethasone may flocculate.
Direct injection: Use only in severe or life-threatening conditions and follow with intermittent infusion. First, dilute dose in 10 ml of diluent. Then inject diluted dose over 5 to 10 minutes into vein or I.V. line that contains a free-flowing, compatible solution.
Intermittent infusion: Dilute in 50 to 100 ml of diluent. Infuse over 20 to 30 minutes into established I.V. line that contains a free-flowing, compatible solution.

- Drug may contain sulfites.
- Watch for signs of infection.
- Discontinue drug gradually and as soon as possible.
- Adrenal function may take 1 week to recover after high-dose therapy lasting 1 to 5 days. It may take up to 1 year after prolonged therapy.

biperiden lactate • Akineton

Class: ***antiparkinsonian*** • *Pregnancy risk category C*

Drug-induced extrapyramidal disorders. *Adults:* 2 mg (0.4 ml), repeated q 30 minutes until symptoms subside. Maximum 8 mg over 24 hr.

Available in 1-ml ampules containing 5 mg/ml. Drug is stable at room temperature. Protect from light.
Incompatibilities: None reported.
Direct injection: Inject drug over at least 1 minute into vein or I.V. tubing that contains a free-flowing, compatible solution.

- Obtain baseline blood pressure and heart rate, and monitor patient for hypotension and tachycardia during and after administration. Keep patient in bed during injection and until blood pressure stabilizes.
- Bradycardia and hypotension can be minimized or avoided by slow I.V. administration.
- Keep room darkened if photophobia develops.
- Use precautions if patient's confused or disoriented.
- Expect to switch to oral route as soon as possible.
- Provide frequent mouth care and monitor bladder and bowel function for urine retention and constipation.
- For overdose, give vasopressors, respiratory support, antipyretics, fluid replacement, and physostigmine, if life-threatening. Don't give phenothiazines because they could cause coma.

COMMON INDICATIONS AND DOSAGES	ADMINISTRATION	SPECIAL CONSIDERATIONS

bleomycin sulfate • Blenoxane◆

Class: ***antineoplastic*** *• Pregnancy risk category D*

COMMON INDICATIONS AND DOSAGES

Malignant lymphoma, lymphosarcoma, or reticulum cell sarcoma; squamous cell carcinoma of skin, head, neck, lips, mouth, palate, sinuses, buccal mucosa, gingivae, tongue, tonsils, nasopharynx, oropharynx, paralarynx, larynx, epiglottis, cervix, vulva, or penis; testicular cancer. *Adults:* 0.25 to 0.5 U/kg once or twice weekly. For lymphoma, give 2 U or less for first two doses to reduce risk of anaphylactoid reactions.
Hodgkin's disease. *Adults:* 0.25 to 0.5 U/kg once or twice weekly. When tumor halved, give 1 U daily or 5 U weekly.

ADMINISTRATION

Drug has carcinogenic, mutagenic, and teratogenic risks. When preparing it, follow facility policy. Vials contain 15 or 30 U of drug. Dilute with at least 5 or 10 ml of 0.9% NaCl, respectively. Don't use with dextrose-containing fluids because drug will lose potency. Diluted solution is stable for 24 hr at room temperature. Manufacturer recommends using it within 24 hr because it has no preservatives. Discard unused portion.
Incompatibilities: Amino acids, aminophylline, ascorbic acid injection, cephalosporins, diazepam, drugs containing sulfhydryl groups, furosemide, hydrocortisone, methotrexate, mitomycin, penicillin, riboflavin, terbutaline, and solutions containing divalent and trivalent cations (especially calcium salts and copper) because drug causes chelation.
Direct injection: Inject reconstituted drug over 10 minutes at a new I.V. site.
Intermittent infusion: Using a secondary line, infuse dose into an established line that contains a free-flowing, compatible solution.

SPECIAL CONSIDERATIONS

- Assess respiratory function carefully before each treatment, especially if patient is at high risk for pulmonary toxicity. Signs include dyspnea, bibasilar crackles, and a nonproductive cough.
- Obtain BUN and creatinine clearance levels, liver and pulmonary function tests, ECG, and chest X-rays before and during treatment. Expect to stop drug if tests show marked deterioration.
- Monitor patient closely, including blood pressure, during infusion and for 1 hr after.
- In patients prone to fever after treatment, give acetaminophen before treatment and for 24 hr after.
- Tell patient to inform anesthesiologist that he's had bleomycin if he ever needs anesthesia.

bretylium tosylate • Bretylate◇

Class: ***ventricular antiarrhythmic*** *• Pregnancy risk category C*

COMMON INDICATIONS AND DOSAGES

Ventricular fibrillation or hemodynamically unstable ventricular tachycardia. *Adults:* 5 mg/kg given undiluted over 1 minute. If persistent, follow with 10 mg/kg q 5 to 30 minutes p.r.n. Maximum 30 to 35 mg/kg/day.

ADMINISTRATION

Supplied as single-dose, 10-ml ampule that contains 500 mg of drug. For infusion, dilute with at least 50 ml of D_5W or 0.9% NaCl injection. Store at 59° to 86° F (15° to 30° C). Diluted drug remains stable for 48 hr at room temperature, 7 days if refrigerated. Prediluted, commercially prepared solutions are also available.

SPECIAL CONSIDERATIONS

- Track ECG, heart rate, pulse, and blood pressure.
- Keep patient supine until he develops tolerance to hypotension, usually after several days of therapy. Notify doctor immediately of significant change.
- Subtherapeutic doses (below 5 mg/kg) may cause hypotension.

Persistent ventricular tachycardia. *Adults:* 5 to 10 mg/kg infused over 8 to 10 minutes. Maintenance dosage is 5 to 10 mg/kg over 8 minutes or more, repeated q 6 to 8 hr, or continuous infusion at 1 to 2 mg/minute.
Other life-threatening arrhythmias. *Adults:* 5 to 10 mg/kg over at least 8 minutes repeated at 1- to 2-hr intervals if persistent. Maintenance dosage is 5 to 10 mg/kg q 6 hr or continuous infusion at 1 to 2 mg/minute.
Dosage adjustment. Increase dosage interval if patient has renal impairment.

Incompatibilities: None reported.
Direct injection: Inject undiluted over 8 to 10 minutes into I.V. line.
Intermittent infusion: After diluting, infuse ordered dose over 8 minutes or more.
Continuous infusion: Give diluted drug at 1 to 2 mg/minute.

- Rapid administration may cause severe nausea and vomiting.
- For overdose, give nitroprusside or another short-acting antihypertensive to treat initial hypertensive effects. Treat hypotension with fluids and dopamine or norepinephrine. Dialysis doesn't remove drug.

brompheniramine maleate • Nasahist B, ND-Stat

Class: ***antihistamine*** • *Pregnancy risk category B*

Moderate to severe allergic reaction. *Adults:* 5 to 20 mg q 6 to 12 hr. Maximum 40 mg daily. *Children under age 12:* 0.5 mg/kg/day or 15 mg/m^2/day divided q 6 to 8 hr.

Available in 1-ml ampules that contain 10 mg of drug. Also available in 10- and 30-ml multiple-dose vials (10 mg/ml). Store brompheniramine injection away from light and at room temperature. Crystals may form in ampules stored below 32° F (0° C) but will dissolve when warmed to 84° F (29° C).
Incompatibilities: Iodipamide meglumine and combinations of diatrizoate meglumine and diatrizoate sodium.
Direct injection: Give undiluted or diluted to a 1:10 concentration in D_5W or 0.9% NaCl over 3 to 5 minutes.
Intermittent infusion: Dilute desired dose with 50 ml D_5W or 0.9% NaCl. Infuse over 20 to 30 minutes into an established I.V. line that contains free-flowing, compatible solution.

- Give drug with patient in recumbent position to ensure safety if hypotension develops.
- Give sugarless gum, hard candy, or ice chips for dry mouth.
- Monitor blood count during long-term therapy; observe for signs of blood dyscrasia.
- Withdraw drug 4 days before skin tests for allergies to avoid misleading results.
- Antihistamine overdose may cause fatal CNS depression or stimulation (most likely in children). Treat symptomatically with artificial respiration, if needed; vasopressors, such as norepinephrine or phenylephrine (not epinephrine); and physostigmine to counteract CNS anticholinergic effects. If it fails to correct seizures, give diazepam. Treat hyperthermia with cold packs or by sponging with tepid water.

COMMON INDICATIONS AND DOSAGES / ADMINISTRATION / SPECIAL CONSIDERATIONS

bumetanide • Bumex

Class: ***diuretic*** • *Pregnancy risk category C*

Common indications and dosages

Edema from heart failure or hepatic or renal disease. *Adults:* Initially, 0.5 to 1 mg daily, repeated q 2 to 3 hr if needed. Maximum 10 mg daily.

Adjunctive treatment to enhance elimination of a drug or toxin. *Adults:* Dosage varies with desired response. Start with small doses, adjust carefully, and use intermittent schedule if possible. Maximum 10 mg daily.

Administration

Available with premixed preservative in 2-ml (0.25 mg/ml) ampules and 2-, 4-, and 10-ml (0.25 mg/ml) vials. Drug can be further diluted for I.V. infusion using D_5W, 0.9% NaCl, or lactated Ringer's solution in glass or plastic containers. Prepare solution for I.V. infusion within 24 hr of use. Protect drug from light to avoid discoloration. Store at room temperature. For large doses, use vials to keep glass particles from ampules out of solution. If ampules must be used, add filter to I.V. tubing.

Incompatibilities: Dobutamine.

Direct injection: Inject desired dose of 0.25 mg/ml solution over 1 to 2 minutes.

Intermittent infusion: Give diluted drug at ordered rate through intermittent infusion device or piggyback into I.V. line that contains a free-flowing, compatible solution.

Special considerations

- Drug may contain benzyl alcohol.
- Check blood pressure and pulse during rapid diuresis. Use cautiously with potassium-wasting drugs.
- Monitor patient's serum electrolytes, BUN, creatinine, and carbon dioxide frequently.
- Watch for signs of hypokalemia, such as weakness, dizziness, confusion, anorexia, vomiting, and cramps. In excessive diuresis or electrolyte imbalance, expect to stop drug or reduce dosage until imbalance reverses.
- For overdose, give replacement fluids and electrolytes, as needed, based on urine output and serum and urine electrolyte levels.

buprenorphine hydrochloride • Buprenex

Class: ***analgesic*** • *Pregnancy risk category C* • *Controlled substance schedule V*

Common indications and dosages

Moderate to severe pain (cancer, postoperative, trigeminal neuralgia, trauma). *Adults and children age 13 or older:* 0.3 mg q 6 hr p.r.n. Can repeat first dose once in 30 to 60 minutes if needed. Can give up to 0.6 mg q 4 hr I.M. if needed in adults not at risk of respiratory depression. Studies have used continuous infusion of 25 to 250 mcg/hr for postoperative pain in adults. *Children ages 2 to 12:*

Administration

Supplied as 0.324 mg (equivalent to 0.3 mg) of drug in 1-ml preservative-free ampules. Prevent prolonged exposure to light and temperatures outside 32° to 104° F (0° to 40° C). Drug can be diluted in D_5W, dextrose 5% and 0.9% NaCl, or lactated Ringer's and 0.9% NaCl.

Incompatibilities: Diazepam, furosemide, and lorazepam.

Direct injection: Inject over at least 2 minutes into an I.V. line that contains a free-flowing, compatible solution. Rapid injection could cause possibly fatal anaphylactoid or cardiopulmonary problems.

Special considerations

- Monitor patient's blood pressure and respirations frequently for at least 1 hr after administration. Keep resuscitation equipment and naloxone readily available. If rate drops below 8 breaths/minute, wake patient to stimulate breathing, then notify doctor.
- Give stool softener, if needed.
- Tell patient to get up slowly and avoid activities that require alertness; he may be dizzy and drowsy.
- Physical and psychological dependence can develop

2 to 6 mcg/kg q 4 to 6 hr. Don't exceed 6 mcg/kg.

Dosage adjustment. Reduce dose by half if risk of respiratory depression.

Continuous infusion: Dilute with 0.9% NaCl to a concentration of 15 mcg/ml. Using a controller, infuse diluted drug at prescribed rate through I.V. line that contains a free-flowing, compatible solution.

with prolonged use, and withdrawal symptoms may occur up to 14 days after drug is stopped. Tell patient not to exceed recommended dose.
- When used after surgery, urge patient to turn, cough, and breathe deeply to prevent atelectasis.

butorphanol tartrate • Stadol

Classes: ***analgesic, adjunct to anesthesia*** • *Pregnancy risk category C (D for prolonged use or high doses at term)*

Pain caused by labor. *Adults:* 1 to 2 mg if fetus is at least 37 weeks' gestation with no signs of distress. Repeat after 4 hr as needed.

Moderate to severe pain from acute and chronic disorders. *Adults:* 1 mg (range 0.5 to 2 mg) q 3 to 4 hr p.r.n. Reduce to 0.5 mg q 6 hr if patient is elderly or has liver or renal impairment.

Adjunct to balanced anesthesia. *Adults:* 2 mg I.V. shortly before induction. During maintenance anesthesia, 0.5 to 1 mg I.V. Total dose varies; few patients require less than 4 mg or more than 12.5 mg.

Available in single- and multiple-dose vials and disposable syringes at concentrations of 1 and 2 mg/ml. No dilution needed. Store at room temperature away from light.

Incompatibilities: Pentobarbital sodium.

Direct injection: Inject drug directly into vein or an established I.V. line over several minutes.

- Determine dose used in labor from initial response, concomitant analgesic or sedative drugs, and expected time of delivery. Don't repeat dose in less than 4 hr and don't give within 4 hr of anticipated delivery.
- Determine preoperative dose from age, body weight, physical status, underlying condition, drugs taken, anesthesia used, and surgery performed.
- Keep patient recumbent to reduce hypotension and dizziness.
- Rapid I.V. injection can cause severe respiratory depression, hypotension, circulatory collapse, and cardiac arrest. Keep emergency resuscitation equipment readily available.
- Periodically monitor postoperative vital signs and bladder function. Because drug decreases rate and depth of respirations, arterial oxygen saturation may help assess respiratory depression.

calcitriol • Calcijex

Class: ***antihypocalcemic*** • *Pregnancy risk category C*

Hypocalcemia during chronic renal dialysis. *Adults:* 0.5 mcg three times weekly, about every other day. May increase by 0.25 to 0.5 mcg at 2- to 4-

Available in ampules or 1 or 2 mcg/ml. Store at room temperature. Avoid freezing. Discard unused drug immediately; it doesn't contain a preservative.

Incompatibilities: None reported.

- Check serum calcium and phosphorus levels at least twice weekly at start of therapy and when adjusting dose.

(continued)

COMMON INDICATIONS AND DOSAGES	ADMINISTRATION	SPECIAL CONSIDERATIONS
calcitriol *(continued)* week intervals. Maintenance dosage 0.5 to 3 mcg three times weekly.	***Direct injection:*** Inject into vein or I.V. tubing that contains a free-flowing, compatible solution.	• Check serum magnesium, alkaline phosphatase, and 24-hr urine calcium and phosphorus levels periodically during treatment. • Avoid vitamin D and metabolites during therapy. • Give calcium supplement P.O. as needed to ensure adequate daily intake of calcium.

calcium chloride, calcium gluceptate, calcium gluconate • Calciject◇

Classes: ***cardiotonic, electrolyte replacement*** • *Pregnancy risk category C*

COMMON INDICATIONS AND DOSAGES	ADMINISTRATION	SPECIAL CONSIDERATIONS
Emergency treatment of hypocalcemia. *Adults:* 7 to 14 mEq. *Children:* 1 to 7 mEq. *Infants:* Less than 1 mEq repeated q 1 to 3 days p.r.n. **Hypocalcemic tetany.** *Adults:* 4.5 to 16 mEq. *Children:* 0.5 to 0.7 mEq/kg t.i.d. or q.i.d. or until controlled. *Infants:* 2.4 mEq/kg daily in divided doses. **Hyperkalemia with cardiac toxicity.** *Adults:* 2.25 to 14 mEq while watching ECG; repeat in 1 to 2 minutes p.r.n. **Advanced cardiac life support.** *Adults:* 0.027 to 0.054 mEq/kg calcium chloride, 4.5 to 6.3 mEq calcium gluceptate, or 2.3 to 3.7 mEq calcium gluconate repeated p.r.n. *Children:* 0.27 mEq/kg calcium chloride repeated in 10 minutes p.r.n. **Magnesium toxicity.** *Adults:* 7 mEq; subsequent doses based on response. **Transfusion of citrated blood.** *Adults:* 1.35 mEq/dl of citrated blood. *Neonates:* 0.45 mEq/dl of citrated blood.	Calcium chloride comes in 10-ml ampule, vial, and syringe of 10% solution containing 1.36 mEq calcium/ml. Calcium gluceptate comes in 5-ml ampule and in 50- and 100-ml bulk containers of 22% solution containing 0.9 mEq calcium/ml. Calcium gluconate comes in 10-ml ampules and vials and 20-ml vials as a 10% solution containing 0.45 to 0.48 mEq calcium/ml. All may be diluted with most I.V. and total parenteral nutrition solutions before infusion. Store between 59° and 86° F (15° and 30° C) unless instructed otherwise. Use only clear solutions. If crystals present, discard calcium gluceptate; warm calcium gluconate to 86° to 104° F (30° to 40° C) to dissolve them. Except in emergency, warm injection to body temperature before giving. ***Incompatibilities:*** All three calcium salts are precipitated by carbonates, bicarbonates, phosphates, sulfates, and tartrates. Mixing with tetracyclines causes chelation. *Calcium chloride* is incompatible with amphotericin B, cephalothin, chlorpheniramine, dobutamine, and magnesium sulfate. *Calcium gluceptate* is incompatible with cefamandole, cephalothin, magnesium sulfate, prednisolone sodium phosphate, and prochlorperazine edisylate. *Calcium gluconate* is incompatible with amphotericin B, cefamandole, cephalothin, dobutamine, indomethacin sodium trihydrate, magnesium	• Hypocalcemia may cause muscle twitching and spasms; hypercalcemia may cause bradycardia, depressed nervous and neuromuscular function, arrhythmias, and impaired renal function. • Calcium chloride is three times as potent as calcium gluconate. • After I.V. injection, keep patient briefly recumbent. • Tell patient he may have tingling, heat waves, and a calcium or chalky taste after drug delivery. • Extravasation may cause burning, sloughing, and necrosis. If it occurs, stop infusion, infiltrate area with 1% procaine and hyaluronidase to reduce vasospasm and dilute calcium, and apply local heat. • If serum calcium level exceeds 12 mg/dl, give 0.9% NaCl, I.V. fluids, and furosemide or ethacrynic acid to promote calcium excretion. Closely monitor serum potassium and magnesium levels, blood pressure, and ECG to detect complications.

sulfate, methylprednisolone sodium succinate, and prochlorperazine edisylate.

Direct injection: Use small needle to deliver into large vein or I.V. line that contains free-flowing, compatible solution. Don't exceed 1 ml/minute (1.5 mEq/minute) for calcium chloride, 1.5 to 5 ml/minute for calcium gluconate, or 2 ml/minute for calcium gluceptate. Don't use scalp vein in child.

Intermittent infusion: Infuse diluted solution using I.V. line with compatible solution. Don't exceed 100 mg/minute for calcium chloride or 200 mg/minute for calcium gluceptate and calcium gluconate.

Continuous infusion: Infuse after addition of large volume of fluid at no more than 100 mg/minute for calcium chloride or 200 mg/minute for calcium gluceptate and calcium gluconate.

carboplatin • Paraplatin◆

Class: ***antineoplastic*** • *Pregnancy risk category D*

Ovarian carcinoma. *Adults:* 360 mg/m^2 on day 1 q 4 weeks. Reduce dose 25% if platelet count below 50,000/mm^3 or neutrophil count below 500/mm^3. May repeat or increase 25% if platelet count above 100,000/mm^3 and neutrophil count above 2,000/mm^3.

Dosage adjustment. For creatinine clearance between 41 and 59 ml/minute, give 250 mg/m^2; if between 16 and 40 ml/minute, give 200 mg/m^2.

Follow facility protocol for handling chemotherapy drugs. Available in 50-, 150-, and 450-mg vials. Store unopened vials at room temperature and protect from light. Just before use, reconstitute with D_5W, 0.9% NaCl, or sterile water for injection to 10 mg/ml. Dilute with 0.9% NaCl injection or D_5W to as low as 0.5 mg/ml. Reconstituted and diluted solutions stable at room temperature for 8 hr. Discard after 8 hr because drug contains no preservatives. Don't use needles or administration sets that contain aluminum because drug may precipitate and lose potency.

Incompatibilities: Aluminum, fluorouracil, mesna, and sodium bicarbonate.

Intermittent infusion: Infuse over 15 minutes or more into vein or free-flowing, compatible I.V. solution.

- Determine serum electrolytes, creatinine, BUN, CBC and platelet count, and creatinine clearance levels before first infusion and before each course.
- Drug can cause severe vomiting; give antiemetic therapy first.
- Watch closely for hypersensitivity reactions, which may occur within minutes. Keep epinephrine, corticosteroids, and antihistamines readily available.
- Monitor patient's vital signs during infusion.
- Tell patient to watch for signs of infection (fever, sore throat, fatigue) or bleeding (bruising, nosebleeds, melena, bleeding gums), and to take temperature daily.

COMMON INDICATIONS AND DOSAGES	ADMINISTRATION	SPECIAL CONSIDERATIONS
carmustine (BCNU) • BiCNU♦		
Class: ***antineoplastic*** • *Pregnancy risk category D*		
Brain and liver tumors, Hodgkin's disease, lymphomas, malignant melanoma, multiple myeloma. *Adults and children:* 150 to 200 mg/m² as single dose or divided into daily doses, such as 75 to 100 mg/m² on two successive days. Repeat full dose q 6 weeks if WBCs exceed 3,000/mm³ and platelets exceed 75,000/mm³. Give 70% of dose if WBC count is 2,000 to 3,000/mm³ and platelet count is 25,000 to 75,000/mm³. Give 50% of previous dose if WBC count below 2,000/mm³ and platelet count below 25,000/mm³.	Follow facility protocol for handling chemotherapy drugs. Drug comes as a powder in 100-mg vials. Discard if oily film visible at bottom of vial (sign of decomposition). Dilute 100 mg with 3 ml of sterile, dehydrated ethyl alcohol supplied with drug. After dissolving, add 27 ml sterile water for injection to make a clear, colorless to yellow solution of 3.3 mg carmustine/ml of 10% alcohol. Stable for 8 hr at room temperature, 24 hr if refrigerated. Protect from light. Reconstituted solution may be diluted with 250 to 500 ml D_5W or 0.9% NaCl for infusion. Stable for 48 hr if refrigerated, protected from light, and prepared in glass container. ***Incompatibilities:*** Sodium bicarbonate. ***Intermittent infusion:*** Infuse diluted solution (250 to 500 ml) over 1 to 2 hr. If patient reports pain, dilute drug further or slow infusion.	• Give antiemetics before carmustine. • Check baseline pulmonary function tests and follow results during therapy. Risk of pulmonary toxicity rises if cumulative dose exceeds 1,400 mg/m². • Giving over less than 2 hr may cause severe pain and burning at injection site and along vein. • Check CBC weekly for at least 6 weeks following dose to monitor extent of myelosuppression. • Avoid vaccinating patient or exposing him to recipients of live-virus vaccines.
cefamandole nafate • Mandol♦		
Class: ***antibiotic*** • *Pregnancy risk category B*		
Severe infections caused by susceptible organisms. *Adults:* 500 mg to 1 g q 4 to 8 hr. *Children age 1 month and older:* 50 to 100 mg/kg/day in divided doses q 4 to 8 hr. **Life-threatening infections; infections caused by less-susceptible organisms.** *Adults:* up to 2 g q 4 hr. Maximum 12 g daily. *Children age 1 month and older:* 150 mg/kg daily in divided doses q 4 to 8 hr. Maximum 12 g daily.	Available in 1- and 2-g vials. Before reconstituting, store at 59° to 86° F (15° and 30° C). Reconstitute just before use because carbon dioxide buildup in syringe can cause leakage. For direct injection, reconstitute with 10 ml of sterile water for injection, D_5W, or 0.9% NaCl. For intermittent infusion, dilute with 100 ml of compatible solution, such as amino acid solutions; dextran; D_5W; $D_{10}W$; 0.9% NaCl; dextrose 5% and Ionosol B; dextrose 5% and Isolyte E; mannitol 5%, 10%, or 20% in water; and 1/6 M sodium lactate. For continuous infusion, dilute with specified amount. Shake until dissolved. Solution stable 24 hr at room temperature, 96 hr if refrigerated.	• Drug may cause pseudomembranous colitis. If patient develops diarrhea, take stool sample and stop administration if it confirms colitis. • Give with vitamin K if patient is elderly, debilitated, or has vitamin K deficiency. • Assess PT and check for evidence of bleeding. • Check BUN, liver enzyme levels, and creatinine clearance if patient has renal impairment. • With large dose or prolonged therapy, watch for superinfection, especially in high-risk patient. • Use a glucose enzymatic test strip to prevent inac-

Surgical prophylaxis. *Adults:* 1 to 2 g 30 to 60 minutes before surgery and 1 to 2 g q 6 hr for 24 to 48 hr after surgery. *Children age 3 months and older:* 50 to 100 mg/kg/day 30 to 60 minutes before surgery and 50 to 100 mg/kg/day in divided doses q 6 hr for 24 to 48 hr after surgery.
Dosage adjustment. Dosage adjustment required if patient has renal impairment.

Incompatibilities: Aminoglycosides, amiodarone, calcium gluceptate, calcium gluconate, cimetidine, hetastarch, Isolyte M, and magnesium and calcium ions (including Ringer's injection and lactated Ringer's injection).
Direct injection: Give over 3 to 5 minutes through large vein or I.V. line that contains free-flowing, compatible solution.
Intermittent infusion: Give 100 ml over 15 to 30 minutes through intermittent infusion device or I.V. line that contains free-flowing, compatible solution.
Continuous infusion: Infuse diluted solution over 24 hr.

curate results when assessing urine glucose levels.
- Tell patient to avoid alcohol during therapy and for 46 to 72 hr afterward to avoid disulfiram-like reaction.

cefazolin sodium • Ancef◆, Kefzol◆

Class: ***antibiotic*** • *Pregnancy risk category B*

Septicemia, endocarditis, and infections of respiratory tract, GU tract, skin, soft tissue, biliary tract, bones, and joints by susceptible organisms. *Adults:* In mild infection, 250 to 500 mg q 8 hr; in moderate to severe infection, 500 mg to 1 g q 6 to 8 hr; in life-threatening infection, 1 to 1.5 g q 6 hr. Maximum 12 g daily. *Children over age 1 month:* 25 to 50 mg/kg daily in three or four divided doses; in life-threatening infection, 100 mg/kg daily may be required.
Surgical prophylaxis. *Adults:* 1 g 30 to 60 minutes before surgery; 0.5 to 1 g q 2 hr during surgery; 0.5 to 1 g q 6 to 8 hr for 24 hr after surgery.
Dosage adjustment. Dosage adjustment required if patient has renal impairment.

Available in 500-mg and 1-g vials. To reconstitute, add 2 ml of 0.9% NaCl, sterile water, or bacteriostatic water to 500-mg vial or 2.5 ml to 1-g vial to obtain 225 and 330 mg/ml, respectively. Shake well. Dilute reconstituted Ancef with 5 ml, and Kefzol with 10 ml, of compatible solution for direct injection. For intermittent infusion, add reconstituted drug to 50 to 100 ml of compatible solution, such as D_5W; dextrose 5% in lactated Ringer's; dextrose 5% in 0.2%, 0.45%, or 0.9% NaCl; dextrose 5% and Normosol-M; or dextrose 5% and Ionosol B or Plasma-Lyte. Reconstituted and diluted drug is stable 24 hr at room temperature, 10 days if refrigerated. Solutions reconstituted with sterile water, bacteriostatic water, or 0.9% NaCl injection are stable 12 weeks at –4° F (–20° C). Don't use cloudy or precipitated solution and don't refreeze thawed solution.
Incompatibilities: Aminoglycosides, amiodarone, amobarbital, ascorbic acid injection, bleomycin, calcium gluceptate, calcium gluconate, cimetidine, colistimethate, erythromycin gluceptate, hydrocortisone, idarubicin, lidocaine, norepinephrine, oxytetracycline, pentobarbital sodium, polymyxin B, ran-

- Check for penicillin or cephalosporin allergy. Keep epinephrine nearby to treat anaphylaxis.
- If seizures occur, promptly stop drug and give anticonvulsants as ordered.
- Monitor patient's BUN and serum creatinine levels to assess renal function.
- Observe patient for fungal and bacterial superinfection with prolonged therapy.
- For overdose, hemodialysis may remove drug.

(continued)

◆ Also available in Canada. ◇ Available in Canada only.

COMMON INDICATIONS AND DOSAGES	ADMINISTRATION	SPECIAL CONSIDERATIONS
cefazolin sodium *(continued)*	itidine, tetracycline, theophylline, and vitamin B complex with C. ***Direct injection:*** Inject into a vein over 3 to 5 minutes or into I.V. tubing that contains free-flowing, compatible solution. ***Intermittent infusion:*** Insert 21G or 23G needle into port of primary tubing and infuse 50 to 100 ml of solution over 30 minutes.	

cefepime hydrochloride • Maxipime

Class: ***antibiotic*** • *Pregnancy risk category B*

COMMON INDICATIONS AND DOSAGES	ADMINISTRATION	SPECIAL CONSIDERATIONS
Mild to moderate uncomplicated or complicated UTI or pyelonephritis. *Adults and children age 12 and older:* 0.5 to 1 g q 12 hr for 7 to 10 days. **Severe uncomplicated or complicated UTI or pyelonephritis.** *Adults and children age 12 and older:* 2 g q 12 hr for 10 days. **Moderate to severe pneumonia.** *Adults and children age 12 and older:* 1 to 2 g q 12 hr for 10 days. **Moderate to severe uncomplicated skin and skin-structure infections.** *Adults and children age 12 and older:* 2 g q 12 hr for 10 days. **Dosage adjustment.** Dosage adjustment required if patient has renal impairment.	Available in 500-mg and 1- and 2-g vials; 1-g ADD-Vantage vials; and 1- and 2-g piggyback bottles. For intermittent infusion, reconstitute the 1- or 2-g piggyback bottle with 50 or 100 ml of 0.9% NaCl injection, 5% or 10% dextrose injection, 1/6 M sodium lactate injection, 5% dextrose and 0.9% NaCl injection, lactated Ringer's and 5% dextrose injection, or Normosol-R and Normosol-M in 5% dextrose injection. Reconstitute 500-mg vial with 5 ml, 1-g vial with 10 ml, or 2-g vial with 10 ml and add appropriate quantity of the resulting solution to I.V. container with compatible fluid. Reconstitute ADD-Vantage only with 50 or 100 ml of 5% dextrose injection or 0.9% NaCl chloride injection in ADD-Vantage flexible diluent container. Reconstituted solution is stable for 24 hr at 68° to 77° F (20° to 25° C), and 7 days at 36° to 46° F (2° to 8° C). ***Incompatibilities:*** Aminophylline, gentamicin, metronidazole, netilmicin, tobramycin, and vancomycin. ***Intermittent infusion:*** Infuse reconstituted solution over 30 minutes.	• Check for penicillin or cephalosporin allergy. • Assess PT if prothrombin changes. • Check BUN, liver enzyme levels, and creatinine clearance if patient has renal or liver impairment. • If diarrhea persists during therapy, collect stool specimens to rule out pseudomembranous colitis. • With large doses or prolonged therapy, monitor for superinfection, especially in high-risk patient. • For overdose, provide supportive treatment. Have patient undergo hemodialysis.

cefmetazole sodium • Zefazone

Class: ***antibiotic*** • *Pregnancy risk category B*

Mild to moderate infections caused by susceptible organisms. *Adults:* 2 g q 6 to 12 hr for 5 to 14 days.
Severe to life-threatening infections caused by susceptible organisms. *Adults:* 2 g q 6 hr.
Complicated and uncomplicated UTI. *Adults:* 2 g q 12 hr.
Perioperative prophylaxis. *Adults:* 1 to 2 g 30 to 90 minutes before surgery. Can repeat 8 and 16 hr after first dose for long procedures.
Prophylaxis in patients undergoing cesarean section. *Adults:* 2 g as single dose after clamping cord or 1 g after clamping cord and after 8 and 16 hr.
Dosage adjustment. Adult dosage in renal failure reflects creatinine clearance.

Available in 1- and 2-g vials. Reconstitute with bacteriostatic water, sterile water, or 0.9% NaCl for injection. Shake to dissolve drug, then let solution stand until clear. Add 3.7 ml to 1-g vial to yield about 250 mg/ml. Add 10 ml to 1-g vial to yield about 100 mg/ml. Add 7 ml to 2-g vial to yield about 250 mg/ml. Add 15 ml to 2-g vial to yield about 125 mg/ml. Store powder at controlled 59° to 86° F (15° to 30° C). Reconstituted solution is stable 24 hr at room temperature, 1 week if refrigerated, up to 6 weeks if frozen at –4° F (–20° C). Thaw at room temperature (not with microwave oven or warm water). If solution is cloudy or precipitated at room temperature, don't use. Thawed solution is stable 24 hr; don't refreeze.
Incompatibilities: Aminoglycoside antibiotics and heparin sodium.
Direct injection: Temporarily stop drugs being given at same site and inject over 3 to 5 minutes.
Intermittent infusion: Reconstituted drug may be diluted to 1 to 20 mg/ml by adding 0.9% NaCl injection, D_5W, or lactated Ringer's injection. Infuse over 10 to 60 minutes.

- Check for cephalosporin or penicillin allergy before giving first dose. Keep epinephrine, corticosteroids, antihistamines, pressor agents, and fluids available to treat anaphylaxis.
- Track PT and administer vitamin K, as ordered.
- Monitor patient with renal impairment frequently for signs of toxicity.
- Tell patient to avoid alcohol during therapy and for 48 to 72 hr after treatment ends.
- Prolonged use may result in overgrowth of nonsusceptible organisms.

cefonicid sodium • Monocid

Class: ***antibiotic*** • *Pregnancy risk category B*

Septicemia and infections of the lower respiratory and urinary tracts, skin and skin structure, and bone and joints by susceptible organisms. *Adults:* 1 g q 24 hr. For uncomplicated infection, 0.5 g q 24 hr; for life-threatening infections, 2 g q 24 hr.
Surgical prophylaxis. *Adults:* 1 g 60

Reconstitute 500-mg vial with 2 ml or 1-g vial with 2.5 ml sterile water for injection to yield 225 or 325 mg/ml, respectively. Shake well. Reconstitute piggyback vial with 50 to 100 ml of compatible solution, such as dextrose 5% and 0.15% potassium chloride; dextrose 5% in 0.2%, 0.45%, or 0.9% NaCl; dextrose 5% in lactated Ringer's; dextrose 5% or 10% in water; Ringer's injection; lactated Ringer's; 0.9% NaCl; and 1/6 M sodium lactate. Solution is stable for 24 hr at

- Check for penicillin or cephalosporin allergy.
- Monitor patent's BUN and serum creatinine levels to assess renal function. Adjust dosage accordingly.
- If diarrhea persists during therapy, collect stool specimens to rule out pseudomembranous colitis.

(continued)

◆ Also available in Canada. ◇ Available in Canada only.

COMMON INDICATIONS AND DOSAGES	ADMINISTRATION	SPECIAL CONSIDERATIONS
cefonicid sodium *(continued)* minutes before surgery; may give 1 g q 24 hr for 2 days. **Prophylaxis for cesarean section.** *Adults:* 1 g after cord is clamped. **Dosage adjustment.** Dosage adjustment required if patient has renal impairment.	room temperature, 72 hr if refrigerated. Protect from light. ***Incompatibilities:*** Hetastarch and sargramostim. ***Direct injection:*** Inject reconstituted drug over 3 to 5 minutes into vein or tubing with free-flowing compatible solution. ***Intermittent infusion:*** Infuse 50 to 100 ml of diluted drug over 20 to 30 minutes into free-flowing, compatible solution.	• Observe patient for fungal and bacterial superinfection during prolonged use. • If patient has dialysis, keep prescribed dosage. Only small amounts of drug are removed by dialysis.

cefoperazone sodium • Cefobid◆

Class: ***antibiotic*** • *Pregnancy risk category B*

COMMON INDICATIONS AND DOSAGES	ADMINISTRATION	SPECIAL CONSIDERATIONS
Septicemia, peritonitis, and gynecologic, skin, urinary tract, and respiratory tract infections by susceptible organisms. *Adults:* 2 to 4 g daily in divided doses q 12 hr. For severe infections, 6 to 12 g daily in divided doses b.i.d, t.i.d., or q.i.d., ranging from 1.5 to 4 g/dose. **Dosage adjustment.** Dosage adjustment required in renal or liver impairment.	Reconstitute 1 g of drug with 5 ml of compatible diluent. Shake vial vigorously until drug dissolves. Let vial stand so foam dissipates before drawing up. For intermittent or continuous infusion, dilute with compatible solution, such as D_5W or dextrose 10% in water, lactated Ringer's, dextrose 5% in lactated Ringer's, dextrose 5% in 0.2% or 0.9% NaCl, Normosol-R, dextrose 5% and Normosol-M, and 0.9% NaCl. Stable 24 hr at room temperature, 72 hr if refrigerated. ***Incompatibilities:*** Aminoglycosides, doxapram, hetastarch, labetalol, meperidine, ondansetron, perphenazine, promethazine hydrochloride, and sargramostim. ***Intermittent infusion:*** Dilute with 20 to 40 ml of compatible diluent, then infuse over 15 to 30 minutes into tubing with compatible solution. ***Continuous infusion:*** Use enough diluent to make a solution of 2 to 25 mg/ml, then infuse at ordered rate.	• Check for cephalosporin or penicillin allergy. • Monitor patient's BUN and serum creatinine levels to assess renal function. • Monitor patient's CBC and PT results to assess bleeding problems. • Culture stool to rule out *Clostridium difficile* infection if patient has persistent diarrhea. • Watch for fungal or bacterial superinfection with prolonged use. • Tell patient to avoid alcohol during therapy and for 48 to 72 hr afterward to avoid disulfiram-like reactions. • If patient needs hemodialysis, give drug afterward. • For overdose, treat symptoms. Patient may undergo hemodialysis to remove drug.

cefotaxime sodium • Claforan ◆

Class: ***antibiotic*** • *Pregnancy risk category B*

Life-threatening infections by susceptible organisms. *Adults:* 2 g q 4 hr; maximum dosage, 12 g daily.
Moderate to severe infections by susceptible organisms. *Adults and children weighing 110 lb (50 kg) or more:* 1 to 2 g q 6 to 8 hr. *Children ages 1 month to 12 years (weighing under 110 lb):* 50 to 180 mg/kg daily in four to six divided doses. *Neonates ages 1 to 4 weeks:* 50 mg/kg q 8 hr. *Neonates under age 1 week:* 50 mg/kg q 12 hr.
Uncomplicated infections by susceptible organisms. *Adults:* 1 g q 12 hr.
Surgical prophylaxis. *Adults:* 1 g 30 to 90 minutes before surgery.
Prophylaxis for cesarean section. *Adults:* 1 g once umbilical cord clamped, then 1 g 6 and 12 hr later.
Dosage adjustment. Dosage adjustment required if patient has renal impairment.

Available in vials containing 500 mg, 1 g, or 2 g and in infusion bottles containing 1 or 2 g. Reconstitute vials with 10 ml of sterile water for injection. Shake well to dissolve. Infusion bottles can be diluted in 50 to 100 ml of D_5W or 0.9% NaCl. For continuous infusion, reconstituted drug can be diluted in 50 to 1,000 ml of compatible solution, such as D_5W or dextrose 10% in water; 0.9% NaCl; dextrose 5% in 0.2%, 0.45%, or 0.9% NaCl; invert sugar 10% in water; lactated Ringer's; and 1/6 M sodium lactate. Reconstituted solution stable 24 hr at 77° F (25° C), 10 days at below 41° F (5° C).
Incompatibilities: Aminoglycosides, aminophylline, doxapram, fluconazole, hetastarch, and sodium bicarbonate injection.
Direct injection: Give over 3 to 5 minutes into intermittent infusion device or I.V. tubing that contains free-flowing, compatible solution.
Intermittent infusion: Infuse diluted solution over 20 to 30 minutes into butterfly or scalp vein needle or through I.V. line with compatible solution. Stop primary I.V. flow if piggyback method is used.
Continuous infusion: Give ordered infusion over 24 hr.

- Check for penicillin or cephalosporin allergy.
- Assess I.V. site for inflammation or phlebitis and change site as needed.
- Monitor patient's CBC if therapy exceeds 10 days.
- If diarrhea persists during therapy, collect stool specimens to rule out pseudomembranous colitis.
- Observe patient for fungal or bacterial superinfection with prolonged use.
- For overdose, treat symptoms. Patient may undergo hemodialysis or peritoneal dialysis to remove drug.

cefotetan disodium • Cefotan ◆

Class: ***antibiotic*** • *Pregnancy risk category B*

Infections (except UTI) by susceptible organisms. *Adults:* 1 to 2 g q 12 hr; in life-threatening infections, 3 g q 12 hr.
Skin and skin-structure infections. *Adults:* 2 g daily or 1 g q 12 hr.
UTI. *Adults:* 500 mg q 12 hr or 1 to 2 g once daily or b.i.d.

Available as white to pale yellow powder in 1- and 2-g vials and infusion vials. Reconstitute vials with 10 to 20 ml sterile water for injection. Reconstitute infusion vials with 50 to 100 ml D_5W or 0.9% NaCl. Solution stable 24 hr at room temperature, 96 hr if refrigerated, 1 week if frozen.
Incompatibilities: Aminoglycosides, doxapram, and heparin sodium.

- Check for penicillin or cephalosporin allergy.
- If diarrhea persists during therapy, collect stool specimens to rule out pseudomembranous colitis.
- Check PT if patient is elderly or has renal or liver impairment, malnutrition, or cancer.

(continued)

◆ Also available in Canada. ◇ Available in Canada only.

COMMON INDICATIONS AND DOSAGES	ADMINISTRATION	SPECIAL CONSIDERATIONS
cefotetan disodium *(continued)* **Surgical prophylaxis.** *Adults:* 1 to 2 g 30 to 60 minutes before surgery. For cesarean, give as soon as umbilical cord is clamped. Maximum 6 g daily. **Dosage adjustment.** Dosage adjustment required if patient has renal impairment.	***Direct injection:*** Inject reconstituted drug directly into vein over 3 to 5 minutes. ***Intermittent infusion:*** Over 20 to 60 minutes, infuse solution through butterfly or scalp vein needle or into tubing of free-flowing, compatible solution. Stop primary I.V. during administration.	• Watch for superinfection with large doses or prolonged use. • Tell patient to avoid alcohol within 72 hr of drug administration. • For overdose, treat symptoms. Patient may undergo hemodialysis or peritoneal dialysis to remove drug.

cefoxitin sodium • Mefoxin◆

Class: ***antibiotic*** • *Pregnancy risk category B*

COMMON INDICATIONS AND DOSAGES	ADMINISTRATION	SPECIAL CONSIDERATIONS
Severe infections by susceptible organisms. *Adults:* 1 to 2 g q 6 to 8 hr; if life-threatening, up to 12 g. *Children age 3 months and older:* 80 to 160 mg/kg daily in four to six divided doses. **Surgical prophylaxis.** *Adults:* 2 g 30 to 60 minutes before surgery, then 2 g q 6 hr for 1 day after surgery. *Children age 3 months and older:* 30 to 40 mg/kg 30 to 60 minutes before surgery, then 30 to 40 mg/kg q 6 hr for up to 24 hr after. **Prophylaxis for cesarean section.** *Adults:* 2 g as single dose after cord is clamped or 2 g after cord is clamped and 2 g 4 and 8 hr later. **Dosage adjustment.** Dosage adjustment required if patient has renal impairment.	Available in 1- and 2-g vials, PVC bags, and infusion bottles. Store vials at 86° F (30° C). Reconstitute 1- and 2-g vials with 10 ml sterile water for injection. For intermittent infusion, reconstitute 1- and 2-g infusion bags or bottles with 50 to 100 ml of compatible solution, such as D_5W or dextrose 10% in water; dextrose 5% in 0.2%, 0.45%, or 0.9% NaCl; Ringer's injection; lactated Ringer's; 0.9% NaCl; 1/6 M sodium lactate; invert sugar 5% or 10% in water; and dextrose 5% and Ionosol B. Stable 24 hr at room temperature, 48 hr if chilled. Powder or solution may turn amber, which doesn't reflect lower potency. ***Incompatibilities:*** Aminoglycosides and hetastarch. ***Direct injection:*** Inject diluted drug over 3 to 5 minutes directly into vein, intermittent infusion device, or I.V. line with free-flowing, compatible solution. ***Intermittent infusion:*** Give 50 to 100 ml solution through butterfly or scalp vein needle, intermittent infusion device, or patent I.V. line at ordered flow rate. Stop primary solution during cefoxitin infusion. Give over 15 to 30 minutes. ***Continuous infusion:*** Add up to 1 liter of compatible solution to reconstituted drug and infuse for prescribed duration.	• Check for penicillin or cephalosporin allergy. • Thrombophlebitis less likely with butterfly or scalp vein needle. • If diarrhea persists during therapy, collect stool specimens to rule out pseudomembranous colitis. • Monitor patient's intake, output, serum creatinine, and BUN levels to help detect nephrotoxicity. • Watch for fungal and bacterial superinfection with large doses or prolonged use. • If patient needs hemodialysis, give loading dose of 1 to 2 g afterward. Maintenance doses should reflect patient's creatinine clearance.

ceftazidime • Ceptaz◆, Fortaz◆, Tazicef, Tazidime◆

Class: ***antibiotic*** • *Pregnancy risk category B*

Uncomplicated infections (except UTI) caused by susceptible organisms. *Adults and children over age 12:* 1 g q 8 to 12 hr; maximum 6 g daily. *Children ages 1 month to 12 years:* 25 to 50 mg/kg q 8 hr; maximum 6 g daily. *Neonates:* 30 mg/kg q 12 hr.
UTI. *Adults and children over age 12:* Uncomplicated infection, 250 mg q 12 hr; severe infection, 500 mg q 8 to 12 hr.
Bone and joint infection. *Adults and children over age 12:* 2 g q 12 hr.
Uncomplicated pneumonia and mild skin and skin-structure infections. *Adults and children over age 12:* 500 mg to 1 g q 8 hr.
Peritonitis, meningitis, severe gynecologic infections, other life-threatening infections. *Adults and children over age 12:* 2 g q 8 hr.
Dosage adjustment. Dosage adjustment required if patient has renal impairment.

Available as white to off-white sterile powder in 500-mg, 1-, and 2-g vials or in 1- and 2-g piggyback vials for infusion. Powder and solution may darken, but potency doesn't usually change. Protect from light. To reconstitute 500-mg vial, add 5 ml of sterile water for injection to yield 100 mg/ml. To reconstitute 1-g vial, add 3 ml of sterile water for injection to yield 280 mg/ml, or 10 ml to yield 95 to 100 mg/ml. To reconstitute a 2-g vial, add 10 ml of sterile water for injection to yield 180 mg/ml. For the 1- or 2-g piggyback vial, reconstitute with 10 ml sterile water for injection and dilute with 90 ml of a compatible solution to yield 10 or 20 mg/ml, respectively. Remain potent 18 to 24 hr at room temperature, 7 to 10 days if refrigerated. See manufacturer's instructions about freezing. For infusing 1 to 40 mg/ml, use these solutions: 0.9% NaCl injection; 1/6 M sodium lactate injection; dextrose 5% in 0.2%, 0.45%, or 0.9% NaCl; or D_5W or dextrose 10% in water. For infusing 1 to 20 mg/ml, use Ringer's injection, lactated Ringer's injection, invert sugar 10% in sterile water for injection, or dextrose 5% and Normosol-M.
Incompatibilities: Aminoglycosides, fluconazole, idarubicin, sargramostim, sodium bicarbonate solutions, and vancomycin.
Direct injection: Inject reconstituted drug into vein over 3 to 5 minutes or give through I.V. line with free-flowing, compatible solution.
Intermittent infusion: Using Y-type administration set, infuse solution over 15 to 30 minutes. Stop primary solution during infusion.
Continuous infusion: Infuse prescribed volume over 24 hr.

- Check for penicillin or cephalosporin allergy.
- Monitor patient's PT and give vitamin K if needed.
- Check I.V. site for inflammation; change if needed.
- If diarrhea persists during therapy, collect stool specimens to rule out pseudomembranous colitis.
- Closely monitor renal function if patient has renal impairment or is receiving aminoglycoside antibiotics or potent diuretics.
- Watch for superinfection with prolonged use.
- For overdose, treat symptoms. Patient may undergo dialysis to remove drug.

◆ Also available in Canada. ◇ Available in Canada only.

ceftizoxime sodium • Cefizox

Class: ***antibiotic*** • *Pregnancy risk category B*

COMMON INDICATIONS AND DOSAGES

Life-threatening infections by susceptible organisms. *Adults:* 3 to 4 g q 8 hr; maximum 12 g daily. *Children over 6 months old:* 200 mg/kg daily in divided doses. Maximum 12 g daily.

Uncomplicated infections (except UTI) to severe infections by susceptible organisms. *Adults:* 1 to 2 g q 8 to 12 hr; maximum 12 g daily. *Children over 6 months old:* 50 mg/kg q 6 to 8 hr. Maximum 12 g daily.

Uncomplicated UTI caused by susceptible organisms. *Adults:* 500 mg q 12 hr. Give higher dosage in *Pseudomonas aeruginosa* infection.

Dosage adjustment. Dosage adjustment required if patient has renal impairment.

ADMINISTRATION

Available as white to pale yellow crystalline powder in 500-mg, 1-, and 2-g vials. Protect from light and store at 59° to 86° F (15° to 30° C). Also supplied as frozen solution in 50-ml single-dose plastic containers, equivalent to 1 or 2 g in D_5W. Store frozen but not below –4° F (–20° C). When reconstituting powder, add 5 ml sterile water for injection to 500-mg vial, 10 ml to 1-g vial, or 20 ml to 2-g vial to yield 95 mg/ml. Reconstitute piggyback vials with 50 to 100 ml of 0.9% NaCl injection or use D_5W, dextrose 10% in water; dextrose 5% in 0.2%, 0.45%, or 0.9% NaCl; Ringer's injection; lactated Ringer's; invert sugar 10% in sterile water for injection; or 5% sodium bicarbonate in sterile water for injection. Shake well. Stable 24 hr at room temperature, 96 hr if refrigerated. May turn yellow to amber, but change doesn't reflect altered potency. Don't use if seal broken or solution leaky, cloudy, or precipitated. Thaw frozen solution at room temperature. After thawing, stable 24 hr at room temperature, 10 days if refrigerated. Don't refreeze.

Incompatibilities: Aminoglycosides.

Direct injection: Inject reconstituted drug over 3 to 5 minutes into vein or I.V. line with compatible solution. Don't inject frozen solutions intended for infusion.

Intermittent infusion: Infuse 50 to 100 ml of diluted drug over 15 to 30 minutes.

Continuous infusion: Add compatible solution to reconstituted drug in amount appropriate for patient's condition and infuse over 24 hr using infusion pump.

SPECIAL CONSIDERATIONS

- Check for penicillin or cephalosporin allergy.
- Frozen solution contains dextrose 5%.
- If patient needs high doses, takes other antibiotics (especially aminoglycosides), or has renal impairment, monitor renal function and intake and output.
- If diarrhea persists during therapy, collect stool specimens to rule out pseudomembranous colitis.
- Observe patient for superinfection with large doses or prolonged use.
- If patient needs hemodialysis, give dose afterward. Supplemental doses not required.

ceftriaxone sodium • Rocephin

Class: ***antibiotic*** • *Pregnancy risk category B*

Severe infections by susceptible organisms. *Adults:* 1 to 2 g once daily or in divided doses q 12 hr. Maximum 4 g daily. Dosage depends on infection type and severity. *Children under age 12:* 50 to 75 mg/kg daily in divided doses q 12 hr. Maximum 2 g daily.
Meningitis. *Adults and children:* 100 mg/kg/day once daily or in divided doses q 12 hr. May give 100-mg/kg loading dose. Maximum 4 g daily.
Disseminated gonococcal infections. *Adults:* 1 g daily.
Surgical prophylaxis. *Adults:* 1 g 30 minutes to 2 hr before surgery.

Available as white to yellowish orange crystalline powder in vials containing 250 mg, 500 mg, 1 g, or 2 g. Also available in 1- and 2-g piggyback vials. When reconstituted, solution turns light yellow to amber depending on diluent, concentration, and storage duration. Reconstitute with sterile water for injection, 0.9% NaCl injection, D_5W, dextrose 10% injection, or a combination of NaCl and dextrose injection and other compatible solutions. These include sodium lactate, invert sugar 10%, sodium bicarbonate 5%, FreAmine III, dextrose 5% and Normosol-M, dextrose 5% and Ionosol B, and mannitol 5% or 10%. Reconstitute by adding 2.4 ml diluent to the 250-mg vial, 4.8 ml to the 500-mg vial, 9.6 ml to the 1-g vial, or 19.2 ml to the 2-g vial. Reconstitute 1-g piggyback vial with 10 ml diluent and 2-g vial with 20 ml diluent. All reconstituted solutions yield average of 100 mg/ml. After reconstitution, dilute to 10 to 40 mg/ml for intermittent infusion. Lower concentrations can be used. Dilutions stable 24 hr to 3 days at room temperature, 3 to 10 days if refrigerated.
Incompatibilities: Aminoglycosides. Don't mix with amsacrine, clindamycin phosphate, fluconazole, or vancomycin.
Direct injection: Inject reconstituted drug over 2 to 4 minutes into vein, intermittent infusion device, or I.V. with compatible solution.
Intermittent infusion: Give diluted drug over 15 to 30 minutes using intermittent infusion device or I.V. line that contains compatible solution. Give over 10 to 30 minutes in neonates or children.

- Check for penicillin or cephalosporin allergy.
- Check PT and give vitamin K if prolonged.
- High doses, fast rates raise risk of cholelithiasis. Stop drug if symptoms of gallbladder disease occur.
- If diarrhea persists during therapy, collect stool specimens to rule out pseudomembranous colitis.
- If patient receives high doses (over 2 g daily) or other antibiotics (especially aminoglycosides) or has renal problems, track renal function, intake, and output.
- Watch for superinfection with large doses or prolonged use.
- Continue giving for at least 2 days after symptoms of infection resolve. Usual 4- to 14-day therapy may be longer in severe infection.

cefuroxime sodium • Kefurox, Zinacef

Class: ***antibiotic*** • *Pregnancy risk category B*

COMMON INDICATIONS AND DOSAGES

Uncomplicated UTI, skin and skin-structure infections; disseminated gonococcal infections; uncomplicated pneumonia caused by susceptible organisms. *Adults:* 750 mg q 8 hr. *Children over 3 months old:* 50 to 100 mg/kg daily in divided doses q 6 to 8 hr.

Severe or complicated infections by susceptible organisms. *Adults:* 1.5 g q 8 hr. Give q 6 hr if life-threatening infection or less susceptible organism.

Bacterial meningitis. *Adults:* up to 3 g q 8 hr. *Children over 3 months old:* 200 to 240 mg/kg/day in divided doses q 6 to 8 hr; after improvement, may reduce to 100 mg/kg/day.

Preoperative prophylaxis. *Adults:* 1.5 g 30 to 60 minutes before surgery and, during long procedures, 750 mg q 8 hr.

Dosage adjustment. Dosage adjustment required if patient has renal impairment.

ADMINISTRATION

Available as sterile powder in 750-mg and 1.5-g vials. Store between 59° and 86° F (15° and 30° C) and protect from light. Reconstitute Zinacef with 8 ml or 16 ml respectively (9 ml or 14 ml for Kefurox) using sterile water for injection. Withdraw 8 ml for 750-mg Kefurox dose or entire amount for other doses. After reconstitution, solutions potent for 24 hr at room temperature, 48 hr if refrigerated. Properly frozen solutions can be stored for 6 months. For infusion, dilute 750 mg or 1.5 g in 50 to 100 ml D_5W for injection. Solution potent 24 hr at room temperature, 7 days if refrigerated. Other compatible solutions include dextrose 5% in 0.2%, 0.45%, or 0.9% NaCl; dextrose 10% in water; invert sugar 10%; Ringer's injection; lactated Ringer's; 0.9% NaCl; and 1/6 M sodium lactate. Reconstitute ADD-Vantage vials according to the manufacturer's directions.

Incompatibilities: Aminoglycosides, doxapram, fluconazole, and sodium bicarbonate injection.

Direct injection: Give directly into vein over 3 to 5 minutes or inject into I.V. line that contains free-flowing, compatible solution.

Intermittent infusion: Infuse over 15 to 60 minutes after stopping primary infusion.

Continuous infusion: Infuse at ordered rate using established I.V. line.

SPECIAL CONSIDERATIONS

- Check for penicillin or cephalosporin allergy.
- Monitor patient's intake, output, serum creatinine, and BUN levels.
- Assess site for phlebitis; change site as needed.
- If diarrhea persists during therapy, collect stool specimens to rule out pseudomembranous colitis.
- Watch for superinfection with large doses or prolonged use.
- For overdose, treat symptoms. Patient may undergo hemodialysis or peritoneal dialysis.

chlordiazepoxide hydrochloride • Librium

Classes: ***anticonvulsant, anxiolytic, sedative-hypnotic*** • *Pregnancy risk category D* • *Controlled substance schedule IV*

Short-term management of acute or severe anxiety. *Adults:* 50 to 100 mg, then 25 to 50 mg t.i.d. or q.i.d., p.r.n. *Children over age 12:* 25 to 50 mg t.i.d. or q.i.d.
Acute alcohol withdrawal and resulting agitation. *Adults:* 50 to 100 mg, repeated q 2 to 4 hr, p.r.n. Maximum 300 mg daily.

Available as a dry powder in an amber ampule containing 100 mg of drug. Don't use the I.M. diluent provided by manufacturer for I.V. reconstitution because air bubbles will form. Instead, dilute powder with 5 ml of sterile 0.9% NaCl or sterile water for injection to yield 20 mg/ml. Gently rotate ampule until powder dissolves. Protect from light. Give immediately and discard unused solution.
Incompatibilities: Benzquinamide. Manufacturer recommends not mixing with any other drug.
Direct injection: Inject reconstituted drug into vein over at least 1 minute or into I.V. tubing directly above needle or cannula insertion site. After injection, flush tubing with 0.9% NaCl.

- Drug may contain benzyl alcohol.
- Check patient's vital signs before therapy and monitor them carefully during and after injection. Keep resuscitation equipment readily available.
- Maintain bed rest for at least 3 hr after injection.
- Take steps to prevent falls and injuries caused by hypotension, confusion, or oversedation.
- Monitor patient's CBC and liver function studies during prolonged therapy. To avoid withdrawal, don't stop drug abruptly after long-term administration.

chlorpromazine hydrochloride • Largactil◇, Thorazine

Classes: ***antiemetic, antipsychotic*** • *Pregnancy risk category C*

Severe hiccups. *Adults:* 25 to 50 mg.
Adjunctive treatment for tetanus. *Adults:* 25 to 50 mg t.i.d. or q.i.d. *Children age 6 months and older:* 0.55 mg/kg q 6 to 8 hr. Maximum daily dose: 40 mg for children under 50 lb (22.7 kg), 75 mg for children 50 to 100 lb (22.7 to 45.5 kg).
Vomiting during surgery. *Adults:* 2 mg q 2 minutes to total dose of 25 mg. *Children:* 1 mg q 2 minutes to total dose of 0.275 mg/kg. May repeat in 30 minutes if hypotension doesn't occur.

Available in 1- and 2-ml ampules and 10-ml multiple-dose vials at 25 mg/ml. Store below 104° F (40° C), best between 59° and 86° F (15° and 30° C). Protect from light and freezing. Discard if darker than light amber or if precipitate forms.
Incompatibilities: Aminophylline, amphotericin B, ampicillin, atropine, chloramphenicol sodium succinate, chlorothiazide, cimetidine, dimenhydrinate, heparin sodium, melphalan, methicillin, methohexital, paclitaxel, penicillin, pentobarbital, phenobarbital, thiopental, and solutions with pH of 4 to 5.
Direct injection: Dilute with 0.9% NaCl to 1-mg/ml and slowly inject ordered amount into tubing of patent I.V. at no less than 1 mg/minute for adult or 0.5 mg/minute for child.
Continuous infusion: Add ordered dose to 500 to 1,000 ml of 0.9% NaCl and infuse slowly.

- Because of possible hypotension, give I.V. only to patients on bed rest or to ambulatory patients who can be closely monitored.
- Give with patient in a supine position. Keep patient supine for at least 30 minutes after injection.
- Find baseline blood pressure and heart rate, and monitor for tachycardia and hypotension.
- Monitor intake and output for urine retention and constipation.
- After stopping drug, notify doctor if patient has dizziness, nausea, vomiting, GI upset, pain, trembling of hands and fingers, or controlled, repetitive movements of the mouth, tongue, and jaw.

◆ Also available in Canada. ◇ Available in Canada only.

COMMON INDICATIONS AND DOSAGES	ADMINISTRATION	SPECIAL CONSIDERATIONS

cidofovir • Vistide

Class: ***antiviral*** • *Pregnancy risk category C*

COMMON INDICATIONS AND DOSAGES

CMV retinitis in patients with AIDS. *Adults:* 5 mg/kg once weekly for 2 weeks, then 5 mg/kg once q 2 weeks. Must give 2 g probenecid P.O. 3 hr before and 1 g at 2 and 8 hr after completing cidofovir infusion.

Dosage adjustment. Dosage adjustment required if patient has renal impairment.

ADMINISTRATION

Available in vials containing 75 mg/ml. Dilute with 100 ml of 0.9% NaCl and give within 24 hr of preparation. If don't use immediately, refrigerate at 36° to 46° F (2° to 8° C) for up to 24 hr. Let solution reach room temperature before use.

Incompatibilities: None reported, but don't mix with other drugs or supplements.

Intermittent infusion: Infuse entire volume of diluted solution over 1 hr at a constant rate with an infusion device.

SPECIAL CONSIDERATIONS

- Because of mutagenic risk, prepare drug in a class II laminar flow biological safety cabinet. Wear surgical gloves and closed-front surgical gown with knit cuffs.
- Administer 1 L of 0.9% NaCl over 1 to 2 hr just before each cidofovir infusion.
- Give probenecid, as ordered.
- Discontinue zidovudine therapy or reduce dosage by 50% on days you give cidofovir.
- Check WBC count and differential, serum creatinine, and urine protein levels before each dose.
- For overdose, patient may receive hemodialysis and hydration. Probenecid may reduce risk of nephrotoxicity.

cimetidine hydrochloride • Tagamet◆

Class: ***antiulcer agent*** • *Pregnancy risk category B*

COMMON INDICATIONS AND DOSAGES

Short-term treatment of duodenal ulcer. *Adults:* 300 mg q 6 to 8 hr (q 12 hr if creatinine clearance under 30 ml/minute). Maximum 2,400 mg daily. Adjust to keep gastric pH above 5. To increase dosage, give 300-mg doses more often to maximum daily dosage. *Children:* 5 to 10 mg/kg q 6 to 8 hr.

Prevention of upper GI bleeding in critically ill patients. *Adults:* 50 mg/hr by continuous infusion for up to 7 days. If creatinine clearance below 30 ml/minute/

ADMINISTRATION

Available in 2-ml single-dose disposable syringes containing 300 mg, in 8-ml multidose vials containing 300 mg/2 ml, and in PVC bags containing 300 mg/50 ml. Compatible solutions include amino acid solution, D_5W, Ringer's injection, lactated Ringer's, invert sugar 5% in water, 0.9% NaCl, or dextrose 5% in 0.2%, 0.45%, or 0.9% NaCl. Use reconstituted solution within 48 hr. Protect from light and store at room temperature. Solutions become cloudy if refrigerated. Discard if discolored or precipitated.

Incompatibilities: Aminophylline, amphotericin B, barbiturates, cefamandole, cefazolin, cephalothin, indomethacin sodium trihydrate, pentobarbital sodium, and combined pen-

SPECIAL CONSIDERATIONS

- Drug may be infused over at least 30 minutes to minimize risk of adverse cardiac effects.
- Elderly patients may have drug-induced confusion.
- Because cimetidine alters gastric pH, it may affect the bioavailability of many oral drugs.
- If cimetidine and coumarin anticoagulants must be given together, closely monitor PT and adjust dosage as needed.
- If patient needs hemodialysis, give drug afterward and every 12 hr during interdialysis period.
- For overdose, treat tachycardia with a beta blocker. Patient may undergo hemodialysis.

1.73 m^2, give 25 mg/hr.

Pathologic hypersecretory conditions or intractable ulcers. *Adults:* 300 mg q 6 hr.

Dosage adjustment. Dosage adjustment may be needed by adults with liver or renal failure.

tobarbital sodium and atropine sulfate.

Direct injection: Dilute (including single-dose form) with 20 ml 0.9% NaCl for injection and give over at least 5 minutes directly into vein or through an I.V. line containing a free-flowing, compatible solution. Rapid injection may increase the risk of arrhythmias and hypotension.

Intermittent infusion: Dilute with 50 to 100 ml of compatible solution and give over 15 to 20 minutes with intermittent infusion device or into I.V. line that contains free-flowing, compatible solution.

Continuous infusion: Dilute 900 mg of drug in 100 to 1,000 ml of compatible solution. Infuse at 37.5 mg/hr with an infusion pump. Patient may need more than 900 mg/day to maintain pH control. Dosage adjustments should be individualized.

ciprofloxacin • Cipro I.V.

Class: ***antibiotic*** • *Pregnancy risk category C*

Mild to moderate UTI. *Adults:* 200 mg q 12 hr.

Severe to complicated UTI; complicated intra-abdominal infection; mild to moderate infection of lower respiratory tract, skin, skin structure, bone, and joint. *Adults:* 400 mg q 12 hr.

Mild to severe nosocomial pneumonia; severe to complicated infections of lower respiratory tract, skin, skin structure, bone, and joint. *Adults:* 400 mg q 8 hr.

Dosage adjustment. Dosage adjustment required if patient has renal impairment.

Available as clear, colorless to slightly yellow solution in 200- and 400-mg vials (injection concentrate). Reconstitute with 0.9% NaCl injection or 5% dextrose injection to yield 1 to 2 mg/ml. Stable for up to 14 days at room temperature or when refrigerated. Premixed solution also available in flexible containers of 200 mg in 100 ml 5% dextrose or 0.9% NaCl, and 400 mg in 200 ml 5% dextrose.

Incompatibilities: Aminophylline and clindamycin phosphate.

Intermittent infusion: Infuse diluted solution over 60 minutes into a large vein after stopping other solutions flowing in I.V. line.

- Make sure patient drinks enough fluids to be well hydrated and avoid crystalluria.
- Carefully monitor ALT, AST, lactic dehydrogenase, CK, serum bilirubin, and eosinophil and platelet counts; also monitor serum creatinine, BUN, uric acid, blood glucose, and triglyceride levels.
- Watch for superinfection with prolonged use.
- Caution ambulatory patient about risk of dizziness.

◆ Also available in Canada. ◇ Available in Canada only.

cisatracurium besylate • Nimbex

Class: ***skeletal muscle relaxant*** • *Pregnancy risk category B*

COMMON INDICATIONS AND DOSAGES	ADMINISTRATION	SPECIAL CONSIDERATIONS
Dosage requirements vary widely. **As adjunct to general anesthesia, to facilitate tracheal intubation, and to provide skeletal muscle relaxation during surgery.** *Adults:* 0.15 to 0.2 mg/kg followed by maintenance dose of 0.03 mg/kg q 40 to 60 minutes, p.r.n. *Children ages 2 to 12:* 0.1 mg/kg followed by 3 mcg/kg/minute maintenance infusion, reduced to 1 to 2 mcg/kg/minute p.r.n. **Maintenance of neuromuscular blockade during mechanical ventilation in ICU.** *Adults:* 3 mcg/kg/minute (range 0.5 to 10.2 mcg/kg/minute).	Available in 2- and 10-mg/ml vials. Reconstitute with 5% dextrose injection, 0.9% NaCl injection, or 5% dextrose and 0.9% NaCl injection to yield 0.1 to 0.2 mg/ml. Solutions may be refrigerated or stored at room temperature for 24 hr. ***Incompatibilities:*** Solutions with pH above 8.5, ketorolac, lactated Ringer's injection, and propofol. ***Direct injection:*** Give reconstituted solution over 5 to 10 seconds into vein or into I.V. line that contains free-flowing, compatible solution. ***Continuous infusion:*** Infuse diluted solution through I.V. line containing a compatible solution.	• Because of intermediate onset, drug isn't recommended for rapid-sequence endotracheal intubation. • Don't give drug before patient is unconscious. • Burn patient may need increased dosages. Administer analgesics, if appropriate. • Measure neuromuscular function with a peripheral nerve stimulator during infusion. • Monitor acid-base balance and electrolyte levels. • Monitor patient for malignant hyperthermia. • For overdose, maintain patent airway and control ventilation until normal neuromuscular function is achieved.

cisplatin (cis-platinum) • Platinol◊, Platinol-AQ♦

Class: ***antineoplastic*** • *Pregnancy risk category D*

COMMON INDICATIONS AND DOSAGES	ADMINISTRATION	SPECIAL CONSIDERATIONS
Metastatic testicular cancer. *Adults:* 20 mg/m^2/day for 5 days q 3 weeks for three or four cycles or 120 mg/m^2 single dose q 3 to 4 weeks for three cycles. **Metastatic ovarian cancer.** *Adults:* In combination, 75 to 100 mg/m^2 q 4 weeks; alone, 100 mg/m^2 q 4 weeks. **Advanced bladder cancer.** *Adults:* 50 to 70 mg/m^2 q 3 to 4 weeks (50 mg/m^2 q 4 weeks if patient's had radiation or other chemotherapy drugs). **Head and neck cancer.** *Adults:* In combi-	Follow facility protocol for handling chemotherapy drugs. Available as white powder in 10- and 50-mg vials or as aqueous solution at 50 mg/50 ml and 100 mg/100 ml. Protect unopened vials from bright sunlight; fluorescent light isn't harmful. Store vials up to 2 years at room temperature. Reconstitute 10-mg vial with 10 ml and 50-mg vial with 50 ml of sterile water. For intermittent infusion, dilute reconstituted drug in 2 liters 5% dextrose and 0.33% or 0.45% NaCl plus 37.5 g mannitol (18.75 g/liter). Precipitation may cause loss of potency. To avoid it, don't use needles, syringes, or I.V. kits containing aluminum and don't refrigerate reconstituted solutions. Stable 20 hr at room temperature. 72	• Perform audiometric tests before each course to detect high-frequency hearing loss. • Hydrate patient with 0.9% NaCl before giving drug. Maintain urine output of 150 to 400 ml/hr at onset of administration and for at least 4 to 6 hr thereafter, then 100 to 200 ml/hr for 18 to 24 hr. • For an antiemetic, administer high doses of metoclopramide, diphenhydramine, or dexamethasone before and after each dose. • Determine serum magnesium, potassium, calcium, creatinine, BUN, creatinine clearance levels before first infusion and each course

nation, 50 to 120 mg/m^2 as in protocol; alone, 80 to 120 mg/m^2 q 3 weeks.
Cervical carcinoma. *Adults:* 50 to 100 mg/m^2 q 3 weeks.
Non-small-cell lung carcinoma. *Adults:* In combination, 40 to 120 mg/m^2 q 3 to 6 weeks; alone, 75 to 120 mg/m^2 q 3 to 6 weeks.
Osteogenic sarcoma, neuroblastoma. *Children:* 90 mg/m^2 q 3 weeks or 30 mg/m^2 weekly.

hr if prepared with bacteriostatic water for injection and benzyl alcohol or parabens.
Incompatibilities: Aluminum, D_5W, 0.1% NaCl, and solutions with chloride content under 2%, sodium bicarbonate, sodium bisulfate, and sodium thiosulfate.
Intermittent infusion: Give diluted solution through separate I.V. line over 6 to 8 hr or according to facility protocol.
Continuous infusion: Infuse diluted solution over 24 hr or 5 days according to facility protocol.

- Monitor CBC and platelet count weekly.
- Monitor liver and kidney function.
- Check neurologic status regularly and stop drug if neurotoxicity occurs.
- Drug can be removed by hemodialysis for 3 hr after administration.

cladribine (2-chlorodeoxyadenosine) • Leustatin

Class: ***antineoplastic*** • *Pregnancy risk category D*

Treatment of active hairy cell leukemia (significant anemia, neutropenia, thrombocytopenia, or disease-related symptoms). *Adults:* 0.09 mg/kg daily by continuous I.V. infusion for 7 consecutive days, total dosage 0.63 mg/kg. Can give daily over 7 consecutive 24-hr periods or as a continuous 7-day infusion. Don't deviate from this dosage regimen. Safety and efficacy undetermined in children.

Available as preservative-free solution of 1 mg/ml (10-mg vial). Refrigerate unopened vial at 36° to 46° F (2° to 8° C) and protect from light. Freezing may cause precipitate; warm solution to room temperature and shake vigorously to return to solution. Don't heat solution or thaw in microwave. Once thawed, solution stable until labeled expiration date if refrigerated. Don't refreeze. For 24-hr infusion, add calculated dose to 500-ml infusion bag of 0.9% NaCl injection and infuse continuously over 24 hr. Don't use solution that contains dextrose. Or, for 7-day infusion, use bacteriostatic NaCl injection, which contains benzyl alcohol (a preservative). Because calculated dose dilutes preservative, its effectiveness may be reduced in patients weighing more than 187 lb (85 kg). To reduce risk of contamination, calculate 7-day dose of cladribine and amount of diluent needed to bring total volume to 100 ml. First add calculated dose to infusion reservoir through sterile 0.22-micron disposable hydrophilic syringe filter; then add calculated amount of bacteriostatic NaCl (also through filter) to bring total volume to 100 ml. Clamp line and discard filter. Using aseptic technique, aspirate any air bub-

- Monitor patient's hematologic function closely, especially during the first 4 to 8 weeks of therapy.
- Monitor patient's renal and hepatic function.
- Stop or interrupt therapy if neurotoxicity or renal toxicity occurs.
- Because drug is a potent antineoplastic agent, use disposable gloves and protective clothing. If drug touches skin or mucosa, wash with copious amounts of water.
- Watch for fever during first month of treatment.

(continued)

COMMON INDICATIONS AND DOSAGES	ADMINISTRATION	SPECIAL CONSIDERATIONS
cladribine *(continued)*	bles from reservoir using syringe with dry sterile filter or sterile vent filter assembly. Reclamp and discard syringe and filter. Physical and chemical stability has been demonstrated with Pharmacia Deltec medication cassettes. Once diluted, administer promptly or store in refrigerator for no more than 8 hr before administration. Discard unused portion using chemotherapy precautions. ***Incompatibilities:*** Don't mix with other I.V. drugs or additives or infuse with other drugs in common I.V. line. Dextrose solutions speed degradation. ***Intermittent infusion:*** Infuse daily over 7 consecutive 24-hr periods. ***Continuous infusion:*** Infuse continuously over 7 days.	

clindamycin phosphate • Cleocin Phosphate, Dalacin C Phosphate ◇

Class: ***antibiotic*** *• Pregnancy risk category B*

Severe infections by susceptible organisms. *Adults:* 600 mg to 2.7 g daily divided q 6, 8, or 12 hr or by continuous infusion to maintain serum levels of 4 to 6 mcg/ml. May increase to 4.8 g daily for life-threatening infections. *Children over 1 month old:* 15 to 40 mg/kg daily divided q 6 to 8 hr. Single dose shouldn't exceed 600 mg. *Children age 1 month or less:* 15 to 20 mg/kg daily divided q 6 to 8 hr. Maximum 300 mg daily.	Available at 150 mg/ml in 2- and 4-ml ampules and 6-ml vials. Store below 104° F (40° C), preferably between 59° and 86° F (15° and 30° C). Protect from freezing. For 6 mg/ml or less, add 25 ml of compatible solution to each 150 mg of drug (300 mg/50 ml). Compatible solutions include D_5W, dextrose 10% in water, Isolyte H, Isolyte M and dextrose 5%, Isolyte P and dextrose 5%, Normosol-R, lactated Ringer's, and 0.9% NaCl. Solutions should be used within 24 hr. ***Incompatibilities:*** Aminophylline, ampicillin, barbiturates, calcium gluconate, ciprofloxacin hydrochloride, idarubicin, magnesium sulfate, phenytoin sodium, and theophylline. Also incompatible with rubber closures, as on I.V. tubing. ***Intermittent infusion:*** Infuse diluted drug (6 mg/ml or less) with intermittent infusion device or into I.V. line that contains free-flowing, compatible solution. Give 300 mg/50 ml over 10 minutes, 600 mg/100 ml over 20 minutes, or	• Drug may contain benzyl alcohol. • Anaphylaxis requires emergency treatment with epinephrine, oxygen, and corticosteroids. • During long-term therapy, monitor patent's kidney and liver function tests and blood cell counts. • If severe, persistent diarrhea occurs, discontinue drug and obtain a stool specimen for culture. • Watch for superinfection with prolonged use. • Colitis may not develop for several weeks after drug has been discontinued.

900 mg/150 ml over 30 minutes. Give 1,200 mg/100 ml over 40 minutes. Don't give more than 1,200 mg in 1 hr.
Continuous infusion: Give a single, rapid infusion followed by continuous infusion using diluted drug (6 mg/ml). For serum levels above 4 mcg/ml, rapidly infuse 10 mg/minute for 30 minutes, then give maintenance dose of 0.75 mg/minute. For serum levels above 5 mcg/ml, rapidly infuse 15 mg/minute for 30 minutes, then give maintenance dose of 1 mg/minute. For serum levels above 6 mcg/ml, rapidly infuse 20 mg/minute for 30 minutes, then give maintenance dose of 1.25 mg/minute.

colchicine

Class: ***antigout*** *• Pregnancy risk category D*

Acute gout, gouty arthritis. *Adults:* 2 mg, followed by 0.5 mg q 6 hr p.r.n. Maximum 4 mg daily.

Available in 1-mg/2 ml ampules. Dilute with 0.9% NaCl injection or sterile water for injection. Store in tight, light-resistant container away from moisture and high temperatures. Don't use if turbid.
Incompatibilities: 5% dextrose injection and bacteriostatic 0.9% NaCl injection.
Direct injection: Give by slow I.V. push over 2 to 5 minutes into vein or I.V. tubing that contains free-flowing, compatible solution.

- Obtain baseline laboratory studies, including CBC, before starting therapy and periodically thereafter.
- Advise patient to report rash, sore throat, fever, unusual bleeding and bruising, tiredness, weakness, numbness, or tingling.
- Stop drug if patient has nausea, abdominal pain, vomiting, or diarrhea — the first signs of toxicity.

corticotropin (ACTH) • Acthar◆

Class: ***diagnostic aid*** *• Pregnancy risk category C*

Diagnosis of adrenocortical insufficiency in otherwise normal patients and those with complete primary adrenal insufficiency. *Adults:* 10 to 25 U over 8 hr.
Evaluation of adrenocortical reserve in

Available as a lyophilized white or near-white, water-soluble solid in 25- or 40-unit vials. Reconstitute with sterile water for injection or 0.9% NaCl for injection so that required dose is contained in 1 to 2 ml of solution. For continuous infusion, dilute in 500 ml of compatible solution, such as lactated Ringer's, 0.9% NaCl, D_5W, or dextrose 5% in 0.9% NaCl.

- Hypersensitivity reactions, including anaphylaxis, have occurred. Keep emergency supplies available.
- Increased dosage prolongs duration of action.
- Drug raises blood glucose level; diabetic patients may need increased insulin dosage.

(continued)

◆ Also available in Canada. ◇ Available in Canada only.

COMMON INDICATIONS AND DOSAGES	ADMINISTRATION	SPECIAL CONSIDERATIONS
corticotropin *(continued)* **secondary adrenocortical insufficiency or hypopituitarism.** *Adults:* 10 to 25 U over 8 hr daily on 4 to 5 successive days. **Rapid screening of adrenocortical insufficiency.** *Adults:* 25 U by rapid injection.	Reconstituted solution stable 1 to 7 days when stored at 36° to 46° F (2° to 8° C). ***Incompatibilities:*** Aminophylline and sodium bicarbonate. ***Direct injection:*** Inject reconstituted drug into vein or I.V. tubing that contains free-flowing, compatible solution. ***Intermittent infusion:*** Infuse diluted solution over 8 hr. ***Continuous infusion:*** Infuse diluted solution q 12 hr for 48 hr.	• Monitor patient's weight and intake and output. • Prolonged therapy may require calorie or sodium restriction or potassium supplement. • Repeated infusions on successive days heighten adrenocortical response to further stimulation.

cosyntropin • Cortrosyn♦

Class: ***diagnostic aid*** • *Pregnancy risk category C*

COMMON INDICATIONS AND DOSAGES	ADMINISTRATION	SPECIAL CONSIDERATIONS
Rapid screening of adrenal function. *Adults and children age 2 and over:* 0.25 mg. *Children under age 2:* 0.125 mg. **Adrenal stimulus.** *Adults:* 0.25 mg at a rate of 0.04 mg/hr for 6 hr.	Available in two-vial packets. Store at 59° to 86° F (15° to 30° C) unless manufacturer specifies otherwise. To reconstitute, add 1 ml of 0.9% NaCl injection to vial containing 0.25 mg of drug to yield 250 mcg/ml. For infusion, dilute with D_5W or 0.9% NaCl. Reconstituted solution stable 24 hr at room temperature, 3 weeks if refrigerated at 36° to 46° F (2° to 8° C). Diluted solution stable 12 hr at room temperature. ***Incompatibilities:*** Blood and plasma (enzymes inactivate drug). ***Direct injection:*** Use intermittent infusion device to give drug over 2 minutes or inject into I.V. tubing with free-flowing, compatible solution. Stop primary infusion during injection. ***Intermittent infusion:*** Give diluted solution at 0.04 mg/hr for 4 to 8 hr.	• Highest plasma cortisol levels occur about 45 to 60 minutes after giving cosyntropin. • Watch patient closely for adverse reactions. Keep emergency resuscitation equipment nearby when giving drug because of risk of anaphylaxis.

co-trimoxazole (trimethoprim-sulfamethoxazole) • Bactrim I.V. Infusion, Septra I.V. Infusion♦

Class: ***antibiotic*** • *Pregnancy risk category C (D near term)*

COMMON INDICATIONS AND DOSAGES	ADMINISTRATION	SPECIAL CONSIDERATIONS
Systemic bacterial infections by susceptible organisms. *Adults and children*	Available in 5-ml ampules and 5-, 10-, and 30-ml vials. Before infusion, add 125 ml of D_5W to dilute 5-ml vial. New concen-	• Closely monitor patients with AIDS because of increased risk of severe adverse reactions.

age 2 months and over: 8 to 10 mg/kg trimethoprim in two to four doses q 6, 8, or 12 hr. Maximum 960 mg/day.
***Pneumocystis carinii* pneumonitis.** *Adults and children age 2 months and older:* 15 to 20 mg/kg trimethoprim in three or four divided doses q 6 to 8 hr.
Dosage adjustment. Dosage in renal failure reflects creatinine clearance.

tration contains 0.64 mg trimethoprim and 3.2 mg sulfamethoxazole. Diluted 1:25 solution stable 6 hr at room temperature. Solutions with 0.64 to 0.83 mg trimethoprim and 3.2 to 4 mg sulfamethoxazole stable for 4 hr; those with 0.8 to 1.1 mg trimethoprim and 4 to 5.3 mg sulfamethoxazole stable 2 hr. Don't refrigerate drug or solutions. Discard cloudy or precipitated solutions.
Incompatibilities: Avoid diluting with any solution but D_5W because drug components lose potency. Manufacturer recommends mixing with no other drugs.
Intermittent infusion: Infuse ordered dose of diluted drug into an I.V. line of free-flowing D_5W over 60 to 90 minutes or into a flushed and patent intermittent infusion device. If the only available site contains incompatible solution, flush tubing with 10 ml sterile water for injection before and after infusion and turn off primary I.V. solution during administration.

- Monitor patient's BUN, serum creatinine, CBC, platelet count, PTT, PT, electrolyte levels, and urinalysis results.
- Tell patient to increase fluids to stay hydrated.
- Watch for superinfection with prolonged use.
- Trimethoprim and active sulfamethoxazole are partially removed by dialysis.

cyclophosphamide • Cytoxan◆, Neosar, Procytox◇

Class: ***antineoplastic*** • *Pregnancy risk category D*

Lymphomas; acute leukemia (in adults); cancers of lung, brain, breast, and reproductive organs; autoimmune diseases; prevention of graft-versus-host disease in organ transplants. Dosage reflects patient's disease, condition, response, and other treatments. *Adults:* 40 to 50 mg/kg in divided doses over 2 to 5 days. Maintenance dosage is 10 to 15 mg/kg q 7 to 10 days or 3 to 5 mg/kg twice weekly. *Children:* 2 to 8 mg/kg or 60 to 250 mg/m² once weekly for 6 weeks, depending on susceptibili-

Follow facility protocol for handling chemotherapy drugs. Available in 100-mg, 200-mg, 500-mg, 1-g, and 2-g vials. Reconstitute with sterile water for injection or bacteriostatic water for injection (parabens-preserved only) to yield 20 mg/ml. If prepared with sterile water for injection, use solution within 6 hr. Powder contains enough NaCl to produce an isotonic solution. Shake vigorously. Unreconstituted drug stable at room temperature; reconstituted drug stable for 24 hr at room temperature, 6 days if refrigerated. Discard unused drug after 24 hr. Other compatible solutions include dextrose 5% in lactated Ringer's, dextrose 5% in 0.9% NaCl, lactated Ringer's, 0.45% or 0.9% NaCl, and 1/6 M sodium lactate.

- Use a new site for each injection or infusion. Heparin locks aren't recommended.
- Infuse slowly to prevent facial flushing.
- To avoid hemorrhagic cystitis, encourage patient to void every 1 to 2 hr while awake and to drink plenty of fluids before, during, and for 72 hr after treatment.
- If cystitis (hematuria, painful urination) occurs, stop drug immediately.
- Monitor patient's CBC, kidney and liver function, and uric acid levels.
- Monitor for infection in patients with leukopenia.
- High I.V. dosage may cause SIADH, leading to hyponatremia.

(continued)

◆ Also available in Canada. ◇ Available in Canada only.

COMMON INDICATIONS AND DOSAGES	ADMINISTRATION	SPECIAL CONSIDERATIONS
cyclophosphamide *(continued)* ty of neoplasm. Maintenance dosage depends on patient tolerance and WBC count of 2,500 to 4,000/mm^3. Recommended maintenance dosage is 10 to 15 mg/kg q 7 to 10 days, or 30 mg/kg q 3 to 4 weeks, or when bone marrow recovers.	***Incompatibilities:*** None known. ***Direct injection:*** Using 23G to 25G winged-tip needle, inject reconstituted drug over 2 to 3 minutes. ***Intermittent infusion:*** Infuse diluted drug over 15 to 20 minutes.	• Tell patient to avoid OTC drugs containing aspirin. • Drug can be removed by dialysis.

cyclosporine • Sandimmune♦

Class: ***immunosuppressant*** • *Pregnancy risk category C*

Prophylaxis and treatment of organ tissue rejection. *Adults and children:* 5 to 6 mg/kg daily beginning 4 to 12 hr before surgery and continuing after surgery until patient can tolerate oral form. Adjust dose to maintain plasma trough levels of 100 to 300 ng/ml.	Available in 5-ml ampules containing 50 mg/ml. For infusion, dilute each ml of drug in 20 to 100 ml of 0.9% NaCl or D_5W. Reconstituted solution stable up to 24 hr in D_5W injection and 6 to 12 hr in 0.9% NaCl injection (6 hr in polyvinyl chloride containers and 12 hr in glass containers). Store below 104° F (40° C), preferably at 59° to 86° F (15° to 30° C). Don't freeze or expose to light. ***Incompatibilities:*** None reported. ***Continuous infusion:*** Infuse diluted drug slowly over 2 to 6 hr or up to 24 hr.	• Always give with a corticosteroid. • Significant amounts of drug are lost when given through polyvinyl chloride tubing. • Monitor patient continuously for first 30 minutes and then at frequent intervals because of risk of anaphylaxis. Keep resuscitation equipment nearby. • Perform liver and renal function tests routinely. • Monitor blood pressure because hypertension can develop within a few weeks after start of therapy.

cytarabine (Ara-C, cytosine arabinoside) • Cytosar◊, Cytosar-U

Class: ***antineoplastic*** • *Pregnancy risk category D*

Induction of remission in acute myelogenous or lymphocytic leukemia. *Adults and children:* 200 mg/m^2 daily for 5 days by continuous infusion, then 2 weeks off; maintenance dosage, 70 to 200 mg/m^2 daily for 2 to 5 days at	Follow facility protocol for handling chemotherapy drugs. Drug is available in 100-mg, 500-mg, 1-g, and 2-g vials. Reconstitute 100-mg vial with 5 ml of bacteriostatic water for injection (with benzyl alcohol) to yield 20 mg/ml. Reconstitute 500-mg vial with 10 ml to yield 50 mg/ml. Reconstitute 1-g vial with 10 ml to yield 100 mg/ml. Reconstitute 2-g vial	• When giving high-dose cytarabine, perform a thorough neurologic assessment before every dose. • Monitor patient's kidney and liver function and WBC and platelet counts. • Prevent or minimize uric acid nephropathy by providing good hydration, alkalinizing urine, or admin-

monthly intervals. Dosage varies with regimen.
Refractory leukemia or malignant lymphoma. *Adults and children:* 3 g/m^2 q 12 hr for up to 12 doses.

with 20 ml to yield 100 mg/ml. However, avoid using benzyl alcohol as a diluent when preparing high-dose cytarabine. Reconstituted solution stable 48 hr at room temperature. Discard if cloudy. For infusion, dilute with D_5W or 0.9% NaCl; solution stable 8 days at room temperature. Other compatible solutions include dextrose 5% in 0.9% NaCl and dextrose 5% in lactated Ringer's.
Incompatibilities: Cephalothin, fluorouracil, heparin sodium, methylprednisolone sodium succinate, nafcillin, oxacillin, and penicillin.
Direct injection: Give directly into vein or through a winged-tip needle, an intermittent infusion device, or an I.V. line containing a free-flowing, compatible solution.
Intermittent infusion: Give diluted drug over 1 hr or as ordered.
Continuous infusion: Give diluted drug as ordered for 5 days.

istering allopurinol.
- If toxicity occurs, withhold next dose of cytarabine and notify doctor.
- Many doctors order prophylactic ophthalmic steroid solutions and pyridoxine (100 mg daily) for patients receiving high-dose therapy.
- Treat skin reactions from high-dose cytarabine with products used in burn therapy.
- If diarrhea develops, give meticulous skin care to avoid or treat perirectal abscess. Be alert for electrolyte imbalance, malabsorption, and pressure ulcers.

cytomegalovirus immune globulin intravenous, human (CMV-IGIV) • CytoGam

Class: ***immune serum*** • *Pregnancy risk category C*

To attenuate primary CMV disease in a seronegative patient who receives a kidney transplant from a seropositive donor. *Adults:* 150 mg/kg within 72 hr of transplant, 100 mg/kg after 2 weeks, 100 mg/kg after 4 weeks, 100 mg/kg after 6 weeks, 100 mg/kg after 8 weeks, 50 mg/kg after 12 weeks, and 50 mg/kg after 16 weeks.

Available in a single-dose vial containing about 2,500 mg of lyophilized immunoglobulin. Refrigerate at 36° to 46° F (2° to 8° C). To prepare, remove tab and swab rubber stopper with 70% alcohol or equivalent. Reconstitute with 50 ml sterile water for injection to yield about 50 mg/ml. Don't shake; avoid foaming. Use double-ended transfer needle or large syringe to add diluent. For the former, insert one end into the vial of water first because the lyophilized powder is in an evacuated vial and the water will transfer by suction. After the water is transferred, release any residual vacuum to hasten

- Begin infusion within 6 hr of reconstitution and end within 12 hr.
- Adverse reactions are usually related to rate of administration. Slow or stop infusion if minor adverse reactions occur.
- Monitor patient's vital signs before infusion, midway, after infusion, and before a rate increase.
- If anaphylaxis or hypotension occurs, stop infusion and give diphenhydramine and epinephrine.

(continued)

COMMON INDICATIONS AND DOSAGES	ADMINISTRATION	SPECIAL CONSIDERATIONS
cytomegalovirus immune globulin intravenous, human *(continued)*	the dissolving process. Gently rotate container to wet any undissolved powder. Allow 30 minutes for dissolution. Reconstituted drug should be colorless and translucent. Don't store or dilute it. ***Incompatibilities:*** Don't mix with other drugs. ***Intermittent infusion:*** Give through separate I.V. line with infusion pump or piggyback into existing line of 0.9% NaCl injection, dextrose 2.5% in water, D_5W, $D_{10}W$, or $D_{20}W$. Dextrose solutions may have NaCl added. Don't dilute more than 1:2. Filter not necessary. Give first dose at 15 mg/kg/hr, increase to 30 mg/kg/hr after 30 minutes if no adverse reaction, then to 60 mg/kg/hr after another 30 minutes. Don't exceed 75 ml/hr. Subsequent doses may be given at 15 mg/kg/hr for 15 minutes, increasing at 15-minute intervals to 60 mg/kg/hr.	• Tell patient to defer live-virus vaccinations for at least 3 months after administration.

dacarbazine • DTIC♦, DTIC-Dome

Class: ***antineoplastic*** • *Pregnancy risk category C*

COMMON INDICATIONS AND DOSAGES	ADMINISTRATION	SPECIAL CONSIDERATIONS
Metastatic malignant melanoma. *Adults:* 2 to 4.5 mg/kg/day for 10 days, repeated q 4 weeks; or 250 mg/m^2/day for 5 days, repeated q 3 weeks. **Hodgkin's disease (second-line therapy).** *Adults:* 150 mg/m^2/day for 5 days with other drugs and repeated q 4 weeks; or 375 mg/m^2 on day 1 with other drugs and repeated q 15 days.	Follow facility protocol for handling chemotherapy drugs. Drug comes as a powder in 100- and 200-mg vials that require refrigeration at 36° to 46° F (2° to 8° C) and protection from light. To reconstitute, add 9.9 ml sterile water to 100-mg vial or 19.7 ml sterile water to 200-mg vial. Reconstituted drug remains stable for 8 hr at room temperature, up to 72 hr if refrigerated. Diluted solution remains stable for 8 hr at room temperature, up to 24 hr if refrigerated. Protect drug from light during infusion. If solution turns pink, drug is decomposing. ***Incompatibilities:*** Cefepime, hydrocortisone sodium succinate, piperacillin, and tazobactam. ***Direct injection:*** Inject drug directly into vein or through an intermittent infusion device over 1 minute. Apply hot packs to site to reduce pain or burning.	• Use cautiously in patients with liver or renal impairment and myelosuppression. • When possible, give by infusion; injection can be painful. • Giving antiemetic first and restricting food and fluids 4 to 6 hr before giving drug may help decrease nausea and vomiting. • Some doctors recommend that patient be well hydrated 1 hr before receiving drug. • Avoid extravasation. If it occurs, stop drug and give at another site. Apply ice to area for 24 to 48 hr. • Monitor hematologic status closely, and avoid I.M. injection when platelet count below 100,000/mm^3.

Intermittent infusion: Mix reconstituted solution with 250 ml of either D_5W or 0.9% NaCl for infusion. Infuse diluted drug over 15 to 30 minutes.

daclizumab • Zenapax

Class: ***immunosuppressant*** • *Pregnancy risk category C*

Prevention of acute organ rejection in renal transplant patients receiving immunosuppression with cyclosporine and corticosteroids. *Adults:* Five doses of 1 mg/kg I.V., first dose given no more than 24 hr before surgery and remaining doses given at 14-day intervals.

Available in single-use vials in concentrations of 25 mg/5 ml. Protect undiluted solution from direct light. Dilute in 50 ml of sterile 0.9% NaCl before administration. To avoid foaming, don't shake. Inspect for particulates and discoloration before use; don't use drug if you see them. Diluted solution should be administered within 4 hr. It may be refrigerated at 36° to 46° F (2° to 8° C) for 24 hr. Discard solution if not used within 24 hr. Don't give by direct I.V. injection.
Incompatibilities: None reported, but don't add or infuse other drugs simultaneously through one I.V. line.
Intermittent infusion: Administer over 15 minutes via a central or peripheral line.

- Protein administration may cause anaphylactoid reactions. Keep emergency drugs readily available.
- Monitor patient for lipoproliferative disorders and opportunistic infections.
- Tell patient to report any wounds that fail to heal, unusual bruising or bleeding, or fever.
- Tell patient to drink lots of fluids and to report bloody or decreased urine and painful urination.
- Tell women of child-bearing age to use birth control before therapy and until 4 months afterward.

dactinomycin (actinomycin D) • Cosmegen◆

Class: ***antineoplastic*** • *Pregnancy risk category C*

Dosage varies with patient tolerance, size and location of tumor, and treatments being used.
Choriocarcinoma, Ewing's sarcoma, rhabdomyosarcoma, testicular cancer, uterine cancer, Wilms' tumor. *Adults:* 500 mcg/day, maximum 5 days. *Children over age 6 months:* 15 mcg/kg/day for 5 days, or total dose of 2.5 mg/m^2 over 1 week. Adults and children may receive

Follow facility protocol for handling chemotherapy drugs. To prepare drug, reconstitute 500-mcg vial with 1.1 ml of preservative-free sterile water to yield 0.5 mg/ml or 2.2 ml to yield 0.25 mg/ml. Discard unused reconstituted solution; it has no preservative. Store intact vials below 85° F (30° C).
Incompatibilities: Filgrastim and diluents that contain preservatives (causes precipitation).
Direct injection: Inject 500 mcg over a few minutes, preferably through side port of I.V. line that contains free-flowing D_5W or 0.9% NaCl. Assess vein patency frequently.

- Track patient's CBC, platelet count, and renal and liver function.
- Alkalinizing urine or giving allopurinol may prevent or minimize uric acid nephropathy.
- Encourage patient to stay adequately hydrated.
- If extravasation occurs, stop infusion and aspirate as much drug as possible. Infiltrate area with 4 ml of isotonic sodium thiosulfate (1 g/10 ml) diluted with 6 ml sterile water for injection, 50 to 100 mg

(continued)

◆ Also available in Canada. ◇ Available in Canada only.

COMMON INDICATIONS AND DOSAGES	ADMINISTRATION	SPECIAL CONSIDERATIONS
dactinomycin *(continued)* second course after 3 weeks if toxic effects have subsided. **Dosage adjustment.** In obese or elderly patients, dosage based on body surface area.	After injection, run I.V. solution 2 to 5 minutes or inject 5 to 10 ml of I.V. solution through tubing to remove residual drug. Some in-line cellulose ester filters may partly remove active drug from I.V. solution. ***Intermittent infusion:*** Dilute clear, gold-colored reconstituted drug with D_5W or 0.9% NaCl. Infuse over 10 to 15 minutes into tubing of free-flowing I.V. solution.	hydrocortisone sodium succinate, or ascorbic acid injection. Cover with sterile gauze and cold compresses.

dantrolene sodium • Dantrium Intravenous◆

Class: ***skeletal muscle relaxant*** • *Pregnancy risk category C*

COMMON INDICATIONS AND DOSAGES	ADMINISTRATION	SPECIAL CONSIDERATIONS
Prevention of malignant hyperthermia crisis. *Adults:* 2.5 mg/kg given over 1 hr, about 1.25 hr before anesthesia. **Adjunctive treatment of malignant hyperthermia crisis.** *Adults and children:* At least 1 mg/kg initially, repeated until symptoms subside or reach maximum total dose of 10 mg/kg. To prevent recurrence, 4 to 8 mg/kg/day P.O. in four divided doses for 1 to 3 days after crisis.	Supplied in 20-mg vials. Reconstitute with 60 ml sterile water (without a bacteriostatic agent) for a concentration of 0.333 mg/ml. Solution remains stable for 6 hr when stored at 59° to 86° F (15° to 30° C). Protect from light. ***Incompatibilities:*** D_5W and 0.9% NaCl. Don't mix with other drugs in a syringe. ***Direct injection:*** Rapidly inject drug directly into vein or through an I.V. line containing a free-flowing, compatible solution.	• Expect to obtain baseline liver function tests at the start of therapy. • Obtain baseline neuromuscular functions for later comparisons. • Because of solution's high pH, avoid extravasation. • Track urine output and serum electrolyte levels. • As ordered, give oxygen, treatments for metabolic acidosis, and cooling measures while giving dantrolene. • Check liver and renal function tests and WBC and platelet count, especially in prolonged therapy.

daunorubicin hydrochloride (daunomycin hydrochloride) • Cerubidine◆

Class: ***antineoplastic*** • *Pregnancy risk category D*

COMMON INDICATIONS AND DOSAGES	ADMINISTRATION	SPECIAL CONSIDERATIONS
To induce remission in acute nonlymphocytic leukemia (adults) and acute lymphocytic leukemia (adults and children) when used with other chemotherapy drugs. *Adults:* 30 or 45 mg/m^2/day on days 1, 2, and 3 of first course; for	Follow facility protocol for handling chemotherapy drugs. Drug available in 20-mg glass vials. Reconstitute with 4 ml of sterile water for injection, then draw desired dose into syringe containing 10 to 15 ml of 0.9% NaCl. Reconstituted solution stable for 24 hr at room temperature and 48 hr if refrigerated and protected from direct sunlight.	• Give antiemetic before treatment, as ordered, to prevent nausea and vomiting. • Watch for signs of infiltration, and tell patient to report changes in sensation, such as burning at the I.V. site. Extravasation can cause slow, progressive skin necrosis and painful ulcers. If it occurs, stop

acute nonlymphocytic leukemia, on days 1 and 2 of subsequent courses. *Children:* 25 mg/m^2 weekly together with other chemotherapy drugs.
To induce remission in acute myelogenous leukemia. *Adults:* 60 mg/m^2/day for 3 days, repeated q 3 to 4 weeks. Maximum total lifetime dose, 550 mg/m^2 (450 mg/m^2 after chest radiation therapy).
Dosage adjustment. Manufacturer suggests giving 75% of daily dose if patient's serum bilirubin levels are 1.2 to 3 mg/dl and 50% if serum bilirubin or creatinine levels exceed 3 mg/dl.

Incompatibilities: Dexamethasone and heparin. Don't mix with other drugs.
Direct injection: Give drug through side port of new I.V. line. Inject 10 to 15 ml over 2 to 3 minutes, then flush vein with primary I.V. solution.
Intermittent infusion: Infuse 100 ml of solution over 30 to 45 minutes. Flush and monitor site as above.

injection and aspirate as much drug as possible. Infiltrate area with 50 to 100 ml of hydrocortisone sodium succinate or sodium bicarbonate and apply cold compresses.
- Drug can reactivate radiation-induced skin lesions.
- Keep patient well hydrated; alkalinizing urine and possibly administering allopurinol can prevent or minimize uric acid nephropathy.
- Monitor ECG (before treatment and monthly during therapy), CBC, and hepatic function.
- Tell patient that urine may turn red for 1 to 2 days, but not from blood.

deferoxamine mesylate • Desferal◆

Class: ***heavy metal antagonist*** • *Pregnancy risk category C*

Acute iron intoxication for patients in CV collapse. (I.M. route preferred for all patients not in shock.) *Adults and children:* 1 g initially, followed by 500 mg q 4 hr for 2 doses, then 500 mg q 4 to 12 hr if needed based on clinical response. Maximum dose 6 g in 24 hr.
Chronic iron overload. *Adults and children:* 0.5 to 1 g I.M. Also 2 g I.V. with, but separate from, each unit of blood, rate not to exceed 15 mg/kg/hr.

Available in 500-mg vials. Reconstitute by adding 2 ml of sterile water for injection to each vial. Further dilute for I.V. infusion by adding 0.9% NaCl, D_5W, or lactated Ringer's solution. Reconstituted solution stable for 1 week when protected from light. Store below 104° F (40° C), preferably between 59° and 86° F (15° and 30° C).
Incompatibilities: All drugs in solution or syringe.
Intermittent infusion: Infuse diluted solution directly into vein or through I.V. line that contains free-flowing, compatible solution at a rate not exceeding 15 mg/kg/hr.
Continuous infusion: Same rate as intermittent infusion.

- Drug is most effective when given early in treatment of iron intoxication. It isn't used in place of standard measures for iron intoxication; rather, it's used only in potentially fatal intoxication (serum iron level above 400 mcg/dl) or when patient has severe symptoms, such as coma, seizures, or CV collapse.
- If giving I.V., change to I.M. as soon as possible.
- Keep epinephrine 1:1,000 readily available in case of allergic reaction.
- Warn patient that urine may turn red.
- Tell patient to report adverse reactions promptly, such as changes in hearing or vision.

◆ Also available in Canada. ◇ Available in Canada only.

COMMON INDICATIONS AND DOSAGES	ADMINISTRATION	SPECIAL CONSIDERATIONS

desmopressin acetate • DDAVP♦, Octostim◊

Classes: ***antidiuretic, hemostatic*** • *Pregnancy risk category B*

COMMON INDICATIONS AND DOSAGES	ADMINISTRATION	SPECIAL CONSIDERATIONS
Nonnephrogenic diabetes insipidus. *Adults and children age 12 and over:* 2 to 4 mcg daily given in two divided doses. Dosage adjustment based on changes in urine volume and osmolality. **Hemophilia A and von Willebrand disease.** *Adults and children age 3 months and older:* 0.3 mcg/kg by slow I.V. infusion.	Available in 10-ml multidose vials, 1-ml ampules (4 mcg/ml), and 1- and 2-ml ampules (15 mcg/ml). Store at 39° F (4° C) unless manufacturer specifies otherwise. Protect from freezing. ***Incompatibilities:*** None reported. ***Intermittent infusion:*** Dilute appropriate dose in 50 ml of 0.9% NaCl if patient weighs more than 22 lb (10 kg) or in 10 ml of 0.9% NaCl if patient weighs 22 lb or less. Infuse diluted drug over 15 to 30 minutes. Rapid administration may produce hypotension.	• During infusion, assess blood pressure and pulse. After, check intake, output, and serum sodium level. • Decrease patient's fluid intake to avoid water intoxication and hyponatremia. • If patient has hemorrhagic disorder, monitor levels of factor VIII, factor VIII:R co-factor, factor VIII antigen levels, and APTT. • If patient has diabetes insipidus, monitor urine volume and osmolality and serum osmolality.

dexamethasone sodium phosphate • Dalalone, Decadron Phosphate♦, Decaject, Dexasone, Dexone, Hexadrol Phosphate, Solurex

Classes: ***anti-inflammatory, immunosuppressant*** • *Pregnancy risk category C*

COMMON INDICATIONS AND DOSAGES	ADMINISTRATION	SPECIAL CONSIDERATIONS
Adjunctive treatment of shock. *Adults:* 1 to 6 mg/kg in a single dose, 40 mg q 2 to 6 hr p.r.n., or 20 mg in a single dose followed by 3 mg/kg over 24 hr in a continuous infusion. **Adjunctive treatment of cerebral edema.** *Adults:* 10 mg I.V. initially, then 4 mg I.M. q 6 hr. For inoperable or recurrent brain tumor, 2 mg I.V. given b.i.d. or t.i.d as maintenance dose.	Available in 4-, 10-, and 24-mg/ml vials and syringes in various sizes. Solution is clear but may look yellow at higher concentrations. Dilute in D_5W or 0.9% NaCl for intermittent or continuous infusion. Protect from light and freezing. ***Incompatibilities:*** Daunorubicin, doxorubicin, and vancomycin. ***Direct injection:*** Give undiluted drug over at least 1 minute. ***Intermittent infusion:*** Give diluted drug as ordered. ***Continuous infusion:*** Infuse diluted drug over 24 hr.	• Keep emergency resuscitation equipment nearby throughout therapy. • I.V. route usually followed by I.M. or P.O. route. • Long-term therapy may retard bone growth in infants and children; they should be monitored closely.

dexrazoxane • Zinecard

Class: ***cardioprotective agent*** • *Pregnancy risk category C*

To prevent and control doxorubicin-induced cardiomyopathy in women with metastatic breast cancer who have received a cumulative dose of 300 mg/m^2 but would benefit from continued doxorubicin therapy. *Adults:* dosage ratio of dexrazoxane to doxorubicin is 10:1 (such as 500 mg/m^2 dexrazoxane to 50 mg/m^2 doxorubicin).

Drug must be diluted with supplied diluent (0.167 M sodium lactate injection) to reach concentration of 10 mg dexrazoxane per 1 ml sodium lactate. Reconstituted drug may be further diluted with either 0.9% NaCl or D_5W to a concentration range of 1.3 to 5 mg/ml in I.V. infusion bags. Solutions are stable for 6 hr at 59° to 86° F (15° to 30° C). Discard unused solutions. When handling and preparing reconstituted solution, wear gloves and use precautions needed for antineoplastic drugs. If drug powder or solution contacts skin or mucosa, immediately wash affected area thoroughly with soap and water.
Incompatibilities: Don't mix with other drugs.
Direct injection: Administer by slow I.V. push. Within 30 minutes of start, give I.V. injection of doxorubicin.
Intermittent infusion: Administer by rapid I.V. infusion over 5 to 15 minutes. Within 30 minutes of the start time, give I.V. injection of doxorubicin.

- Take precautions against infection and use CBC results to guide precautions against bleeding.
- Tell patient to report signs of infection and bleeding.
- Take patient's temperature daily.
- For overdose, give supportive care until myelosuppression and related conditions resolve.

dextran • Low-molecular-weight dextran 40: Dextran 40, Gentran 40, LMD 10%, Rheomacrodex; High-molecular-weight dextran 70 and 75: Dextran 70, Dextran 75, Gentran 70, Macrodex

Class: ***plasma volume expander*** • *Pregnancy risk category C*

Adjunctive treatment of shock from hemorrhage, burns, surgery, or other trauma. *Adults and children:* Dosage corresponds to fluid loss and resulting hemoconcentration. For 10% low-molecular-weight solution, don't exceed 2 g/kg (20 ml/kg) for first 24 hr, then 1 g/kg (10 ml/kg) daily for 4 days. For 6% high-molecular-weight solution, don't exceed

Available in 500-ml bottles as a 6% (high molecular weight) or 10% (low molecular weight) solution diluted in 0.9% NaCl or D_5W. Store at a constant temperature, preferably 77° F (25° C). Crystals may form at low temperatures. Place bottle in warm water to dissolve them before infusing. Don't use cloudy solution. Discard partly used bottles because solution has no preservatives.
Incompatibilities: Ascorbic acid, phytonadione, promethazine, and protein hydrolysate. Don't add any drug to a bottle of dextran.

- Check patient's pulse, blood pressure, central venous pressure, and urine output every 5 to 15 minutes for first hr and then hourly.
- Stop infusion at first sign of allergic reaction. Keep I.V. access open and resuscitation equipment available.
- Maintain hydration with additional I.V. fluids.
- Slow or stop infusion if central venous pressure rises rapidly (normal is 7 to 14 cm H_2O) or if patient is

(continued)

◆ Also available in Canada. ◇ Available in Canada only.

COMMON INDICATIONS AND DOSAGES	ADMINISTRATION	SPECIAL CONSIDERATIONS
dextran *(continued)* 1.2 g/kg (20 ml/kg) for first 24 hr, then 0.6 g/kg (10 ml/kg) daily, p.r.n. **Prevention of venous thrombosis and pulmonary embolism.** *Adults:* 50 to 100 g (500 to 1,000 ml) of 10% low-molecular-weight solution during surgery, then 50 g daily for 2 to 3 days, then 50 g q 2 or 3 days up to 2 weeks.	***Intermittent infusion:*** Give 500 ml of low-molecular-weight dextran over 15 to 30 minutes. Slowly infuse remainder based on patient response. In an emergency, infuse high-molecular-weight dextran at 1.2 to 2.4 g (20 to 40 ml)/minute. Don't exceed 0.24 g (4 ml)/minute in normovolemic patient. ***Continuous infusion:*** Infuse over 24 hr based on patient condition and response.	anuric or oliguric after receiving 500 ml of dextran. Give mannitol to help increase urine flow. • Change I.V. tubing or flush well with 0.9% NaCl before transfusing blood. Dextran may cause blood to coagulate in the tubing.

dextrose in NaCl solutions

Class: ***fluid volume replacement*** • *Pregnancy risk category C*

COMMON INDICATIONS AND DOSAGES	ADMINISTRATION	SPECIAL CONSIDERATIONS
Temporary treatment of circulatory insufficiency and shock when plasma volume expander isn't available; fluid replacement, especially in patients with burns or dehydration. *Adults and children:* Concentration and rate reflect patient's age, weight, condition, and fluid, electrolyte, and acid-base balance.	Available in 250-, 500-, and 1,000-ml bottles and polyvinyl chloride bags. Dextrose 5% in 0.2% NaCl also comes in 150-ml containers. Concentrations include 2.5% dextrose in 0.45% NaCl; 5% dextrose in 0.11%, 0.2%, 0.225%, 0.3%, 0.45%, or 0.9% NaCl; and 10% dextrose in 0.2% or 0.9% NaCl. Store solutions in a cool, dry place and protect from freezing or extreme heat. Don't give cloudy solution. ***Incompatibilities:*** Amphotericin B, ampicillin sodium, amsacrine, diazepam, erythromycin lactobionate, mannitol, and phenytoin. ***Continuous infusion:*** Infuse through peripheral or central vein at ordered rate.	• Solutions of dextrose 2.5% or 5% and 0.45% NaCl are hypotonic. Others are isotonic. • Assess changes in fluid balance, electrolyte levels, and acid-base balance during prolonged parenteral therapy. • Give electrolyte supplements as needed. • Watch for fluid overload (increased hypertension, signs of heart failure or pulmonary edema), especially in elderly patients or those with renal or cardiac disease.

dextrose in water solutions (glucose solutions)

Classes: ***caloric agent, fluid volume replacement, total parenteral nutrition component*** • *Pregnancy risk category C*

COMMON INDICATIONS AND DOSAGES	ADMINISTRATION	SPECIAL CONSIDERATIONS
To provide calories and water for metabolism and hydration. *Adults and children:* 2.5%, 5%, or 10% solution.	Available in 50-, 100-, 150-, 250-, 500-, and 1,000-ml bottles or polyvinyl chloride bags in the following concentrations: 2.5%, 5%, 7.7%, 10%, 11.5%, 20%, 25%, 30%, 38%,	• Solutions of 2.5% are hypotonic, solutions of 5% are isotonic, and solutions over 10% are hypertonic. • Extravasation can cause tissue sloughing and

Hyperkalemia and conditions that require calories but little water. *Adults and children:* 20% solution.
To promote diuresis. *Adults and children:* 20% to 50% solution.
Base solution for I.V. hyperalimentation. *Adults and children:* 10% to 70% solution.
Adjunctive treatment of shock. *Adults and children:* 40% to 70% solution.
Cerebral edema, pregnancy-induced hypertension, renal disease, acute hypoglycemia, and as sclerosing agent. *Adults and children:* 50% solution.
Acute symptomatic hypoglycemia. *Infants and neonates:* 10% to 25% solution.

38.5%, 40%, 50%, 60%, and 70%. Because dextrose is an excellent medium for bacterial growth, store solutions in a cool, dry place. Protect from freezing and extreme heat. Don't give cloudy solution.
Incompatibilities: Ampicillin sodium, cisplatin, diazepam, erythromycin lactobionate, fat emulsions (10% and 25%), phenytoin, procainamide, thiopental (10% and above), and whole blood.
Direct injection: Give 50 ml of 50% solution at 3 ml/minute.
Continuous infusion: Give isotonic solutions through peripheral vein, hypertonic solutions through central venous line. Rate depends on concentration and patient's age and condition. Hourly rate above 0.5 g/kg may cause glycosuria in healthy people. Don't exceed 0.8 g/kg/hr.

necrosis. Rapid infusion of hypertonic solution can cause hyperglycemia and fluid shift.
- Monitor patient's serum glucose levels and electrolyte and acid-base balance during prolonged therapy. Give electrolyte supplements, as needed.
- Monitor patient's intake, output, and weight, and watch for signs of fluid overload.
- To avoid rebound hypoglycemia, substitute dextrose 5% or 10% after stopping hypertonic solution.

diazepam • Valium ◆

Classes: ***amnesic, anticonvulsant, anxiolytic, sedative-hypnotic*** • *Pregnancy risk category D* • *Controlled substance schedule IV*

Short-term relief of acute anxiety or as skeletal muscle relaxant in patients who can't take oral medication. *Adults and children over age 12:* 2 to 10 mg (0.4 to 2 ml) q 3 to 4 hr. May repeat in 1 hr. Maximum 30 mg in 8 hr. Give 2 to 5 mg to elderly patients or when another sedative has been given.
Cardioversion. *Adults:* 5 to 15 mg (1 to 3 ml) just before procedure as amnesic.
Endoscopy. *Adults:* Up to 20 mg before procedure, titrated for desired effect. May produce anterograde amnesia.
Tetanus. *Adults and children age 5 and*

Available in 10-ml vials (5 mg/ml), prefilled syringes, and 2-ml ampules. Protect vials from light. Manufacturer warns against diluting drug because of incompatibility, but studies have used diazepam infusions prepared using 0.9% NaCl injection. Concentration shouldn't exceed 10 mg/100 ml, and only glass bottles should be used. Avoid polyvinyl chloride infusion sets, and use an in-line filter. Don't store in plastic syringes. Check with a pharmacist for more information.
Incompatibilities: All other drugs and most I.V. solutions.
Direct injection: Slowly inject undiluted drug into large vein or catheter at less than 5 mg/minute for adults and 0.25 mg/kg of body weight over 3 minutes for children. Avoid extravasation. If drug is injected into tubing, choose a site di-

- Obtain baseline blood pressure and respiratory rate.
- If patient is receiving a narcotic, expect to reduce its dosage by at least one-third.
- Keep emergency resuscitation equipment nearby.
- Stop drug if paradoxical reaction occurs: anxiety, acute excitation, hallucinations, increased muscle spasticity, insomnia, or rage.
- Abrupt withdrawal after high doses or extended use can cause seizures and delirium.
- Keep patient in bed for 3 hr after parenteral use.
- For overdose, provide supportive care. Maintain airway patency and give I.V. fluids. Give dopamine, norepinephrine, and metaraminol for hypotension.

(continued)

◆ Also available in Canada. ◇ Available in Canada only.

COMMON INDICATIONS AND DOSAGES	ADMINISTRATION	SPECIAL CONSIDERATIONS
diazepam *(continued)* *older:* 5 to 10 mg. May repeat dose in 3 to 4 hr. *Infants over age 1 month:* 1 to 2 mg q 3 to 4 hr. **Status epilepticus and recurrent seizures.** *Adults:* 5 to 10 mg by slow I.V. push at 2 to 5 mg/minute. May repeat q 10 to 15 minutes up to 30 mg. Give 2 to 5 mg to elderly or debilitated patients; in recurrent seizures, may repeat dose in 20 to 30 minutes. *Children age 5 and older:* 0.5 to 1 mg q 2 to 5 minutes to total of 10 mg. May repeat in 2 to 4 hr. *Infants over age 1 month:* 0.2 to 0.5 mg q 2 to 5 minutes to total of 5 mg. May repeat in 2 to 4 hr.	rectly above the needle or catheter insertion site. Afterward, flush with 0.9% NaCl.	

diazoxide • Hyperstat IV

Classes: ***antihypertensive, antihypoglycemic*** • *Pregnancy risk category C*

COMMON INDICATIONS AND DOSAGES	ADMINISTRATION	SPECIAL CONSIDERATIONS
Emergency treatment of severe malignant and nonmalignant hypertension. *Adults and children:* 1 to 3 mg/kg (maximum 150 mg) as single injection repeated q 5 to 15 minutes until response is adequate. Maintenance doses q 4 to 24 hr p.r.n. until oral antihypertensive therapy can start.	Available in 20-ml ampules of 300 mg. Store between 36° and 86° F (2° and 30° C), and protect from freezing, heat, and light. ***Incompatibilities:*** Hydralazine and propranolol. ***Direct injection:*** Inject undiluted drug over 10 to 30 seconds. Avoid extravasation because drug is extremely alkaline. Slow injection causes a reduced response because of drug's extensive protein binding. ***Intermittent infusion:*** Usually not recommended; however, some investigators have used intermittent infusions of 7.5 to 30 mg/minute for 30 minutes.	• Record blood pressure during and after rapid infusion to monitor rapid fall. Monitor every 5 minutes until blood pressure is stable, then hourly. • Monitor intake and output for fluid retention. Weigh patient daily. • Watch diabetic patient for signs of severe hyperglycemia or hyperosmolar nonketotic coma. Give insulin, as needed. • Keep patient supine during infusion and for 15 to 30 minutes after. If he becomes hypotensive, keep him supine for at least 1 hr. If he receives furosemide with diazoxide, keep him supine for 8 to 10 hr.

- If extravasation occurs, infiltrate the area with NaCl solution, then apply warm compresses. Relieve pain by infiltrating a local anesthetic.
- I.V. diazoxide usually lasts no longer than 5 days before oral antihypertensive therapy starts. Don't give drug for more than 10 days.
- Long-term monitoring is necessary because drug has a long half-life.

diethylstilbestrol diphosphate • Honvol◇, Stilphostrol

Classes: ***estrogen replacement, antineoplastic*** • *Pregnancy risk category X*

Palliative treatment of prostatic cancer. *Adults:* 0.5 g on first day, then 1 g/day for 5 or more days as needed based on patient's therapeutic response. Maintenance dosage is 0.25 to 0.5 g once or twice weekly.

Available in 5-ml vials containing 250 mg of colorless to straw-colored drug. Dilute with 300 ml D_5W or 0.9% NaCl. Store at 59° to 86° F (15° to 30° C); avoid freezing.
Incompatibilities: None reported.
Intermittent infusion: Infuse diluted drug at 1 to 2 ml/minute for 10 to 15 minutes into an I.V. line that contains a free-flowing, compatible solution. Adjust rate so remaining solution infuses within 1 hr. Go slowly; rapid rate can cause perineal or vaginal burning.

- If specimens must be analyzed by a pathologist, indicate that patient is receiving estrogen therapy.
- Watch closely for signs of hypercalcemia (polyuria, polydipsia, weakness, constipation, mental changes). Tell patient to report these signs immediately; hypercalcemia can rapidly progress to coma and death.
- Instruct patient to report leg pain, chest pain, or dyspnea promptly. High-dose therapy causes an increased risk of thrombophlebitis and other thromboembolic complications (pulmonary embolism, MI, and CVA).

digoxin • Lanoxin◆

Classes: ***antiarrhythmic, intropic*** • *Pregnancy risk category C*

Heart failure, atrial flutter and fibrillation, atrial tachycardias (including paroxysmal atrial tachycardia). *Adults and children over age 10:* loading dose 0.5 to 1 mg (or 0.008 to 0.012 mg/kg); maintenance 0.125 to 0.5 mg daily (usu-

Available in 1- and 2-ml ampules (0.25 mg/ml) for adults and in 1-ml ampules (0.1 mg/ml) for children. Store at room temperature. Give undiluted or dilute with 10 ml D_5W, 0.9% NaCl, or sterile water. Drug can precipitate at less than a fourfold dilution. Give diluted drug immediately.

- Divide the loading dose over 24 hr, as ordered.
- Check patient's apical pulse for 1 minute before each dose. Report significant changes (irregular beats or pulse outside 60 to 100 beats/minute). Report blood pressure changes and expect an order for 12-lead ECG.

(continued)

◆ Also available in Canada. ◇ Available in Canada only.

COMMON INDICATIONS AND DOSAGES	ADMINISTRATION	SPECIAL CONSIDERATIONS
digoxin *(continued)* ally 0.25 mg). *Children ages 5 to 10:* loading dose 0.015 to 0.03 mg/kg; maintenance 25% to 35% of loading dose. *Children ages 2 to 5:* loading dose 0.025 to 0.035 mg/kg; maintenance 25% to 35% of loading dose. *Children 1 month to 2 years old:* loading dose 0.03 to 0.05 mg/kg; maintenance 25% to 35% of loading dose. *Full-term neonates under 1 month old:* loading dose 0.02 to 0.03 mg/kg; maintenance 25% to 35% of loading dose. *Premature infants:* loading dose 0.015 to 0.025 mg/kg; maintenance 20% to 30% of loading dose.	***Incompatibilities:*** Dobutamine, doxapram, fluconazole, and foscarnet. Manufacturer recommends not mixing digoxin with other drugs or giving in the same I.V. line. ***Direct injection:*** Inject undiluted drug over at least 5 minutes as close to I.V. insertion site as possible.	• Use a continuous ECG to monitor patient for development or improvement of arrhythmias. • Stop drug at first sign of toxicity (anorexia, diarrhea, nausea, and vomiting in adults; in children, the most common sign is cardiac arrhythmias). • Keep serum potassium level at 3.5 to 5 mEq/L. • Therapeutic serum levels are 0.5 to 2 ng/ml. Measure peak serum levels at least 4 hr after a dose and trough levels just before the next dose.

digoxin immune Fab • Digibind

Class: ***cardiac glycoside antidote*** • *Pregnancy risk category C*

COMMON INDICATIONS AND DOSAGES	ADMINISTRATION	SPECIAL CONSIDERATIONS
Potentially life-threatening cardiac glycoside toxicity. *Adults and children:* For digoxin tablets, solution, or I.M. injection, find antidote dose (in mg) by multiplying ingested amount by 0.8; divide answer by 0.5 and multiply by 38. For digitoxin tablets, digoxin capsules, or I.V. digoxin or digitoxin, find antidote dose (in mg) by dividing ingested dose (in mg) by 0.5 and multiplying by 38. If serum digoxin or digitoxin level is known, multiply serum digoxin level (in ng/ml) by patient's weight (in kg); divide by 100 and multiply by 38. Or, multiply serum digitoxin level	Available in 38-mg vials. For injection, reconstitute with 4 ml sterile water. For infusion, dilute reconstituted drug with 0.9% NaCl to convenient volume. For children or patients who need small doses, reconstitute 38-mg vial with 34 ml of 0.9% NaCl for 1 mg/ml concentration. Use reconstituted solution promptly or refrigerate for up to 4 hr. ***Incompatibilities:*** None reported. ***Direct injection:*** If cardiac arrest is imminent, use a 0.22-micron filter needle to rapidly inject into vein or I.V. line that contains a free-flowing, compatible solution. ***Continuous infusion:*** Infuse diluted solution over 15 to 30 minutes through a 0.22-micron filter needle.	• If patient is allergic to sheep proteins or has reacted to digoxin immune FAB and condition isn't life-threatening, consider skin testing. Dilute 0.1 ml reconstituted drug in 10 ml sterile NaCl. Inject 0.1 ml of solution intradermally and check site in 20 minutes. Urticarial wheal and erythema is positive result. • Obtain serum digoxin or digitoxin levels before giving digoxin immune FAB because serum studies will be difficult to interpret afterward. • Don't try redigitalization until Digibind is eliminated (which can take up to 1 week). • Overly high doses can cause allergic reaction, febrile reaction, or delayed serum sickness.

(in ng/ml) by patient's weight (in kg), divide by 1,000, and multiply by 38.
In acute toxicity or if ingested amount or serum digoxin level is unknown. *Adults and children:* Give 20 vials (760 mg) as ordered and watch patient's response. Dosage should be effective in most life-threatening ingestions in adults and children, but may cause volume overload in young children.

dihydroergotamine mesylate • D.H.E. 45

Class: ***vasoconstrictor*** • *Pregnancy risk category X*

Rapid control of vascular headaches (including migraine and cluster).
Adults: 1 mg I.M. at start of attack, then 1 mg I.M. in 1 hr p.r.n. until headache relieved; don't exceed 3 mg/day. For faster response, give I.V. to maximum of 2 mg. Don't exceed 6 mg weekly.

Available in 1 mg/ml vials. Doesn't need dilution for I.V. use. Protect from light, freezing, and heat. Store at 59° to 86° F (15° to 30° C). Don't give discolored solution.
Incompatibilities: None reported.
Direct injection: I.M. or I.V. at the first warning sign of vascular headache.

- Give drug when prodromal signs occur or as soon as possible after headache begins. Dosage and speed of relief may be directly related to prompt administration.
- Tell patient to report immediately numbness or tingling in limbs, weakness, chest pain, changes in heart rate, edema, or itching.
- For overdose, provide symptomatic care. Treat seizures with I.V. diazepam or barbiturates, as ordered. Support respirations. For severe vasospasm, apply warmth to ischemic limbs to prevent tissue damage. Give vasodilators carefully (nitroprusside, prazosin, or tolazoline) because they can cause hypotension.

diltiazem hydrochloride • Cardizem

Classes: ***antianginal, antiarrhythmic*** • *Pregnancy risk category C*

Temporary control of rapid ventricular rate in atrial fibrillation or atrial flutter;

Available as a 5-mg/ml in 5- and 10-ml single-dose vials. Refrigerate at 36° to 46° F (2° to 8° C). Drug may be stored

- Monitor patient's ECG continuously and blood pressure frequently during continuous infusion. Keep

(continued)

◆ Also available in Canada. ◇ Available in Canada only.

COMMON INDICATIONS AND DOSAGES	ADMINISTRATION	SPECIAL CONSIDERATIONS
diltiazem hydrochloride *(continued)* **rapid conversion of paroxysmal supraventricular tachycardia.** *Adults:* Initially, 0.25 mg/kg bolus over 2 minutes; if inadequate, second bolus of 0.35 mg/kg given after 15 minutes. Subsequent I.V. bolus doses should be individualized. For continued reduction of heart rate, continuous infusion of 10 mg/hr may be started immediately after bolus doses. Initial rate may be increased by 5 mg/hr up to 15 mg/hr p.r.n. Avoid infusions longer than 24 hr or over 15 mg/hr.	at room temperature for up to 1 month; afterward, discard it. ***Incompatibilities:*** Furosemide, heparin, phenytoin, and rifampin when mixed directly. ***Direct injection:*** Withdraw ordered dose from vial and inject into patent I.V. line. Don't inject with incompatible drugs or solutions. ***Continuous infusion:*** Transfer ordered dose to desired volume of 0.9% NaCl, D_5W, or dextrose 5% in 0.45% NaCl. Mix thoroughly and use within 24 hr. Refrigerate until ready to use. Using an infusion control device, infuse over 24 hr at a rate not exceeding 15 mg/hr.	defibrillator and emergency equipment nearby. • Infusion shouldn't exceed 24 hr. Instead, expect to shift patient to other antiarrhythmic drugs. • Don't give I.V. diltiazem and I.V. beta blockers together or within a few hr of each other. • Stop drug if erythema multiforme or exfoliative dermatitis occur or persist.

dimenhydrinate • Dinate, Dramanate, Dymenate, Gravol◇, Hydrate

Classes: ***antihistamine, antiemetic, antivertigo*** • *Pregnancy risk category B*

To prevent or treat nausea, vomiting, and dizziness from motion sickness. *Adults:* 50 mg; repeat q 4 hr p.r.n.	Available in 5- and 10-ml ampules of 50 mg/ml. Dilute each 50 mg (1 ml) with 10 ml of 0.9% NaCl before injection. Store diluted solution for up to 10 days at 59° to 86° F (15° to 30° C); avoid freezing. ***Incompatibilities:*** Aminophylline, ammonium chloride, amobarbital, butorphanol, chlorpromazine, glycopyrrolate, heparin, hydrocortisone sodium succinate, hydroxyzine hydrochloride, midazolam, pentobarbital sodium, phenobarbital sodium, phenytoin, prochlorperazine edisylate, promazine, promethazine hydrochloride, and thiopental. ***Direct injection:*** Inject diluted drug over 2 minutes.	• Keep patient supine during drug administration. • CNS depression and hypotension are more common in elderly patients. • Most preparations (except Gravol) contain benzyl alcohol. • Drug can interfere with diagnosis of appendicitis. • Like other antiemetics, drug may mask symptoms of ototoxicity, brain tumor, or intestinal obstruction. Closely monitor high-risk patient. • For overdose, treat symptoms. For respiratory depression, provide mechanical ventilation and oxygen. Treat seizures with diazepam as ordered.

diphenhydramine hydrochloride • Benadryl◆, Hyrexin-50

Classes: ***antihistamine, antiemetic, antivertigo, antidyskinetic, sedative-hypnotic, antitussive*** • *Pregnancy risk category B*

Parkinsonism and drug-induced extrapyramidal reaction in elderly patients unable to tolerate stronger drugs; mild cases of parkinsonism (including drug-induced) with centrally acting anticholinergic agents; treatment of allergic reactions, nausea, and vertigo. *Adults:* 10 to 50 mg, up to 100 mg if required. Maximum 400 mg daily. *Children:* 5 mg/kg/day or 150 mg/m^2 divided into four doses. Maximum 300 mg daily.

Available in 10- and 50-mg/ml vials. Store in light-resistant containers at 59° to 86° F (15° to 30° C), and avoid freezing. Further dilution isn't required for direct injection.
Incompatibilities: Compatibility depends on concentration of drugs, diluent used, pH, and temperature. Consult specialized references for specific compatibility information.
Direct injection: Inject drug over 3 to 5 minutes into vein or I.V. line that contains free-flowing, compatible solution.
Intermittent infusion: After diluting appropriate dosage, infuse slowly.

- Keep patient in supine position during administration.
- Monitor patient's vital signs and level of consciousness during infusion.
- Withdraw drug 4 days before skin tests.

dobutamine hydrochloride • Dobutrex◆

Class: ***inotropic*** • *Pregnancy risk category B*

Short-term treatment of cardiac decompensation caused by depressed contractility in heart disease or cardiac surgery. *Adults:* 2.5 to 15 mcg/kg/minute.

Supplied in 20-ml vials containing 250 mg of drug. Before reconstitution, store at room temperature. Reconstitute with 10 ml sterile water or D_5W (25 mg/ml). Reconstituted solution stays potent for 6 hr at room temperature, 48 hr if refrigerated. Before administration, dilute with at least 50 ml of one of following diluents: D_5W, dextrose 5% in 0.45% NaCl, 0.9% NaCl, 10% dextrose injection, Isolyte M with 5% dextrose injection, Ringer's injection, Normosol-M in D_5W, 20% Osmitrol in water for injection, or sodium lactate injection. For a concentration of 250 mcg/ml, mix 250 mg of drug in 1,000 ml of solution; for 500 mcg/ml, mix 250 mg in 500 ml of solution; for 1 mg/ml, mix 250 mg in 250 ml of solution. Maximum concentration for infusion is 5 mg/ml. Use diluted solution within 24 hr. Solution may turn pink from slight drug oxidation, but this doesn't significantly affect potency. Avoid freezing; solution may crystallize.

- Before treatment, correct hypovolemia with a volume expander and, as ordered, digitalize patient who has rapid ventricular response to atrial fibrillation.
- Monitor patient's blood pressure and heart rate and rhythm continuously. Also monitor cardiac output and pulmonary artery wedge pressure.
- Signs of overdose include tachycardia or excessive alteration in blood pressure. Reduce rate or discontinue therapy until patient is stable.

(continued)

◆ Also available in Canada. ◇ Available in Canada only.

COMMON INDICATIONS AND DOSAGES	ADMINISTRATION	SPECIAL CONSIDERATIONS
dobutamine hydrochloride *(continued)*	***Incompatibilities:*** Acyclovir, alkaline solutions, alteplase, aminophylline, bretylium, bumetanide, calcium chloride, calcium gluconate, cefamandole, cefazolin, diazepam, doxapram, ethacrynate sodium, foscarnet, hydrocortisone, indomethacin sodium trihydrate, insulin (regular), magnesium sulfate, penicillin, phenytoin, phytonadione, sodium bicarbonate, and verapamil. ***Continuous infusion:*** Administer via central I.V. line using an infusion pump. Titrate appropriately diluted infusion.	

docetaxel • Taxotere

Class: ***antineoplastic*** *• Pregnancy risk category D*

COMMON INDICATIONS AND DOSAGES	ADMINISTRATION	SPECIAL CONSIDERATIONS
Treatment of patients with locally advanced or metastatic breast cancer who have progressed during anthracycline-based therapy or have relapsed during anthracycline-based adjuvant therapy. *Adults:* 60 to 100 mg/m^2 I.V. q 3 weeks.	Follow facility protocol for handling chemotherapy drugs. Available as a 20-mg vial with 1.83-ml diluent vial or 80-mg vial with 7.33-ml diluent vial. Store unopened vials at 36° to 46° F (2° to 8° C) and protect from light. Reconstitute drug vial with contents of diluent vial to yield 10 mg/ml. Let drug and diluent stand 5 minutes at room temperature before mixing. After mixing, let foam settle before diluting. Dilute solution for infusion in 250 ml of 0.9% NaCl or 5% dextrose for a final concentration of 0.3 to 0.9 mg/ml. Don't exceed 0.9 mg/ml. For a dose greater than 240 mg, use a larger volume of infusion solution. Mix infusion thoroughly by rotating. ***Incompatibilities:*** None reported. ***Intermittent infusion:*** Administer as 1-hr infusion at room temperature and under ambient light.	• Don't give drug if patient's bilirubin is above upper limit of normal. Patient with ALT or AST above 1.5 times or alkaline phosphatase above 2.5 times the upper limit of normal usually won't receive drug either. • Premedicate patient with oral corticosteroid, such as dexamethasone 8 mg twice daily for 5 days, starting 1 day before docetaxel administration, to reduce fluid retention and hypersensitivity reactions. • Bone marrow toxicity is the most frequent and dose-limiting toxicity. Monitor patient's blood count often during therapy.

dolasetron mesylate • Anzemet

Classes: ***antinausea agent, antiemetic*** *• Pregnancy risk category B*

COMMON INDICATIONS AND DOSAGES	ADMINISTRATION	SPECIAL CONSIDERATIONS
Prevention of nausea and vomiting from chemotherapy. *Adults and children ages*	Available in concentrations of 20 mg/ml in 12.5 mg/0.625 ml single-use ampules or 100 mg/5 ml single-use vials. Dilute	• Give cautiously to patients who have or could develop prolonged cardiac conduction intervals: those

2 to 16: 1.8 mg/kg (or fixed dose of 100 mg in adults) as single I.V. dose 30 minutes before chemotherapy starts. Maximum 100 mg for children.
Prevention of postoperative nausea and vomiting. *Adults:* 12.5 mg as single I.V. dose about 15 minutes before anesthesia stops. *Children ages 2 to 16:* 0.35 mg/kg as single I.V. dose about 15 minutes before anesthesia stops. Maximum 12.5 mg.
Treatment of postoperative nausea and vomiting. *Adults:* 12.5 mg as single I.V. dose as soon as nausea or vomiting starts. *Children ages 2 to 16:* 0.35 mg/kg as single I.V. dose as soon as nausea or vomiting starts. Maximum 12.5 mg.

with 50 ml of 0.9% NaCl, D_5W, D_5W and 0.45% NaCl, D_5W and lactated Ringer's, or lactated Ringer's. After dilution, don't use beyond 24 hr at room temperature, 48 hr if refrigerated.
Incompatibilities: Don't mix with other drugs. Flush the infusion line before and after administration.
Direct injection: Give as rapidly as 100 mg/30 seconds.
Continuous infusion: Can be diluted in 50 ml compatible solution and infused over 15 minutes.

with electrolyte abnormalities, history of arrhythmia, and cumulative high-dose anthracycline therapy.
- Tell patient to report nausea or vomiting.

dopamine hydrochloride • Intropin♦

Classes: ***inotropic, vasopressor*** • *Pregnancy risk category C*

Infusion must be carefully adjusted to patient response.
Adjunctive treatment of shock that persists after adequate fluid volume replacement or in which oliguria is refractory to other vasopressors; to increase cardiac output, blood pressure, and urine flow. *Adults:* Initially, 1 to 5 mcg/kg/minute, increased by 1 to 4 mcg/kg/minute or less at 10- to 30-minute intervals until desired response achieved. Maintenance dosage usually under 20 mcg/kg/minute.
Chronic refractory heart failure. *Adults:* 0.5 to 2 mcg/kg/minute until desired response achieved.

Available in 5-ml vials, single-dose vials, and prefilled syringes of 200 mg (40 mg/ml), 400 mg (80 mg/ml), and 800 mg (160 mg/ml). Because injectable solution is light-sensitive, it comes in protective vials. Also comes premixed with D_5W for infusion in concentrations of 0.8, 1.6, and 3.2 mg/ml in 250- and 500-ml glass or polyvinyl chloride containers. Don't use solution if discolored or darker than light yellow. Dilute dopamine concentrate to 200 mg/250 ml or 200 mg/500 ml using 0.9% NaCl, D_5W, dextrose 5% in 0.9% NaCl, lactated Ringer's solution, dextrose 5% in lactated Ringer's solution, or 1/6 M sodium lactate. Dilution with 250 ml yields an 800-mcg/ml solution. Protect the diluted concentration from light. It's stable for 24 hr.
Incompatibilities: Acyclovir sodium, alteplase, amphotericin B, ampicillin sodium, cephalothin, gentamicin, in-

- Correct hypovolemia before dopamine therapy.
- Before and during therapy, monitor heart rate, blood pressure, urine output, peripheral perfusion, central venous pressure or pulmonary artery wedge pressure, and cardiac output.
- Watch infusion site closely for extravasation. If it occurs, use a small-gauge needle to promptly infiltrate area with 10 to 15 ml of 0.9% NaCl containing 5 to 10 mg of phentolamine.
- When discontinuing drug, reduce infusion rate gradually to prevent severe hypotension.

(continued)

♦ Also available in Canada. ◇ Available in Canada only.

COMMON INDICATIONS AND DOSAGES | **ADMINISTRATION** | **SPECIAL CONSIDERATIONS**

dopamine hydrochloride

(continued)

Occlusive vascular disease. *Adults:* 1 mcg/kg/minute or less to start therapy.
Severe illness. *Adults:* Initially, 5 mcg/kg/minute, increased by 5 to 10 mcg/kg/minute at 10- to 30-minute intervals up to 50 mcg/kg/minute until desired response achieved.

domethacin sodium trihydrate, iron salts, oxidizing agents, penicillin G potassium, and sodium bicarbonate or other alkaline solutions. Don't mix additives with a dopamine and dextrose solution because of the risk of incompatibility.
Continuous infusion: Using an infusion control device to avoid boluses, give diluted drug through a long I.V. catheter in a large vein, such as the antecubital fossa, rather than in a hand or ankle because of risk of extravasation.

doxacurium chloride • Nuromax

Class: ***skeletal muscle relaxant*** • *Pregnancy risk category C*

All onset and duration times are averages; expect wide variation.
To relax skeletal muscle during surgery as an adjunct to general anesthesia. *Adults:* 0.05 mg/kg rapid I.V. allows endotracheal intubation in 5 minutes in about 90% of patients when used with thiopental and narcotic induction technique. Neuromuscular blockade lasts about 100 minutes. Higher doses (0.08 mg/kg) allow intubation within about 4 minutes, but blockade lasts 160 minutes or more. If given during anesthesia with enflurane, halothane, or isoflurane, consider reducing dose by 33%. *Children over age 2:* 0.03 mg/kg given with halothane anesthesia causes a block in 7 minutes lasting 30 minutes; 0.05 mg/kg causes a block in 4 minutes lasting 45 minutes.
Maintenance of skeletal muscle paraly-

Available in 5-ml vials containing 1 mg/ml. Reconstitute with D_5W, 0.9% NaCl injection, dextrose 5% in 0.9% NaCl injection, lactated Ringer's injection, or dextrose 5% in lactated Ringer's injection. Diluted solutions are stable for 24 hr at room temperature, but because the preservative is diluted, there is a risk of contamination. Give right after reconstituting. Discard unused solution after 8 hr.
Incompatibilities: Alkaline solutions (such as barbiturate solutions). Don't give through the same I.V. line because precipitate may form.
Direct injection: Inject ordered dose directly into a vein or tubing that contains a free-flowing I.V. solution.

- Drug has no effect on consciousness or pain threshold. Don't give it until consciousness is obtunded by general anesthetic.
- Give only under direct medical supervision and only if familiar with using neuromuscular blockers and techniques needed to maintain patent airway. Don't give drug unless equipment for artificial respiration, mechanical ventilation, oxygen therapy, intubation, and antagonist are available.
- When diluted as directed, drug is compatible with alfentanil hydrochloride, fentanyl citrate, and sufentanil citrate.
- Acid-base or electrolyte imbalance may influence drug action. Alkalosis may counteract paralysis, and acidosis may enhance it.
- Maintain patent airway and control ventilation. As ordered, give an anticholinesterase agent with an anticholinergic.
- Monitor for bradycardia during anesthesia; drug has minimal vagolytic action.

sis during general anesthesia. *Adults and children:* After initial dose of 0.05 mg/kg, maintenance of 0.005 to 0.01 mg/kg prolongs neuromuscular blockade for 30 to 45 minutes. Children may need more frequent maintenance doses.
Dosage adjustment. Adjust dose for obesity, burns, or liver or renal failure.

- A nerve stimulator and train-of-four monitoring is recommended to assess recovery of muscle strength. Don't try pharmacologic reversal with neostigmine without evidence of spontaneous recovery.

doxapram • Dopram◆

Classes: ***CNS stimulant, respiratory stimulant*** • *Pregnancy risk category B*

Postanesthesia respiratory depression unrelated to muscle relaxant drugs. *Adults and children over age 12:* 0.5 to 1 mg/kg as single injection (maximum 1.5 mg/kg) or q 5 minutes (maximum 2 mg/kg total dose). Or give infusion at 5 mg/minute. Then reduce to 1 to 3 mg/minute. Maximum total dose by infusion, 4 mg/kg.
Drug-induced CNS depression. *Adults and children over age 12:* For injection, 1 to 2 mg/kg repeated in 5 minutes, then 1 to 2 mg/kg q 1 to 2 hr until patient wakes. Maximum dose of 3 g daily. For infusion, priming dose of 2 mg/kg, repeated in 5 minutes and again in 1 to 2 hr, p.r.n. If response occurs, infuse 1 mg/ml at 1 to 3 mg/minute until patient wakes. Don't infuse longer than 2 hr or give more than 3 g/day. May resume infusion p.r.n.
COPD and acute hypercapnia. *Adults:* 1 to 2 mg/minute (maximum 3 mg/minute) infused up to 2 hr. Don't give additional infusions.

Available in 20-ml multidose vials at 20 mg/ml. Store between 59° and 86° F (15° and 30° C); avoid freezing. Compatible with most I.V. fluids. For postanesthesia or drug-induced CNS depression, add 250 mg of drug to 250 ml of D_5W, dextrose 10% in water, or 0.9% NaCl. In COPD, add 400 mg of drug to 180 ml of D_5W, dextrose 10% in water, or 0.9% NaCl.
Incompatibilities: Aminophylline, ascorbic acid, cefoperazone, cefotaxime, cefotetan, cefuroxime sodium, dexamethasone sodium phosphate, diazepam, digoxin, dobutamine, folic acid, furosemide, hydrocortisone sodium phosphate, hydrocortisone sodium succinate, ketamine, methylprednisone sodium succinate, monocycline, and ticarcillin disodium.
Direct injection: Inject drug into a vein or an I.V. line that contains free-flowing, compatible solution.
Intermittent infusion: Give diluted solution at ordered rate (usually 1 to 2 mg/minute, but not more than 3 mg/minute) for up to 2 hr. If necessary, repeat in 30 minutes to 2 hr. Rapid infusion may cause hemolysis.

- Establish adequate airway before giving drug.
- Delay giving drug for at least 10 minutes after stopping general anesthetics, which affect the myocardium.
- Drug has a narrow margin of safety. Don't use as an analeptic or with mechanical ventilation.
- For postanesthesia use, reduce infusion rate when response occurs or adverse reactions develop.
- Stop doxapram if sudden hypotension or dyspnea develops.
- Monitor patient's blood pressure, pulse rate, and deep tendon reflexes.
- If patient has COPD, draw samples for arterial blood gas analysis before doxapram and oxygen administration, then at least every 30 minutes.
- Tell patient to report musculoskeletal adverse reactions or shortness of breath promptly.
- Avoid extravasation or extended use of single injection site; either may lead to thrombophlebitis or local skin irritation.

◆ Also available in Canada. ◇ Available in Canada only.

COMMON INDICATIONS AND DOSAGES	ADMINISTRATION	SPECIAL CONSIDERATIONS

doxorubicin hydrochloride (hydroxydaunomycin hydrochloride) • Adriamycin PFS, Adriamycin RDF, Rubex

Class: ***antineoplastic*** • *Pregnancy risk category D*

Solid tumors, including carcinomas, soft-tissue and osteogenic sarcomas, breast and ovarian carcinoma, transitional-cell bladder carcinoma, small-cell lung carcinoma, gastric carcinoma, neuroblastoma, Wilms' tumor, lymphomas, acute lymphocytic leukemia, acute myelocytic leukemia. *Adults:* 60 to 75 mg/m^2 as single dose every 21 days; 20 mg/m^2 weekly; or 25 to 30 mg/m^2/day for 2 or 3 consecutive days q 3 to 4 weeks. Maximum total lifetime dose 550 mg/m^2 because of cumulative cardiotoxicity. *Children:* 30 mg/m^2 for 3 consecutive days q 4 weeks.

Dosage adjustment. If serum bilirubin level is 1.2 to 3 mg/dl, reduce dosage by 50%; if above 3 mg/dl, reduce by 75%.

Follow facility protocol for handling chemotherapy drugs. Drug supplied as powder in 10-, 20-, 50-, 100-, and 150-mg vials. Store in a dry place away from sunlight. Reconstitute with 0.9% NaCl, D_5W, or sterile water for injection. Avoid diluents with preservatives or a pH below 3 or above 7. To reconstitute, add 5 ml of diluent to 10-mg vial, 10 ml to 20-mg vial, 25 ml to 50-mg vial, 50 ml to 100-mg vial, or 75 ml to 150-mg vial. When using sterile water for injection, add 2 to 3 volumes of 0.9% NaCl to drug to make solution isotonic. Shake vial to dissolve drug. Reconstituted drug stable for 24 hr at room temperature, 48 hr at 39° to 50° F (4° to 10° C). Use it within 8 hr. Discard unused drug.

Incompatibilities: Aluminum, aminophylline, bacteriostatic diluents, cephalothin, dexamethasone sodium phosphate, diazepam, fluorouracil, furosemide, heparin sodium, and hydrocortisone sodium succinate.

Direct injection: Using a 21G or 23G winged-tip needle, inject drug into a large vein over 3 to 5 minutes or inject into tubing of I.V. line with free-flowing 0.9% NaCl or D_5W. Avoid injecting into veins over joints or into limbs with compromised venous return or impaired lymphatic drainage. Flush administration set with 0.9% NaCl after use.

- Prevent or minimize uric acid nephropathy through hydrating, alkalinizing urine, or giving allopurinol.
- Reduce rate if patient develops facial flushing or local erythema.
- Some degree of toxicity occurs with a therapeutic response.
- Cardiotoxicity may be more common in children under age 2, in elderly patients, in patients who have had chest radiation therapy, and in patients whose cumulative dose exceeds 550 mg/m^2.
- Regularly monitor ECG in patients who have received 300 mg/m^2 or more of drug. Also monitor CBC and liver function tests for signs of toxicity.
- Watch for early signs of heart failure; drug-induced condition commonly fails to respond to therapy.

doxycycline hyclate • Doxy 100, Doxy 200, Doxychel Hyclate, Vibramycin IV

Class: ***antibiotic*** • *Pregnancy risk category D*

Infections caused by susceptible organisms when oral route can't be used. *Adults and children over age 8 weighing more than 99 lb (45 kg):* 100 mg q 12 hr

Available as sterile powder in 100- and 200-mg vials. Store at room temperature. Reconstitute with sterile water for injection or other compatible solution. Use 10 ml/100 mg of drug. Further dilute to 0.1 to 1 mg/ml using suitable diluent, such

- Obtain specimens for culture and sensitivity before giving first dose. Therapy may start before results are available.
- If syphilis is also suspected, a dark-field examina-

on day 1, then 100 to 200 mg/day, depending on severity of infection. *Children over age 8 weighing 99 lb or less:* 2.2 mg/kg q 12 hr on day 1, then 2.2 to 4.4 mg/kg/day, depending on severity of infection.

Acute pelvic inflammatory disease when gonorrhea or chlamydia suspected. *Adults:* 100 mg q 12 hr (plus cefoxitin 2 g q 6 hr or cefotetan 2 g q 12 hr) daily for at least 2 days after clinical improvement. Then substitute oral doxycycline to complete 14 day course.

as 0.9% NaCl, D_5W, Ringer's injection, invert sugar 10% in water, lactated Ringer's injection, dextrose 5% in lactated Ringer's injection, Normosol-M in dextrose 5%, Normosol-R in dextrose 5%, Plasma-Lyte 56 in dextrose 5%, or Plasma-Lyte 148 in dextrose 5%. After reconstitution, dilutions using 0.9% NaCl or D_5W remain stable for 48 hr at room temperature when protected from direct sunlight. Other diluted solutions retain potency for 12 hr at room temperature, up to 72 hr if refrigerated and protected from light. To ensure stability, complete infusions within 6 hr. When frozen immediately after reconstitution, solutions of 10 mg/ml are stable for 8 weeks. Once thawed, don't refreeze.

Incompatibilities: Riboflavin and drugs that aren't stable in acidic solutions, such as barbiturates, erythromycin lactobionate, methicillin, nafcillin, oxacillin, penicillin G potassium, and sulfonamides.

Intermittent infusion: Infuse 100 mg (0.5 mg/ml) over 1 to 4 hr depending on dose. Avoid extravasation.

tion should be performed before therapy. Blood serology should be repeated monthly for at least 4 months.
- If diarrhea persists during therapy, collect stool specimens to check for pseudomembranous colitis.
- Watch for signs of overgrowth. Check patient's tongue for signs of *Candida* infection, and stress careful oral hygiene.
- Tell patient to avoid direct sunlight and ultraviolet light because of possible photosensitivity.
- If patient is taking oral contraceptives for birth control, suggest an alternate form.

droperidol • Inapsine◆

Class: ***tranquilizer*** • *Pregnancy risk category C*

Preoperative sedation and prevention or treatment of nausea and vomiting. *Adults and children over age 12:* 2.5 to 10 mg given 30 to 60 minutes before surgery. *Children ages 2 to 12:* 0.088 to 0.165 mg/kg given 30 to 60 minutes before surgery.

Adjunct to induction in general anesthesia. *Adults and children over age 12:* 0.22 to 0.275 mg/kg.

Maintenance in general anesthesia. *Adults and children over age 12:* 1.25 to

Available in concentrations of 2.5 mg/ml in 1-, 2-, and 5-ml ampules and 10-ml multidose vials. Protect from light and store at room temperature. Drug is compatible with all I.V. solutions.

Incompatibilities: Barbiturates, fluorouracil, foscarnet, furosemide, heparin, leucovorin, methotrexate sodium, and nafcillin.

Direct injection: Inject directly into vein in small incremental boluses or into an established I.V. line containing a free-flowing solution.

- Keep resuscitation equipment available during administration.
- When giving an opioid analgesic with droperidol, reduce narcotic dosage by one-fourth to one-third for up to 12 hr or until patient becomes fully alert.
- Watch for signs of an extrapyramidal reaction, such as akathisia or dystonia. Call doctor immediately if such signs occur.
- Monitor patient's vital signs frequently.

(continued)

◆ Also available in Canada. ◇ Available in Canada only.

COMMON INDICATIONS AND DOSAGES	ADMINISTRATION	SPECIAL CONSIDERATIONS
droperidol *(continued)* 2.5 mg. *Children ages 2 to 12:* 0.088 to 0.165 mg/kg. **Conscious sedation for diagnostic procedures.** *Adults and children over age 12:* After I.M. premedication, 1.25 to 2.5 mg I.V. titrated to response. **Adjunct in regional anesthesia.** *Adults:* 2.5 to 5 mg.		

edetate calcium disodium (calcium EDTA) • Calcium Disodium Versenate◆

Class: ***heavy metal antagonist*** • *Pregnancy risk category B*

COMMON INDICATIONS AND DOSAGES	ADMINISTRATION	SPECIAL CONSIDERATIONS
Diagnosis of lead poisoning (calcium EDTA mobilization test). *Adults and children:* 500 mg/m². Maximum 1 g by I.V. infusion. **Acute and chronic lead poisoning and lead encephalopathy.** *Adults and children:* 1 g/m²/day for 3 to 5 days for serum lead levels from 25 to 70 mcg/dl; 1.5 g/m²/day for 3 to 5 days with dimercaprol for serum lead levels above 70 mcg/dl. Children may need more than two courses of therapy.	Available in 5-ml ampules at 200 mg/ml. For infusion, dilute with D_5W or 0.9% NaCl to 2 to 4 mg/ml. Store at room temperature. ***Incompatibilities:*** Amphotericin B, dextrose 10% in water, hydralazine, invert sugar 10% in water, invert sugar 10% in 0.9% NaCl, lactated Ringer's solution, Ringer's injection, and 1/6 M sodium lactate. ***Intermittent infusion:*** Infuse diluted drug into an established I.V. line at a rate guided by patient's condition. If patient has no symptoms, infuse half the daily dose over at least 1 hr every 12 hr. If patient has symptoms, infuse half the daily dose over at least 2 hr and give the second dose after 6 or more hr. ***Continuous infusion:*** Infuse single daily dose over 8 to 24 hr.	• Follow dosage schedule strictly because drug has potentially fatal effects. Each course of therapy should last no more than 7 days, with a 2-week interval between courses. • Before first dose, confirm urine flow by giving I.V. fluids if necessary. Stop drug when urine flow ceases. • To avoid toxic effects, give with dimercaprol. • Force oral fluids (except in lead encephalopathy) to encourage lead excretion. • Monitor patient's ECG, BUN level, and urinalysis as ordered. • Stop continuous infusion for 1 hr before drawing serum lead level.

edetate disodium (EDTA) • Disotate, EDTA, Endrate, Meritate

Class: ***heavy metal antagonist*** • *Pregnancy risk category C*

Emergency treatment of hypercalcemia. *Adults:* 50 mg/kg/day to maximum of 3 g/day. *Children:* 40 to 70 mg/kg/day or 50 mg/kg as single dose.
Cardiac glycoside–induced arrhythmias. *Adults and children:* 15 mg/kg/hr, not to exceed 60 mg/kg/day.

Available in 20-ml ampules as 150 mg/ml. Dilute in 500 ml of D_5W or 0.9% NaCl. Store at room temperature; don't freeze. For children, don't exceed final concentration of 30 mg/ml once mixed in D_5W or 0.9% NaCl.
Incompatibilities: Dextrose 5% and 5% alcohol.
Continuous infusion: Infuse diluted solution over 4 to 6 hr (3 hr if necessary).

- Before infusion, evaluate patient's renal function.
- Monitor patient's ECG, BUN level, and urinalysis as ordered.
- Avoid extravasation because drug is highly irritating.
- Check serum calcium levels after each dose because they may drop suddenly.
- Tell patient to report muscle cramps, irregular heartbeat, and muscle weakness — symptoms of electrolyte imbalance.
- After infusion, keep patient supine to avoid orthostatic hypotension.

edrophonium chloride • Enlon, Reversol, Tensilon◆

Classes: ***cholinergic, diagnostic aid*** • *Pregnancy risk category C*

Diagnosis of myasthenia gravis. *Adults and children over 75 lb (34 kg):* 2 mg, then up to 8 mg more depending on response. *Children up to 75 lb:* 1 mg, then up to 5 mg more depending on response.
Evaluation of anticholinesterase therapy in myasthenia gravis. *Adults:* 1 to 2 mg given 1 hr after last oral dose of anticholinesterase drug.
Differentiation of myasthenic from cholinergic crisis. *Adults:* 1 mg, repeated once if bradycardia or hypotension fails to occur. Maximum 2 mg. Patient with myasthenic crisis shows improved muscle strength.

Available in 1-, 10-, and 15-ml vials at 10 mg/ml.
Incompatibilities: None reported.
Direct injection: *To diagnose myasthenia gravis,* draw 10 mg (1 ml) of drug into tuberculin syringe with 21G or 23G needle. Inject 2 mg (0.2 ml) directly into vein or tubing of free-flowing I.V. line over 15 to 30 seconds. If patient shows no cholinergic effects after 45 seconds, give remaining 8 mg slowly in 2-mg increments. If cholinergic response occurs, stop giving drug and give atropine. *To evaluate anticholinesterase therapy in myasthenia gravis or to differentiate myasthenic from cholinergic crisis,* draw 2 mg (0.2 ml) into tuberculin syringe and give slowly over 30 to 45 seconds in 1-mg increments. *To antagonize neuromuscular blocking drugs,* inject over 30 to 45 seconds.

- Drug may contain sulfites, a possible cause of allergic reaction in some patients.
- Before giving drug, have 1 mg atropine available for immediate injection. Keep emergency equipment readily available.
- If drug is being used to differentiate myasthenic from cholinergic crisis or to antagonize neuromuscular blocking drugs, start mechanical ventilation before administration.
- In patients over age 50, give 0.4 to 0.6 mg atropine sulfate, as ordered, together with edrophonium because of heightened risk of bradycardia and hypotension.

(continued)

◆ Also available in Canada. ◇ Available in Canada only.

COMMON INDICATIONS AND DOSAGES	ADMINISTRATION	SPECIAL CONSIDERATIONS
edrophonium chloride *(continued)* **Antagonism of neuromuscular blocking drugs (such as curare) after surgery.** *Adults:* 10 mg; may repeat q 5 to 10 minutes p.r.n. Maximum total dose, 40 mg.		• Monitor patient's vital signs, ECG rhythm, vital capacity, and muscle strength before and during administration.

enalaprilat • Vasotec I.V.

Class: ***antihypertensive*** • *Pregnancy risk category C*

COMMON INDICATIONS AND DOSAGES	ADMINISTRATION	SPECIAL CONSIDERATIONS
Mild to severe hypertension. *Adults:* 1.25 mg q 6 hr (also for patients being converted from P.O. to I.V. dose). **Concurrent diuretic therapy.** *Adults:* 0.625 mg q 6 hr. Dose may be repeated if poor response after 1 hr. **Dosage adjustment.** For adults with creatinine clearance below 30 ml/minute, initial dose is 0.625 mg titrated gradually based on response. If patient needs hemodialysis, give a supplemental dose on dialysis days.	Available as clear, colorless solution in 1- and 2-ml vials containing 1.25 mg/ml. May be diluted with compatible solution: 5% dextrose injection, 0.9% NaCl injection, 0.9% NaCl injection in 5% dextrose, 5% dextrose in lactated Ringer's injection, or Isolyte E. Diluted solution fully active for 24 hr at room temperature. Store below 86° F (30° C). ***Incompatibilities:*** Amphotericin B and phenytoin sodium. ***Direct injection:*** Administer as provided over at least 5 minutes. ***Intermittent infusion:*** Dilute with up to 50 ml of compatible diluent and infuse slowly over at least 5 minutes.	• If patient becomes hypotensive, place him in supine position and infuse 0.9% NaCl, as ordered. • If patient develops angioedema — trouble breathing or swelling of face, throat, or limbs — stop treatment immediately and begin appropriate therapy. • Monitor patient's WBC count and liver and kidney function.

ephedrine sulfate

Classes: ***bronchodilator, vasopressor*** • *Pregnancy risk category C*

COMMON INDICATIONS AND DOSAGES	ADMINISTRATION	SPECIAL CONSIDERATIONS
Bronchospasm. *Adults:* 12.5 to 25 mg. Subsequent doses based on response. Maximum 150 mg q 24 hr. *Children:* 0.5 to 0.75 mg/kg q 4 to 6 hr. **Hypotension and temporary support of ventricular rate in bradycardia, AV**	Available in 1-ml vials at 50 mg/ml. Store between 59° and 86° F (15° and 30° C) in light-resistant containers; light causes drug to darken and gradually decompose. Discard unused, cloudy, or precipitated solutions. Drug is compatible with most common I.V. fluids. ***Incompatibilities:*** Fructose; hydrocortisone sodium succi-	• Correct hypovolemia before giving drug. • Monitor patient's blood pressure and cardiac status before, during, and after therapy. • Hypoxia, hypercapnia, and acidosis may reduce drug's effectiveness.

block, carotid sinus syndrome, or Stokes-Adams syndrome. *Adults:* 5 to 25 mg repeated in 5 to 10 minutes p.r.n. Maximum 150 mg q 24 hr.

nate; Ionosol B solution; meperidine; pentobarbital sodium; phenobarbital sodium; secobarbital; and thiopental.
Direct injection: Slowly inject drug directly into vein or I.V. line containing free-flowing, compatible solution.

- A sedative or tranquilizer may combat CNS stimulation.

epinephrine hydrochloride • Adrenalin Chloride, EpiPen Auto-Injector, EpiPen Jr., Sus-Phrine

Classes: ***bronchodilator, cardiac stimulant, vasopressor*** • *Pregnancy risk category C*

Bronchospasm and hypersensitivity reactions. *Adults:* 0.1 to 0.25 mg (1.0 to 2.5 ml of 1:10,000 dilution) over 5 to 10 minutes. May be followed by infusion of 1 to 4 mcg/minute. *Children:* 0.1 mg (10 ml of 1:100,000 dilution) over 5 to 10 minutes. May be followed by infusion of 0.1 mcg/kg/minute, increased p.r.n. to maximum of 1.5 mcg/kg/minute.
Cardiac arrest. *Adults:* 0.1 to 1 mg (1 to 10 ml of 1:10,000 dilution) repeated q 5 minutes p.r.n. May be followed by infusion of 1 mcg/minute, increased p.r.n. to 4 mcg/minute. *Children:* 0.01 mg/kg (0.1 ml/kg of a 1:10,000 dilution) repeated q 5 minutes p.r.n. May be followed by infusion of 0.1 mcg/kg/minute, increased p.r.n. by 0.1 mcg/kg/minute to maximum of 1 mcg/kg/minute. *Neonates:* 0.01 to 0.03 mg/kg (0.1 to 0.3 ml/kg of 1:10,000 dilution) repeated q 5 minutes p.r.n.

Available in 1- and 30-ml vials at 0.1 mg/ml (1:10,000), 0.5 mg/ml (1:2,000), and 1 mg/ml (1:1,000). Also available in prefilled syringes of 1 to 2 ml at 1 mg/ml, 5 ml at 0.01 mg/ml, and 10 ml at 0.1 mg/ml. For a solution of 4 mcg/ml, add 1 mg of drug to 250 ml D_5W, 0.9% NaCl, dextrose 10% in water, dextrose 5% in lactated Ringer's injection, or dextrose 5% in Ringer's injection. Compatible with most other I.V. solutions. Protect epinephrine from light. Discard solution that turns brown or contains precipitate.
Incompatibilities: Aminophylline, ampicillin sodium, cephapirin, furosemide, hyaluronidase, and mephentermine. Drug rapidly destroyed by alkalies or oxidizing agents, including halogens, nitrates, nitrites, permanganates, sodium bicarbonate, and salts of easily reducible metals (such as iron, copper, and zinc).
Direct injection: Slowly inject 0.1 mg of drug over 5 to 10 minutes, directly into a vein or into an I.V. line containing free-flowing, compatible solution.
Intermittent infusion: Piggyback diluted drug into compatible solution and infuse over 5 to 10 minutes.
Continuous infusion: Infuse diluted solution at 0.1 to 1.5 mg/kg/minute using an infusion pump.

- Carefully check type, dosage, and concentration of solution prescribed before administration.
- Use with caution in infants and children.
- Monitor patient's urine output and vital signs. Drug can widen pulse pressure.
- Diabetic patient may need increased dosage of antidiabetic drug.

◆ Also available in Canada. ◇ Available in Canada only.

COMMON INDICATIONS AND DOSAGES	ADMINISTRATION	SPECIAL CONSIDERATIONS

epoetin alfa (erythropoietin) • Epogen, Eprex♦, Procrit

Class: ***antianemic*** • *Pregnancy risk category C*

COMMON INDICATIONS AND DOSAGES	ADMINISTRATION	SPECIAL CONSIDERATIONS
Anemia from chronic renal failure. *Adults:* 50 to 100 U/kg three times weekly. Individualize maintenance dosage. Dialysis patients should receive drug I.V.; those with chronic renal failure not on dialysis may receive it S.C. **Anemia from zidovudine (AZT) therapy in patients with HIV infection and low endogenous erythropoietin levels.** *Adults:* 100 U/kg three times weekly for 8 weeks. If response inadequate, 150 or 200 U/kg three times weekly. Reevaluate q 1 to 2 months and increase by 50 to 100 U/kg three times weekly, p.r.n. Response unlikely at more than 300 U/kg three times weekly. Adjust doses cautiously based on concurrent infections or changes in AZT therapy.	Available in 2,000-, 3,000-, 4,000-, and 10,000-U/ml vials that also contain 2.5 mg human albumin. Store at 36° to 46° F (2° to 8° C). Don't shake to avoid denaturing glycoprotein. Don't dilute. Use only one dose per vial. Single-dose vials contain no preservative, although a 2-ml multidose vial is available that contains 10,000 U/ml and preservative. ***Incompatibilities:*** Don't mix with other drugs. ***Direct injection:*** Administer through the I.V. access site after dialysis.	• Before giving to patient with AZT-induced anemia, determine his endogenous erythropoietin levels. If they exceed 500 milliunits/ml, he's unlikely to respond. • Rapidly rising hematocrit can cause loss of blood pressure control. Reduce dosage so hematocrit increases by no more than 4 points in two weeks. • Stop drug if hematocrit rises beyond target range of 30% to 33%. • Hemodialysis patients may need increased heparin to reduce risk of clogging dialysis machine.

epoprostenol sodium • Flolan

Classes: ***vasodilator, antiplatelet aggregator*** • *Pregnancy risk category B*

COMMON INDICATIONS AND DOSAGES	ADMINISTRATION	SPECIAL CONSIDERATIONS
Long-term treatment of primary pulmonary hypertension (New York Heart Association classes III and IV). *Adults:* 2 ng/kg/minute, increased by 2 ng/kg/minute q 15 or more minutes until dose-limiting effects occur. Start maintenance at 4 ng/kg/minute below highest rate tolerated during initial dosing. (If less than	Follow directions strictly when reconstituting. Use sterile diluent. Don't reconstitute or mix with other parenteral medications or solutions. Make sure that prescribed concentration is compatible with infusion pump's minimum and maximum flow rates and reservoir capacity, and with other criteria recommended by the manufacturer. For maintenance infusion, prepare drug in drug delivery reservoir appropriate for the infusion pump, with a total reservoir volume of at least 100 ml.	• For extended use at temperatures above 77° F (25° C), use a cold pouch with frozen gel packs to keep drug at 36° to 46° F (2° to 8° C) for 12 hr. Use reconstituted solution for more than 24 hr. • Give an anticoagulant during maintenance infusion unless contraindicated. • Monitor patient's standing and supine blood pressure and heart rate for several hr to ensure tolerance.

5 ng/kg/minute, start maintenance infusion at half the maximum tolerated rate.) Adjust gradually in increments of 1 to 2 ng/kg/minute q 15 or more minutes. If adverse effects develop, reduce gradually by 2 ng/kg/minute q 15 or more minutes.

Prepare drug with two vials of sterile diluent for 24 hr. Store reconstituted solution at 36° to 46° F (2° to 8° C); don't freeze. Protect from light. Discard if frozen or refrigerated more than 48 hr.
Incompatibilities: Don't infuse with other drugs or I.V. solutions.
Continuous infusion: Administer by ambulatory infusion pump via central catheter. May use peripheral infusion until central access established.

- Avoid abrupt withdrawal of drug or sudden large reductions in infusion rate.

eptifibatide • Integrilin

Class: ***antiplatelet*** • *Pregnancy risk category B*

Acute coronary syndrome (unstable angina or non-Q-wave MI) managed medically or by percutaneous coronary intervention. *Adults:* 180 mcg/kg (maximum 22.6 mg) by I.V. bolus as soon as possible after diagnosis, followed by 2 mcg/kg/minute (maximum 15 mg/hr) by continuous infusion for up to 72 hr. Rate may be decreased to 0.5 mcg/kg/minute during percutaneous intervention and then continued for 20 to 24 hr afterward for total of up to 96 hr.
Percutaneous coronary intervention without acute coronary syndrome. *Adults:* 135 mcg/kg by I.V. bolus just before procedure, followed by 0.5 mcg/kg/minute for 20 to 24 hr by continuous infusion.

Available in 10-ml (2 mg/ml) and 100-ml (0.75 mg/ml) vials. Store at 36° to 46° F (2° to 8° C). Protect from light until administration. If particles appear, solution may not be sterile; discard it. Also discard any drug left in vial after administration.
Incompatibilities: Don't give in same I.V. line as furosemide. May give in same I.V. line as alteplase, atropine, dobutamine, heparin, lidocaine, meperidine, metoprolol, midazolam, morphine, 0.9% NaCl and 5% dextrose, nitroglycerin, or verapamil. No compatibility studies performed with polyvinyl chloride bags.
Direct injection: Withdraw bolus dose from 10-ml vial into a syringe and administer by I.V. push over 1 to 2 minutes.
Continuous infusion: Administer I.V. infusion undiluted directly from 100-ml vial using an infusion pump.

- Drug may contain up to 60 mEq/L of potassium chloride.
- Use cautiously in patients at increased risk of bleeding and patients who weigh over 315 lb (143 kg).
- Obtain baseline laboratory tests before drug therapy starts: hematocrit, hemoglobin, platelet count, serum creatinine level, PT, INR, and APTT.
- Drug is intended for use with heparin and aspirin. If patient's platelet count is below 100,000/mm^3, discontinue eptifibatide and heparin.
- Avoid noncompressible I.V. sites and minimize punctures and other invasive therapies.
- Monitor patient for bleeding.
- Stop infusion before coronary artery bypass graft surgery.

COMMON INDICATIONS AND DOSAGES | **ADMINISTRATION** | **SPECIAL CONSIDERATIONS**

ergonovine maleate • Ergotrate Maleate

Class: ***oxytocic*** • *Pregnancy risk category NR*

Emergency treatment of postpartum or postabortion hemorrhage caused by uterine atony or subinvolution. *Adults:* 0.2 mg in a single dose, repeated q 2 to 4 hr p.r.n. for up to five doses.

Available in 1-ml ampules containing 0.2 mg/ml. Dilute with 5 ml of 0.9% NaCl before infusion. Store below 46° F (8° C) in light-resistant containers. Discard if drug discolors or precipitate develops. Don't freeze.

Incompatibilities: None reported, but don't mix with any I.V. infusions.

Direct injection: Inject diluted drug directly into vein over at least 60 seconds.

- Avoid rapid injection because it raises the risk of severe CV effects.
- Closely monitor patient's blood pressure and pulse.
- Tell patient to report tingling in fingers or toes or other sensory alterations. They reflect vasoconstriction.
- Closely monitor contractions and uterine tone after administration. If appropriate, give analgesics.
- If patient is hypocalcemic, uterus may not respond until calcium is administered I.V.

esmolol hydrochloride • Brevibloc

Classes: ***antiarrhythmic, antihypertensive*** • *Pregnancy risk category C*

Supraventricular tachycardia; to lower heart rate and blood pressure in patients with acute myocardial ischemia; to produce controlled hypotension during anesthesia. *Adults:* 500 mcg/kg/minute by I.V. infusion over 1 minute as a loading dose, followed by a 4-minute maintenance infusion of 50 mcg/kg/minute. If response inadequate after 5 minutes, repeat loading dose and give maintenance infusion of 100 mcg/kg/minute for 4 minutes. Repeat loading dose and increase maintenance infusion in increments, p.r.n. Maximum maintenance infusion for tachycardia is 200 mcg/kg/minute.

Available in 10-ml ampules containing 250 mg/ml. Before infusion, reconstitute 2 ampules with 20 ml of diluent to yield 10 mg/ml. A ready-to-use formulation containing 10 mg/ml in a 10-ml single-dose vial is also available. Compatible solutions include D_5W, dextrose 5% in lactated Ringer's, lactated Ringer's, dextrose 5% in 0.45% NaCl, potassium chloride 40 mEq in 5% dextrose injection, and 0.45% or 0.9% NaCl. Diluted solution is stable for 24 hr at room temperature. Freezing doesn't alter drug effect, but don't expose to high temperatures.

Incompatibilities: Diazepam, furosemide, procainamide, sodium bicarbonate, and thiopental.

Direct injection: Inject intraoperative dose over 30 seconds. (Don't use 250-mg/ml ampule.)

Continuous infusion: Using an I.V. catheter and infusion pump, give loading dose over 1 minute and maintenance

- Concentrations of 20 mg/ml or higher may cause vein irritation and thrombophlebitis.
- Monitor patient's ECG and blood pressure continuously during infusion, and assess frequently for signs of neurologic deficit.
- Tell patient to report respiratory or cardiac symptoms promptly.
- Hypotension usually can be reversed within 30 minutes by decreasing the dose or, if necessary, stopping the infusion.
- Once patient's heart rate stabilizes, substitute a longer-acting antiarrhythmic, as ordered, and reduce esmolol infusion over 1 hr.

Perioperative hypertension. *Adults:* 80 mg injected over 30 seconds for immediate intraoperative control. If needed, follow with infusion of 150 mcg/kg/minute. For gradual control of hypertension, follow dosing schedule for supraventricular tachycardia.

dose over 4 minutes. If reaction occurs at infusion site, stop infusion and resume at another site. Don't use a winged infusion set.

estrogens, conjugated • Premarin Intravenous

Class: ***estrogen replacement*** • *Pregnancy risk category X*

Abnormal uterine bleeding (hormonal imbalance) in the absence of disease. *Adults:* 25 mg repeated in 6 to 12 hr, if necessary.

Available as a 25-mg vial of drug and a 5-ml ampule of sterile water for injection with 2% benzyl alcohol. To reconstitute, withdraw air from vial and slowly inject provided diluent against inside wall of vial. Swirl gently; don't shake. Intact vial stable for 5 years if refrigerated. Reconstituted drug stable for 60 days if refrigerated and protected from light, although manufacturer recommends immediate use. Don't use if drug darkens or precipitates. Compatible with dextrose, saline, and invert sugar solutions.

Incompatibilities: Ascorbic acid and any solution with an acid pH.

Direct injection: Inject reconstituted drug directly into a vein over 1 to 5 minutes or into established I.V. line containing free-flowing, compatible solution. Inject just distal to the infusion needle.

- If pathology specimens are collected, note that patient is receiving estrogen.
- Monitor patient's endocrine and liver function tests.
- If patient has diabetes, measure blood glucose levels.

etidronate disodium • Didronel IV

Class: ***antihypercalcemic*** • *Pregnancy risk category C*

Hypercalcemia from malignant tumor. *Adults:* 7.5 mg/kg by I.V. infusion for 3 consecutive days. If hypercalcemia recurs, retreatment may be needed. Allow at least 7 days between courses of therapy.

Available in 6-ml ampules containing 300 mg (50 mg/ml). Dilute in at least 250 ml of 0.9% NaCl or 5% dextrose injection before administration. Store between 59° and 86° F (15° and 30° C). Diluted solutions may be stored at controlled room temperatures for 48 hr.

- Hydration with NaCl and use of a loop diuretic increases renal excretion of calcium and reduces serum calcium concentrations.

(continued)

◆ Also available in Canada. ◇ Available in Canada only.

COMMON INDICATIONS AND DOSAGES	ADMINISTRATION	SPECIAL CONSIDERATIONS
etidronate disodium *(continued)*	***Incompatibilities:*** Don't mix with other drugs unless compatibility data is available. ***Intermittent infusion:*** Infuse each dose over at least 2 hr.	• Monitor patient's serum albumin and serum calcium levels periodically during therapy. • Some patients may be treated for up to 7 consecutive days, but risk of hypocalcemia rises after 3 days. • On first day after the last dose of I.V. therapy, start oral etidronate at 20 mg/kg daily for 30 to 90 days.

etoposide (VP-16, VP-16-213) • VePesid♦
etoposide phosphate • Etopophos

Class: ***antineoplastic*** • *Pregnancy risk category D*

COMMON INDICATIONS AND DOSAGES	ADMINISTRATION	SPECIAL CONSIDERATIONS
The following dosages are for etoposide; when giving etoposide phosphate, use equivalent dosages. **Induction of remission in refractory testicular cancer.** *Adults:* 50 to 100 mg/m^2/day on days 1 to 5 or 100 mg/m^2/day on days 1, 3, and 5. Repeat q 3 to 4 weeks. **Small-cell lung cancer.** *Adults:* 35 mg/m^2/day for 4 days or 50 mg/m^2/day for 5 days. Repeat q 3 to 4 weeks.	Follow facility protocol for handling chemotherapy drugs. *Etoposide* available in 5-ml ampules of 20 mg/ml. Stable at room temperature for 2 years unopened, up to 48 hr when diluted. Dilute with D_5W or 0.9% NaCl to yield 0.2 or 0.4 mg/ml. Discard discolored or precipitated solution. *Etoposide phosphate* available as 113.6-mg vials equivalent to 100 mg etoposide. Reconstitute each vial with 5 or 10 ml of sterile water for injection, 5% dextrose injection, 0.9% NaCl injection, bacteriostatic water for injection with benzyl alcohol, or bacteriostatic NaCl for injection with benzyl alcohol. Reconstitution with 5 ml diluent yields equivalent of 20 mg/ml; 10 ml of diluent yields 10 mg/ml. Reconstituted solution may be given or diluted to as little as 0.1 mg/ml using 5% dextrose injection or 0.9% NaCl injection. Discard discolored or precipitated solution. After reconstitution, etoposide phosphate can be stored at controlled room temperature from 68° to 77° F (20° to 25° C) or refrigerated at 36° to 46° F (2° to 8° C) for 24 hr. ***Incompatibilities:*** Idarubicin. ***Intermittent infusion:*** Give diluted etoposide over 30 to 60 minutes or more. Avoid extravasation. Etoposide phosphate may be given over 5 to 210 minutes.	• Keep emergency equipment readily available in case of anaphylaxis. • Don't administer through a membrane-type in-line filter because diluent may dissolve it. • Monitor patient's blood pressure before and every 15 minutes during infusion. • Monitor patient's CBC throughout therapy. • Give antiemetics to control nausea and vomiting. • Therapeutic response to drug usually also includes toxic effects. • Patients with low serum albumin may be at increased risk for toxic reactions.

factor IX complex • AlphaNine SD, BeneFix, Hemonyne, Konyne 80, Mononine, Profilnine SD, Proplex T

Class: ***hemostatic*** • *Pregnancy risk category C*

Hemostasis in factor IX deficiency (hemophilia B). *Adults and children:* Dosage depends on patient and type of bleeding episode. Consult product-specific package inserts. To find units needed to raise blood level percentages with recombinant factor IX, multiply 1.2 IU/kg by body weight (kg) by desired increase (% of normal). For human-derived factor IX, multiply 1 IU/kg by body weight (kg) by desired increase (% of normal). Doses usually given q 24 hr.
Hemostasis in patients with factor VIII inhibitors. *Adults and children:* Usually 75 IU/kg repeated q 12 hr p.r.n.
Hemostasis in factor VII deficiency (Proplex T only). *Adults and children:* To find IUs required, multiply 0.5 of body weight (kg) by desired percentage of increase. Dose is repeated q 4 to 6 hr p.r.n.

Available in kit that includes concentrate, diluent (from 10 to 30 ml, depending on manufacturer), and filter needle. Refrigerate but don't freeze because diluent bottle will break. After warming concentrate and diluent to room temperature, reconstitute using aseptic technique. Add diluent and swirl bottle to dissolve. Using filter needle, draw into syringe. Administer within 3 hr. Don't refrigerate after reconstitution.
Incompatibilities: All drugs and solutions except 0.9% NaCl.
Direct injection: Using a 21G or 23G winged infusion set, inject slowly at 2 ml/minute. Slow injection reduces risk of thrombosis. If facial flushing or tingling occurs, stop momentarily and resume at a slower rate.

- Obtain coagulation assays before and during treatment.
- To reduce risk of thrombosis, add 5 units of heparin per milliliter of diluent as ordered when treating factor IX-deficient patients — not for patients with factor VIII inhibitors.
- About 15 minutes after giving 2 IU/kg of factor IX, plasma levels rise by about 3% and factor VII levels by about 4%. Minor bleeding episodes require a circulating factor IX level of 20% to 40% of normal; major bleeding episodes require 20% to 60% of normal.

famotidine • Pepcid I.V.

Class: ***antiulcer*** • *Pregnancy risk category B*

Active duodenal ulcer in patients who can't take oral drug. *Adults:* 20 mg q 12 hr.
Hypersecretory conditions, including Zollinger-Ellison syndrome and multiple endocrine adenomas. *Adults:* 20 mg q 6 hr. May require up to 160 mg q 6 hr.

Available in 2-ml single-dose vials and 4- and 20-ml multi-dose vials at 10 mg/ml. Also available premixed as 20 mg/50 ml in 0.9% NaCl. Refrigerate vials, but don't freeze. For injection, reconstitute with 5 or 10 ml of diluent; for infusion, use 100 ml of diluent. Drug is compatible with sterile water for injection, 0.9% NaCl, D_5W, dextrose 10% in water, lactated Ringer's, or 5% sodium bicarbonate. Diluted solution re-

- Gastric cancer must be ruled out before starting famotidine therapy.
- Check I.V. site for irritation.
- Closely monitor patient with gastric ulcers.
- Use cautiously in patients with renal failure.

(continued)

COMMON INDICATIONS AND DOSAGES	ADMINISTRATION	SPECIAL CONSIDERATIONS
famotidine *(continued)*	mains stable for 48 hr at room temperature. ***Incompatibilities:*** Cefepime, piperacillin, and tazobactam. ***Direct injection:*** Inject 5 or 10 ml of reconstituted drug over at least 2 minutes at no more than 10 mg/minute. ***Intermittent infusion:*** Infuse drug diluted in 100 ml over 15 to 30 minutes.	• Discontinue drug for 24 hr before diagnostic skin tests.

fat emulsions, intravenous • Intralipid 10%♦, Intralipid 20%, Liposyn II 10%, Liposyn II 20%, Liposyn III 10%, Liposyn III 20%

Class: ***parenteral nutrition*** • *Pregnancy risk category C*

COMMON INDICATIONS AND DOSAGES	ADMINISTRATION	SPECIAL CONSIDERATIONS
Source of calories and fatty acids with I.V. hyperalimentation. *Adults:* Using 10% solution, give 1 ml/minute for 15 to 30 minutes, then 2 ml/minute up to 500 ml on day 1. Gradually increase on following days to 60% of daily caloric intake. Using 20% solution, give 0.5 ml/minute for 15 to 30 minutes, up to 500 ml (Intralipid) or 250 ml (Liposyn) on day 1. Gradually increase on following days. Maximum 2.5 g/kg Intralipid daily, 3 g/kg Liposyn daily. *Children:* Using 10% solution, give 0.1 ml/minute for 15 to 30 minutes, 1 g/kg of Intralipid; or 100 ml/hr of Liposyn on day 1, gradually increased to 5 to 10 ml/kg daily. Using 20% solution, give 0.05 ml/minute for 15 to 30 minutes, 1 g/kg of Intralipid given over 4 hr on day 1 and gradually increased to 4 g/kg daily; or 100 ml/hr of Liposyn on day 1, gradually increased to 2.5 to 5 ml/kg daily. *Neonates:* Give	Ready-to-use, sterile, nonpyrogenic emulsions are available in single-dose glass bottles of 10% to 20% concentrations in varying volumes. Store at room temperature and discard if frozen. Inspect bottle for cracks or separation at seams; check expiration date and integrity of closure. Discard bottle for any problem. ***Incompatibilities:*** Aminophylline, ampicillin sodium, ascorbic acid injection, calcium chloride, calcium gluconate, cephalothin, gentamicin, magnesium chloride, penicillin G, phenytoin sodium, potassium chloride, sodium bicarbonate, NaCl, and vitamin B complex. Can be mixed with amino acid solution, dextrose, electrolytes, or vitamins in the same I.V. container as part of total nutrient admixture. Check with pharmacist for specific compatibilities. ***Intermittent infusion:*** Give daily as part of parenteral nutrition. Once adult tolerance is known, infuse 500 ml of 10% solution or 250 ml of 20% solution over 4 to 6 hr. ***Continuous infusion:*** Administer through the non-phthalate infusion set provided by manufacturer because product may extract phthalates from phthalate-plasticized polyvinyl chloride tubing. Don't use in-line filter because fat particles are larger than the 0.22-micron filter holes. Use a	• If patient develops fever, chills, or other reactions, or if infusion bottle shows evidence of contamination or instability, stop infusion and notify doctor. • During administration, frequently check the infusion site for signs of inflammation or infection. • Monitor patient's CBC, coagulation studies, liver function tests, and serum lipid levels. • After 4 to 6 hr of infusion, collect serum samples to check triglycerides and cholesterol because transient lipemia must clear after each daily dose. • Neonates and premature infants receive fat emulsions over 24 hr because they metabolize fats more slowly than adults. Check triglyceride and free fatty acid levels daily. Obtain daily platelet counts during the first week because neonates are susceptible to thrombocytopenia. Later, obtain platelet counts on alternate days.

0.5 g/kg/24 hr and increase as tolerated. Maximum 3 g/kg/24 hr.
Fatty acid deficiency. *Adults and children:* 8% to 10% of caloric intake.

new I.V. line for each bottle, infusing solution through peripheral or central venous line. Control flow rate with infusion pump.

fenoldopam mesylate • Corlopam

Class: ***antihypertensive*** • *Pregnancy risk category B*

Short-term (up to 48 hr) hospital management of severe hypertension. *Adults:* 0.025 to 0.3 mcg/kg/minute by continuous infusion, titrated to desired blood pressure no more frequently than q 15 minutes. Titrate at increments of 0.05 to 0.1 mcg/kg/minute.

Available in 5-ml, single-dose ampules at 10 mg/ml. Follow manufacturer's instructions for diluting in 0.9% NaCl or D_5W. Diluted solution stable at room temperature for at least 24 hr.
Incompatibilities: None reported.
Continuous infusion: Administer with an infusion pump.

- Drug contains sodium metabisulfite, which may cause severe allergic reactions.
- Use with caution in patients with glaucoma or ocular hypertension and in those with acute cerebral infarction or hemorrhage.
- Check vital signs q 15 minutes until patient is stable. May stop abruptly or gradually taper infusion. Oral antihypertensives can be added once blood pressure is stable during infusion or after infusion stops.
- Drug causes dose-related tachycardia that declines over time but remains substantial at higher doses.
- Monitor patient's serum electrolytes and watch for hypokalemia.

fentanyl citrate • Sublimaze◆

Classes: ***analgesic, anesthetic, adjunct to anesthesia*** • *Pregnancy risk category C* • *Controlled substance schedule II*

Dosage varies with patient status.
Short-term perioperative analgesia. *Adults:* Up to 2 mcg/kg in divided doses.
General anesthesia (alone, with 100% oxygen). *Adults:* 50 to 100 mcg/kg, up to 150 mcg/kg if needed.
Induction and maintenance of general anesthesia. *Children ages 2 to 12:* 1.7 to 3.3 mcg/kg.

Available in 2-, 5-, 10-, 20-, 30-, and 50-ml containers at 50 mcg/kg. Store at room temperature, avoid excessive heat or freezing, and protect from light. Drug is compatible with most common I.V. solutions.
Incompatibilities: Methohexital, pentobarbital sodium, and thiopental.
Direct injection: Inject drug over at least 1 minute to avoid muscle rigidity.

- Drug may cause muscle rigidity in the chest wall, leading to problems with ventilation. A neuromuscular blocker may be required.
- After recovery from anesthesia, patient may experience delayed respiratory depression, respiratory arrest, bradycardia, asystole, arrhythmias, and hypotension.

(continued)

◆ Also available in Canada. ◇ Available in Canada only.

COMMON INDICATIONS AND DOSAGES	ADMINISTRATION	SPECIAL CONSIDERATIONS
fentanyl citrate *(continued)* **Adjunct in general anesthesia.** *Adults:* For low dose, 2 mcg/kg in divided doses. For moderate dose before major surgery, 2 to 20 mcg/kg, then 25 to 100 mcg p.r.n. For high dose before complicated surgery, 20 to 50 mcg/kg, then 25 mcg to half initial dose p.r.n. **Adjunct in regional anesthesia.** *Adults:* 50 to 100 mcg.		• After high doses, respiratory depression may persist for several hr after the patient awakens, making ventilatory support necessary.

fentanyl citrate with droperidol • Innovar

Classes: ***analgesic, anesthetic, adjunct to anesthesia, antiemetic*** • *Pregnancy risk category C* • *Controlled substance schedule II*

COMMON INDICATIONS AND DOSAGES	ADMINISTRATION	SPECIAL CONSIDERATIONS
Dosage varies with patient status. **Adjunct in induction of general anesthesia.** *Adults:* 1 ml/20 to 25 lb (9 to 11 kg) body weight. *Children over age 2:* 0.5 ml/20 lb body weight. **Adjunct in regional anesthesia.** *Adults:* 1 to 2 ml.	Available in 2- and 5-ml ampules containing 50 mcg/ml of fentanyl and 2.5 mg/ml of droperidol. For infusion, dilute 10 ml in 250 ml of D_5W. Store at room temperature and protect from light. Discard if discolored or precipitated. ***Incompatibilities:*** Barbiturates, diazepam, heparin, and nafcillin. ***Direct injection:*** Inject undiluted drug directly into vein or into I.V. tubing containing free-flowing, compatible solution. ***Continuous infusion:*** Rapidly infuse diluted drug until onset of drowsiness. Then infuse slowly (or stop drip) and give general anesthetic, as ordered.	• Keep resuscitation equipment nearby and monitor patient's neurologic, CV, and respiratory status. • Move and position patient slowly during anesthesia because of risk of orthostatic hypotension. • After recovery from anesthesia, patient may experience delayed respiratory depression, respiratory arrest, bradycardia, asystole, arrhythmias, and hypotension. • When used in high doses, respiratory depression may persist for several hr after patient awakens, making ventilatory assistance necessary.

filgrastim • Neupogen

Class: ***colony stimulating factor*** • *Pregnancy risk category C*

COMMON INDICATIONS AND DOSAGES	ADMINISTRATION	SPECIAL CONSIDERATIONS
To decrease infections caused by myelosuppressive effects of chemotherapy used for nonmyeloid tumors. *Adults and*	Available in 1- and 1.6-ml single-dose vials (300 mcg/ml). For infusion, drug may be diluted in 5% dextrose solution to yield 5 to 15 mcg/ml. Add albumin at a final concentration of	• Let vial reach room temperature before injection. Use only one dose per vial; don't reenter vial. • Obtain patient's CBC and platelet count before ther-

children: 5 mcg/kg/day as a single daily injection. Increase by 5 mcg/kg/day for each cycle if needed. Begin at least 24 hr after the last dose of chemotherapy and continue beyond nadir until neutrophil count reaches 10,000/mm^3. Discontinue at least 24 hr before next dose of chemotherapy.

To reduce duration of neutropenia and related sequelae in patients with nonmyeloid cancer who receive myeloablative chemotherapy and bone marrow transplantation. *Adults:* 10 mcg/kg/day infused over 4 to 24 hr. Give first dose at least 24 hr after chemotherapy and at least 24 hr after bone marrow infusion.

To reduce occurrence and duration of sequelae in symptomatic patients with congenital, cyclic, or idiopathic neutropenia. *Adults:* 2 to 60 mcg/kg/day infused over 30 minutes for congenital neutropenia. 0.5 to 11.5 mcg/kg daily infused over 30 minutes for idiopathic or cyclic neutropenia. Chronic administration is required.

2 mg/ml to prevent adsorption to plastic. Don't shake. Refrigerate but don't freeze. Drug stable at room temperature for 24 hr.

Incompatibilities: NaCl solutions.

Intermittent infusion: Infuse over 15 to 30 minutes using an established I.V. line containing dextrose solution.

Continuous infusion: Infuse over 24 hr or at 10 mcg/kg/day.

apy and twice weekly during therapy. Track hematocrit level.

- Adult respiratory distress syndrome may occur in septic patients because of influx of neutrophils at inflammation site. MI and arrhythmias have occurred; closely monitor patients with preexisting cardiac conditions.
- Tell patient to report promptly fever, chills, and sore throat, which may indicate infection.

fluconazole • Diflucan

Class: ***antifungal*** • *Pregnancy risk category C*

Oropharyngeal candidiasis. *Adults:* 200 mg on day 1, then 100 mg once daily. Continue for 2 weeks. *Children:* 6 mg/kg on day 1, then 3 mg/kg once daily.

Esophageal candidiasis. *Adults:* 200 mg on day 1, then 100 mg once daily. Higher

Available in glass bottles or plastic I.V. bags containing 200 mg/100 ml or 400 mg/200 ml. Store bottles at 41° to 86° F (5° to 30° C) and bags at 41° to 77° F (5° to 25° C). Don't freeze. Don't remove overwrap from bag until just before use to protect sterility. The plastic container may show some opacity from moisture absorbed during sterilization; it

- To prevent air embolism, don't connect in series with other infusions.
- Closely monitor any patient who develops a rash from drug. Discontinue it if rash worsens.

(continued)

◆ Also available in Canada. ◇ Available in Canada only.

COMMON INDICATIONS AND DOSAGES	ADMINISTRATION	SPECIAL CONSIDERATIONS
fluconazole *(continued)* doses (up to 400 mg/day) have been used. Patient should receive drug for at least 3 weeks or 2 weeks after symptoms resolve. *Children:* 6 mg/kg on day 1, then 3 mg/kg once daily. Doses up to 12 mg/kg/day may be used. **Systemic candidiasis.** *Adults:* 400 mg on day 1, then 200 mg once daily. Continue for at least 4 weeks or 2 weeks after symptoms resolve. *Children:* 6 to 12 mg/kg/day. **Cryptococcal meningitis.** *Adults:* 400 mg/day. Continue for 10 to 12 weeks after CSF cultures are negative. *Children:* 12 mg/kg/day on day 1, then 6 mg/kg once daily. **Suppression of relapse of cryptococcal meningitis in patients with HIV infection.** *Adults:* 200 mg/day. *Children:* 6 mg/kg/day. **Dosage adjustment.** Adjust dosage in renal failure.	doesn't affect drug and diminishes over time. ***Incompatibilities:*** Amphotericin B, ampicillin sodium, calcium gluconate, cefotaxime, ceftazidime, ceftriaxone, cefuroxime sodium, chloramphenicol sodium succinate, clindamycin phosphate, co-trimoxazole, diazepam, digoxin, erythromycin lactobionate, furosemide, haloperidol lactate, hydroxyzine hydrochloride, imipenem-cilastatin, pentamidine, piperacillin sodium, and ticarcillin disodium. Manufacturer recommends not mixing with other drugs. ***Intermittent infusion:*** Give ordered dose at about 200 mg/hr.	• Adverse reactions may be worse in patients with severe underlying disease or HIV infection, especially if they take other hepatotoxic drugs or have an exfoliative skin disorder. • If patient needs hemodialysis, give drug after each dialysis session.

fludarabine • Fludara

Class: ***antineoplastic*** • *Pregnancy risk category D*

B-cell chronic lymphocytic leukemia in patients with poor response to at least one standard alkylating agent regimen. *Adults:* 25 mg/m^2 over 30 minutes for 5 consecutive days. Repeat cycle q 28	Available as a 50-mg single-dose vial of lyophilized solid cake. Store at 36° to 45° F (2° to 7° C). To prepare, add 2 ml of sterile water for injection to the solid cake. It should dissolve within 15 seconds. Each ml of solution contains 25 mg of drug. Use within 8 hr of reconstitution. Can be diluted in	• Monitor patient's CBC during and after therapy. • Severe irreversible neurologic effects can result from high doses used to treat acute leukemia, such as delayed blindness, coma, and death. No specific antidote exists. Stop drug and give supportive treatment.

days. Continue for three additional cycles after reaching maximal response, then stop drug.

100 or 125 ml of D_5W or 0.9% NaCl.
Incompatibilities: Acyclovir, amphotericin B, chlorpromazine, daunorubicin, ganciclovir, hydroxyzine hydrochloride, miconazole, and prochlorperazine edisylate. Consult specialized references; compatibility varies.
Intermittent infusion: Infuse 25 mg/m^2 over 30 minutes.

- Tell patient to report promptly symptoms of infection or bleeding.

flumazenil • Romazicon

Class: ***antidote*** • *Pregnancy risk category C*

Complete or partial reversal of sedative effects of benzodiazepines after anesthesia or conscious sedation. *Adults:* 0.2 mg over 15 seconds. If patient doesn't reach the desired level of consciousness after 45 seconds, repeat. If needed, repeat at 1-minute intervals to cumulative dose of 1 mg.
Management of suspected benzodiazepine overdose. *Adults:* 0.2 mg over 30 seconds. If patient doesn't reach desired level of consciousness after 30 seconds, give 0.3 mg over 30 seconds. If patient still doesn't respond adequately, give 0.5 mg over 30 seconds. Repeat 0.5-mg doses at 1-minute intervals to cumulative dose of 3 mg. Don't give more than 5 mg over 5 minutes initially.
Dosage adjustment. In resedation, dosage may be repeated after 20 minutes; however, give no more than 1 mg at any one time and no more than 3 mg/hr.

Available in 5- and 10-ml vials at 0.1 mg/ml. Compatible with D_5W, lactated Ringer's, and 0.9% NaCl. If drawn into a syringe or mixed with any of these solutions, discard after 24 hr.
Incompatibilities: None reported.
Direct injection: Inject over 15 to 30 seconds into an I.V. line in a large vein with free-flowing solution.

- Patient needs a secure airway and I.V. access before administration, and should be awakened gradually.
- To control patient response, don't give as a single bolus dose.
- Monitor patient closely for resedation after reversal of benzodiazepine effects. Duration of monitoring depends on the specific drug being reversed. Resedation is unlikely if patient shows no signs of it 2 hr after receiving 1 mg of flumazenil.
- Excessive flumazenil may produce anxiety, agitation, and possibly seizures. Treat with barbiturates, benzodiazepines, and phenytoin.

fluorouracil (5-FU) • Adrucil ◆

Class: ***antineoplastic*** • *Pregnancy risk category D*

COMMON INDICATIONS AND DOSAGES	ADMINISTRATION	SPECIAL CONSIDERATIONS
Dosage varies with protocol and patient weight. **Palliative treatment of colorectal, stomach, pancreatic, and advanced breast cancer.** *Adults:* 12 mg/kg/day for 4 days, maximum 800 mg/day. If no toxic effects occur, may give 6 mg/kg on days 6, 8, 10, and 12. (No drug on days 5, 7, 9, and 11.) For maintenance, repeat initial dose after 30 days, then give 10 to 15 mg/kg weekly. Don't exceed 1 g/week. *High-risk adults:* 6 mg/kg/day for 3 days, maximum 400 mg/day. If no toxic effects occur, can give 3 mg/kg on days 5, 7, and 9. (No drug on days 4, 6, or 8.) Maintenance dosage is reduced.	Follow facility protocol for handling chemotherapy. Available in 10-ml glass ampules containing 500 mg of drug in a clear yellow aqueous solution. Also available in 10-, 20-, and 100-ml vials containing 50 mg/ml solution. Store at room temperature and protect from direct sunlight. Don't use dark yellow solution because potency may be altered. For injection, drug requires no further dilution. For infusion, dilute with D_5W or 0.9% NaCl at volume appropriate to patient's condition. Use a filtered needle to prevent injection of glass fragments from ampule. ***Incompatibilities:*** Carboplatin, cisplatin, cytarabine, diazepam, doxorubicin, droperidol, epirubicin, filgrastim, methotrexate, and ondansetron. ***Direct injection:*** Using 23G or 25G winged infusion set, give at convenient rate. Consider using distal veins to allow repeated venipunctures. Use new site for each injection. ***Continuous infusion:*** Infuse diluted drug via central line over 2 to 24 hr.	• Expect toxic effects with therapeutic doses. • Observe site for signs of extravasation. • Treat anorexia and nausea with antiemetics. Stop drug if patient has GI bleeding or intractable vomiting or diarrhea. • Monitor patient's CBC for at least 4 weeks. • Tell patient to report bleeding or bruising.

folic acid • Folvite ◆

Class: ***vitamin supplement*** • *Pregnancy risk category A (C if greater than RDA)*

COMMON INDICATIONS AND DOSAGES	ADMINISTRATION	SPECIAL CONSIDERATIONS
Megaloblastic and macrocytic anemias as seen in tropical sprue, anemia of nutritional origin, pregnancy, infancy, or childhood. *Adults and children:* 250 mcg to 1 mg daily.	Available in 10-ml vials containing 5 or 10 mg/ml. Store at 59° to 86° F (15° and 30° C). Protect from light and freezing. For direct injection, dilute 1 ml of 5 mg/ml concentration with 49 ml of sterile water for injection to yield 0.1 mg/ml. ***Incompatibilities:*** Calcium gluconate, 40% dextrose in water, 50% dextrose in water, doxapram, oxidizing and reducing agents, and heavy metal ions. ***Direct injection:*** Slowly inject directly into vein or into tubing of a free-flowing, compatible I.V. solution.	• Use I.V. route only when you can't use the oral route, such as with GI surgery or malabsorption syndromes. • Monitor patient's CBC to measure effectiveness of drug treatment.

foscarnet sodium • Foscavir

Class: ***antiviral*** • *Pregnancy risk category C*

CMV retinitis in patients with AIDS; acyclovir-resistant mucocutaneous herpes simplex virus infection in immunocompromised patients. *Adults:* 60 mg/kg as an induction in patients with normal renal function. Administer as infusion q 8 hr for 2 to 3 weeks based on response. Maintenance infusion is 90 mg/kg/day. May increase to 120 mg/kg/day if disease progresses.
Herpes simplex virus infection. *Adults:* 40 mg/kg either q 8 or 12 hr for 2 to 3 weeks or until infection resolves.
Dosage adjustment. Dosage adjustment required in patients with renal failure.

Available in 250- and 500-ml glass bottles at 24 mg/ml for infusion. Store at 59° to 86° F (15° to 30° C). Undiluted drug stable for 24 months at 77° F (25° C). At 12 mg/ml in 0.9% NaCl, drug is stable for 30 days at 41° F (5° C). Don't freeze because precipitation likely. Discard if frozen. For peripheral use, dilute with an equal amount of 5% dextrose injection or 0.9% NaCl injection for a final concentration of 12 mg/ml. Use only 5% dextrose or 0.9% NaCl for dilution.
Incompatibilities: 30% dextrose, lactated Ringer's, or solution containing calcium (such as total parenteral nutrition). Immediate precipitation occurs with acyclovir, amphotericin B, co-trimoxazole, ganciclovir, pentamidine, trimetrexate, and vancomycin. Delayed precipitation occurs with dobutamine, droperidol, haloperidol, and phenytoin. Gas production occurs with diazepam, digoxin, lorazepam, midazolam, and promethazine. Cloudiness or color change occurs with diphenhydramine, leucovorin, and prochlorperazine.
Intermittent infusion: 60 mg/kg or less infused over at least 1 hr. Infuse higher doses over at least 2 hr. Give undiluted solutions through a central line and diluted solutions through a peripheral line. Use an infusion pump.

- Drug is highly toxic. Use lowest effective maintenance dosage.
- Hydrate patient well before and during therapy.
- About one-third of patients develop anemia and may need transfusion.
- Drug may cause electrolyte imbalance, such as hypocalcemia, hypophosphatemia, hyperphosphatemia, hypomagnesemia, and hypokalemia. Tell patient to report tingling sensation, especially around the mouth, and numbness in limbs.
- Urge regular ophthalmologic examinations.

fosphenytoin • Cerebyx

Class: ***anticonvulsant*** • *Pregnancy risk category D*

Status epilepticus. *Adults:* 15 to 20 mg phenytoin sodium equivalent (PE)/kg at 100 to 150 mg PE/minute as a loading dose, then 4 to 6 mg PE/kg/day as maintenance. Phenytoin may be used instead of fosphenytoin as maintenance at

Available as 2-ml vial containing 150 mg (equivalent to 100 mg of phenytoin sodium) and 10-ml vial containing 750 mg (equivalent to 500 mg phenytoin sodium). Before infusion, dilute in 5% dextrose or 0.9% NaCl for injection to 1.5 to 25 mg PE/ml. Store unopened vials at 36° to 46° F (2° to 8° C). Don't store at room temperature for more than 48 hr.

- Drug should always be prescribed and dispensed in phenytoin sodium equivalent units.
- Phosphate load supplied by fosphenytoin will affect patients on severe phosphate restriction.
- If rash occurs, stop infusion and notify doctor.

(continued)

◆ Also available in Canada. ◇ Available in Canada only.

COMMON INDICATIONS AND DOSAGES	ADMINISTRATION	SPECIAL CONSIDERATIONS
fosphenytoin *(continued)* appropriate dose. **Prevention and treatment of seizures during neurosurgery.** *Adults:* 10 to 20 mg PE/kg infused as loading dose, then maintenance dose of 4 to 6 mg PE/kg/day. **Short-term substitution for oral phenytoin therapy.** *Adults:* Total daily dosage equivalent to oral phenytoin sodium therapy infused as a single daily dose. Some patients need more frequent dosing.	Discard if you see precipitates. ***Incompatibilities:*** Don't infuse with other drugs. ***Intermittent infusion:*** Infuse diluted drug at 150 mg PE/minute or less. Typical infusion for 110-lb (50-kg) patient takes 5 to 7 minutes.	• Monitor serum phosphate levels and liver function tests. • Monitor patient's vital signs and ECG continuously when serum phenytoin reaches maximal levels (about 10 to 20 minutes after infusion ends). • Don't check serum phenytoin levels until conversion of fosphenytoin to phenytoin is complete: About 2 hr after I.V. administration. • Abrupt drug withdrawal may cause status epilepticus.

furosemide • Lasix♦, Lasix Special◇

Classes: ***diuretic, antihypertensive*** • *Pregnancy risk category C*

COMMON INDICATIONS AND DOSAGES	ADMINISTRATION	SPECIAL CONSIDERATIONS
Edema. *Adults:* 20 to 40 mg, increased in 20-mg increments q 2 hr until response is achieved. Then effective dose given once or twice daily p.r.n. **Pulmonary edema.** *Adults:* 40 mg, increased to 80 mg in 1 hr, p.r.n. *Infants and children:* 1 mg/kg, increased by 1 mg/kg q 2 hr, p.r.n. Maximum 6 mg/kg/day. **Hypertensive crisis with pulmonary edema or renal failure.** *Adults:* 100 to 200 mg. **Heart failure and chronic renal failure.** *Adults:* for I.V. bolus injection, maximum should not exceed 1 g/day given over 30 minutes.	Available in 2-, 4-, and 10-ml ampules, single-use vials, and syringes at 10 mg/ml. For infusion, dilute in D_5W, lactated Ringer's, dextrose 5% in lactated Ringer's, dextrose 5% in Ringer's injection, or 0.9% NaCl. Filter solution to remove any glass fragments from opening of ampule. Store at room temperature and protect from light. Discard discolored (yellow) solution or solution that contains precipitate. ***Incompatibilities:*** Acidic solutions ($pH < 5.5$), aminoglycosides, amiodarone, amsacrine, bleomycin, buprenorphine, chlorpromazine, diazepam, dobutamine, doxapram, doxorubicin, droperidol, erythromycin, esmolol, fluconazole, fructose 10% in water, gentamicin, hydralazine, idarubicin, invert sugar 10% in electrolyte #2, isoproterenol, meperidine, metoclopramide, milrinone, morphine, netilmicin, ondansetron, prochlorperazine, promethazine, quinidine, vinblastine, and vincristine. ***Direct injection:*** Inject directly into vein or through tubing	• Give slowly; overly rapid injection or infusion can cause ototoxicity. • Drug may cause hypochloremic metabolic alkalemia and a compensatory respiratory acidemia (increased partial pressure of carbon dioxide). • Monitor patient's BUN, serum uric acid, glucose, and electrolyte levels. Also check liver and kidney function tests, body weight, intake and output, and vital signs. • Tell patient to change positions slowly to minimize orthostatic hypotension. • Tell patient to report immediately changes in hearing, abdominal pain, sore throat, and fever, which may indicate toxic reaction to furosemide.

of free-flowing, compatible solution over 1 to 2 minutes.
Intermittent infusion: Infuse diluted drug at appropriate rate, but not exceeding 4 mg/minute.

ganciclovir • Cytovene

Class: ***antiviral*** • *Pregnancy risk category C*

Treatment of CMV retinitis. *Adults:* 5 mg/kg q 12 hr for 14 to 21 days, then maintenance at 5 mg/kg/day for 7 days/week or 6 mg/kg/day for 5 days/week.
Prevention of CMV disease in transplant recipients. *Adults:* 5 mg/kg q 12 hr for 7 to 14 days, then 5 mg/kg/day for 7 days/week or 6 mg/kg/day for 5 days/week. Duration of therapy varies.
Dosage adjustment. Adjust dosage in patients with renal impairment.

Follow facility protocol for handling cytotoxic drugs. Available in 500-mg vials. Store between 59° and 86° F (15° and 30° C). Add 10 ml of sterile water without preservative to 500-mg vial to yield 50 mg/ml. Shake vial until solution is clear to ensure complete dissolution. After reconstitution, solution retains potency for 12 hr at room temperature. Don't refrigerate. Dilute to final concentration of 10 mg/ml with 100 ml of 0.9% NaCl, D_5W, Ringer's injection, or lactated Ringer's injection. Refrigerate diluted solution and use within 24 hr. Don't freeze.
Incompatibilities: Amsacrine, cytarabine, doxorubicin, fludarabine, foscarnet, ondansetron, parabens, piperacillin sodium, sargramostim, tazobactam, and vinorelbine. Don't mix with other drugs.
Intermittent infusion: Give drug over 1 hr.

- Monitor patient's CBC to detect neutropenia, usually after about 10 days of therapy.
- Tell patient to immediately report signs or symptoms of infection or bleeding.
- If patient receives hemodialysis, give dose after dialysis session.

gemcitabine hydrochloride • Gemzar

Class: ***antineoplastic*** • *Pregnancy risk category D*

Locally advanced or metastatic adenocarcinoma of the pancreas and in patients previously given fluorouracil. *Adults:* 1,000 mg/m^2 once weekly for up to 7 weeks, unless toxic reactions occur. A 1-week rest period follows 7-week treatment course. Subsequent treatment cycles include one infusion weekly for 3 of 4 consecutive weeks.

Follow facility protocol for handling chemotherapy. Available as powder, either 200 mg in 10-ml, single-use vial or 1 g in 50-ml, single-use vial. Add 5 ml preservative-free 0.9 % NaCl injection to 200-mg vial or 25 ml to 1-g vial to yield 40 mg/ml. Shake to dissolve. May dilute with 0.9% NaCl injection to as low as 0.1 mg/ml. Inspect solution before administering and discard if discolored or contains particulates. Reconstituted solution stable at 68° to 77° F (20° to 25° C) for 24 hr. Don't refrigerate. Discard unused solution.

- Evaluate patient's renal and hepatic function before therapy starts.
- Obtain patient's CBC, including differential and platelet counts, before each infusion to assess for myelosuppression.
- Prolonged infusion time or administering more than once weekly may increase toxic reactions.

(continued)

◆ Also available in Canada. ◇ Available in Canada only.

COMMON INDICATIONS AND DOSAGES	ADMINISTRATION	SPECIAL CONSIDERATIONS
gemcitabine hydrochloride *(continued)* **Dosage adjustment.** Adjust dosage if patient has bone marrow suppression.	***Incompatibilities:*** No known incompatibility with infusion bottles, polyvinyl chloride bags, or administration sets. No data on other drugs. ***Intermittent infusion:*** Infuse over 30 minutes; don't prolong infusion time beyond 60 minutes.	• Tell patient to report signs of infection and bleeding promptly.

gentamicin sulfate • Garamycin◆

Class: ***antibiotic*** • *Pregnancy risk category B*

COMMON INDICATIONS AND DOSAGES	ADMINISTRATION	SPECIAL CONSIDERATIONS
Life-threatening infections caused by susceptible organisms. *Adults:* 5 mg/kg/day in divided doses q 6 to 8 hr. Adjust based on serum levels and decrease to 3 mg/kg/day in divided doses as soon as possible. **Severe infections caused by susceptible organisms.** *Adults:* 3 mg/kg/day in divided doses q 8 hr. *Children age 1 and older:* 2 to 2.5 mg/kg q 8 hr. *Infants:* 2.5 mg/kg q 8 hr. *Neonates age 1 week and less:* 2.5 mg/kg q 12 hr. **Prevention of endocarditis in GI or GU procedures.** *Adults:* 1.5 mg/kg with 2 g ampicillin, given separately 30 to 60 minutes before surgery. Give ampicillin P.O. after procedure. *Children:* 2 mg with 50 mg/kg ampicillin 30 to 60 minutes before procedure. Give ampicillin P.O. as ordered after procedure. **Dosage adjustment.** Adjust dosage according to peak and trough levels if patient has renal failure.	Available as clear, colorless to slightly yellow aqueous solution in 2-ml vials at 10 or 40 mg/ml, in 20-ml vials at 40 mg/ml, in 1.5-ml disposable syringes at 40 mg/ml, and in 2-ml disposable syringes at 10 mg/ml. Also available in 60-, 80-, and 100-ml containers at 1 mg/ml (diluted with D_5W for intermittent infusion) and in 50- and 100-ml bags at 0.4 to 2.4 mg/ml (diluted with 0.9% NaCl for intermittent infusion). Intrathecal preparation available as 2 mg/ml preservative-free solution. Containers and bags have no preservatives and must be used promptly after seal is broken. Discard unused portions. Don't use discolored or precipitated solution. Store at 36° to 86° F (2° to 30° C). Solution stable for 24 hr at room temperature. ***Incompatibilities:*** Ampicillin, cefamandole, cefazolin, cefuroxime, cephalothin, cephapirin, cytarabine, dopamine, fat emulsions, furosemide, heparin, hetastarch, idarubicin, nafcillin, certain parenteral nutrition formulations, and ticarcillin. Manufacturer recommends not mixing with other drugs. ***Intermittent infusion:*** Infuse at 1 mg/ml or less over 30 minutes to 2 hr.	• Weigh patient and test renal function before therapy. • During therapy, monitor renal function and intake and output. Keep patient well hydrated to minimize toxic effects and chemical irritation of renal tubules. • Beta-lactam antibiotics (such as penicillins and cephalosporins) may inactivate aminoglycosides. Separate these infusions by several hr. • Risk of neuromuscular blockade is greatest after rapid, direct injection or if given soon after anesthesia or muscle relaxants. • If patient receives hemodialysis, measure serum levels after each session because dialysis may remove half the drug.

glucagon

Classes: ***antihypoglycemic, diagnostic aid*** • *Pregnancy risk category B*

Severe hypoglycemia. *Adults:* 0.5 to 1 mg. Larger doses may be necessary. *Children who weigh under 44 lb (20 kg):* 0.5 mg or equivalent of 20 to 30 mcg/kg. If patient doesn't respond, may repeat dose twice.
Diagnostic aid for GI, urologic, and radiologic examinations. *Adults:* 0.25 to 2 mg, depending on desired onset time and duration of effect.

Potency of glucagon is expressed in USP units. One USP unit equals 1 IU and about 1 mg. Available as powder in 1- and 10-unit vials. Store at room temperature. Reconstitute with provided diluent, which is clear, sterile, and contains 0.2% phenol as a preservative and 1.6% glycerin. Preparation contains lactose.
Although reconstituted solution should be used immediately, it is stable for up to 3 months when stored at 36° to 46° F (2° to 8° C).
Incompatibilities: NaCl solution and other solutions with a pH of 3 to 9.5 because drug may cause precipitation.
Direct injection: Give directly into vein or into I.V. tubing of free-flowing, compatible solution over 2 to 5 minutes. Interrupt primary infusion during glucagon injection if using the same I.V. line.

- Monitor patient's blood pressure and serum glucose levels.
- Glucagon causes a smooth, gradual termination of insulin coma. When used to terminate insulin shock therapy in a psychiatric patient, give dose 1 hr after coma induction.
- Once hypoglycemia resolves, give carbohydrate- and protein-containing foods to prevent recurrence.
- If hypoglycemic patient doesn't respond to glucagon, give dextrose I.V.

glycopyrrolate • Robinul ♦

Classes: ***antispasmodic, antimuscarinic*** • *Pregnancy risk category B*

Adjunctive treatment of peptic ulcers. *Adults and children age 12 and over:* 0.1 to 0.2 mg q 6 to 8 hr.
As an intraoperative antiarrhythmic. *Adults:* 0.1 mg, repeated q 2 to 3 minutes, p.r.n. *Children:* 0.0044 mg/kg (maximum 0.1 mg), repeated q 2 to 3 minutes, p.r.n.
Blockage of adverse muscarinic effects of neostigmine or pyridostigmine. *Adults and children:* 0.2 mg for each 1 mg of neostigmine or 5 mg of pyridostigmine, given in same syringe.

Available as a clear, colorless sterile solution in 1-, 2-, 5-, and 20-ml vials at 0.2 mg/ml. May be diluted. Store at room temperature. For infusion, solutions 0.8 mg/L remain stable at room temperature for 48 hr when mixed with D_5W, dextrose 5% in 0.45% NaCl, 0.9% NaCl, or Ringer's injection. When using lactated Ringer's injection, prepare admixture just before use.
Incompatibilities: Alkaline drugs, chloramphenicol sodium succinate, dexamethasone sodium phosphate, diazepam, dimenhydrinate, methohexital sodium, methylprednisolone sodium succinate, pentazocine lactate, pentobarbital sodium, secobarbital sodium, sodium bicarbonate, and thiopental

- Give cautiously, if at all, to patients with asthma or glaucoma.
- Avoid giving drug for 24 hr before gastric acid secretion tests.
- Older or debilitated patients usually require lower doses.
- High doses over a prolonged period may cause CNS stimulation, resulting in a curare-like action.
- Monitor patient's intake, output, vital signs, and bowel habits.
- Tell patient to report urinary problems (frequency or

(continued)

♦ Also available in Canada. ◇ Available in Canada only.

COMMON INDICATIONS AND DOSAGES	ADMINISTRATION	SPECIAL CONSIDERATIONS
glycopyrrolate *(continued)*	sodium. Drug has a pH of 2 to 3 and is unstable in solutions with a pH over 6. ***Direct injection:*** Inject drug at ordered rate into vein or tubing containing free-flowing, compatible solution. ***Intermittent infusion:*** Infuse at ordered rate or according to hospital guidelines.	urgency), and that drug may cause drowsiness or blurred vision.

gonadorelin hydrochloride • Factrel ◆

Class: ***diagnostic gonadotropic*** *• Pregnancy risk category B*

COMMON INDICATIONS AND DOSAGES	ADMINISTRATION	SPECIAL CONSIDERATIONS
Evaluation of functional capacity and response of anterior pituitary gonadotropin to aid diagnosis of hypogonadism. *Adults and children over age 12:* 100 mcg as a single dose. In females, try to give early in follicular phase of menstrual cycle.	Available in 100- and 500-mcg vials. Just before use, add 1 ml of diluent provided by manufacturer to 100-mcg vial or 2 ml to 500-mcg vial. Reconstituted mixture remains stable for 24 hr at room temperature. Discard unused portions. ***Incompatibilities:*** None reported. ***Direct injection:*** Inject directly into vein.	• Collect serum samples to check luteinizing hormone 15 minutes before drug injection, immediately before injection, and at regular intervals after injection (usually 15, 30, 45, 60, and 120 minutes). • A subnormal response may indicate impaired function of the pituitary, hypothalamus, or both. • Hypersensitivity and anaphylactic reactions have occurred following multiple doses. • Antibody formation has occurred (rarely) after long-term administration of large doses.

granisetron hydrochloride • Kytril

Classes: ***antiemetic, antinausea*** *• Pregnancy risk category B*

COMMON INDICATIONS AND DOSAGES	ADMINISTRATION	SPECIAL CONSIDERATIONS
Prevention of nausea and vomiting from chemotherapy, including high-dose cisplatin therapy. *Adults:* 10 mcg/kg over 5 minutes given 30 minutes before chemotherapy. *Children ages 2 to 16:* 10 mcg/kg.	Available as a 1-ml single-dose vial at 1 mg/ml. May be given undiluted. For infusion, dilute just before use with 0.9% NaCl or 5% dextrose injection to a total volume of 20 to 50 ml. Solution is stable up to 24 hr at room temperature under normal lighting. Don't freeze, and protect from light. ***Incompatibilities:*** Don't mix in solution with other drugs. ***Direct injection:*** Give over 30 seconds. ***Intermittent infusion:*** Infuse over 5 minutes.	• Don't use solution if discolored or precipitated. • Hypotension is more likely to occur in older patients. • Warn patient against activities that require alertness until the drug's CNS effects are known.

heparin sodium • Hepalean◆, Hep-Lock

Class: ***anticoagulant*** • *Pregnancy risk category C*

Dosage varies with patient status.

Venous thrombosis or pulmonary embolism. *Adults:* 5,000 U initially, then continuous infusion of 20,000 to 40,000 U in 1,000 ml of 0.9% NaCl over 24 hr. As alternative, 10,000 U initially, then 5,000 to 10,000 U q 4 to 6 hr. *Children:* 50 U/kg initially, then infusion of 100 U/kg q 4 hr or 20,000 U/m^2 over 24 hr. As alternative, 100 U/kg initially, then 50 to 100 U/kg q 4 hr.

Disseminated intravascular coagulation. *Adults:* 50 to 100 U/kg q 4 hr. Stop after 4 to 8 hr if no improvement. *Children:* 25 to 50 U/kg q 4 hr. Stop after 4 to 8 hr if no improvement.

I.V. flush to maintain indwelling catheter patency. *Adults and children:* 10 to 100 U after catheter use or at designated intervals.

Available in 0.5- to 1-ml ampules, vials, or prefilled syringes and also in 1-, 2-, 4-, 5-, 10-, and 30-ml multidose vials ranging from 1,000 to 40,000 U/ml. Heparin flush ranges from 10 to 100 U/ml. For infusion, dilute with 0.9% NaCl, a dextrose and Ringer's combination, dextrose 2.5% in water, D_5W, fructose 10%, Ringer's injection, or lactated Ringer's to achieve prescribed concentration and volume. When diluting for continuous infusion, invert the container at least six times to keep heparin from pooling in the solution. Store commercially available heparin preparations at room temperature. Avoid excessive heat, and don't freeze. Discard if solution contains particles or is markedly discolored. Slight discoloration doesn't affect potency.

Incompatibilities: Alteplase, amikacin, amsacrine, amiodarone, ampicillin sodium, atracurium, cephalothin, codeine, chlorpromazine, ciprofloxacin, cytarabine, dacarbazine, daunorubicin, diazepam, diltiazem, dobutamine, doxorubicin, droperidol, ergotamine tartrate, erythromycin gluceptate or lactobionate, fentanyl citrate with droperidol, filgrastim, gentamicin, haloperidol, hyaluronidase, hydrocortisone sodium succinate, hydroxyzine, idarubicin, kanamycin, levorphanol, meperidine, methadone, methicillin, methotrimeprazine, methylprednisolone sodium succinate, morphine, netilmicin, penicillin G potassium or sodium, pentazocine, phenytoin, polymyxin B sulfate, prochlorperazine, promethazine, quinidine gluconate, 1/6 M sodium lactate, streptomycin, tobramycin, trifluoperazine, triflupromazine, vancomycin, and vinblastine. Drug may also be incompatible with solutions containing a phosphate buffer or sodium carbonate.

Direct injection: Give diluted or undiluted drug through intermittent infusion device or into I.V. tubing containing free-flowing, compatible solution.

- Frequently monitor patient's platelet count and coagulation tests, such as PT, APTT, and activated clotting time.
- Observe bleeding precautions and monitor patient for bleeding.
- If you see signs of acute adrenal hemorrhage and insufficiency, stop heparin, give I.V. corticosteroids, and draw samples for plasma cortisol determinations.
- If white clot syndrome or severe thrombocytopenia occurs, promptly stop heparin and substitute a coumarin anticoagulant.

(continued)

◆ Also available in Canada. ◇ Available in Canada only.

COMMON INDICATIONS AND DOSAGES	ADMINISTRATION	SPECIAL CONSIDERATIONS
heparin sodium *(continued)*	***Intermittent infusion:*** Give undiluted or diluted drug in 50 to 100 ml of 0.9% NaCl. Administer through a peripheral or central venous line using infusion pump for prescribed duration. ***Continuous infusion:*** Give diluted solution over 24 hr using an infusion pump.	

hetastarch • HES, Hespan

Class: ***plasma volume expander*** • *Pregnancy risk category C*

COMMON INDICATIONS AND DOSAGES	ADMINISTRATION	SPECIAL CONSIDERATIONS
Dosage reflects amount of fluid loss and hemoconcentration. **Plasma volume expansion and fluid replacement.** *Adults:* 500 to 1,000 ml. Maximum 20 ml/kg or 1,500 ml daily. In hemorrhagic shock, maximum 20 ml/kg/hr. Lower dosages used in burns and septic shock. After initial dose, later doses reduced by 50% to 75% for patients with creatinine clearance below 10 ml/minute. **Continuous flow centrifugation leukapheresis.** *Adults:* 250 to 700 ml infused at a fixed ratio of 1 part hetastarch to 8 parts whole blood.	Available in 500-ml, ready-to-use, sterile, nonpyrogenic bottles. Each contains 6% hetastarch in 0.9% NaC1 injection with no preservative. Store at room temperature. Avoid excessive heat, and don't freeze. Discard solution if it turns a turbid deep brown or contains crystalline precipitate. Discard unused solution. ***Incompatibilities:*** Amikacin, ampicillin sodium, cefamandole, cefoperazone, cefotaxime, cefoxitin, cephalothin, gentamicin, ranitidine hydrochloride, theophylline, and tobramycin sulfate. ***Continuous infusion:*** Infuse at rate determined by patient's condition and therapeutic response.	• Monitor patient's blood pressure and vital signs frequently, and check for signs of circulatory overload. • Monitor patient's CBC, including hematocrit, and notify doctor if it drops appreciably. Also check PT, and PTT. • Measure intake and output, and report significant changes in their ratio. Also report oliguria. • Observe patient for bruising or bleeding.

hydralazine hydrochloride • Apresoline◆, Novo-Hylazin◇

Class: ***antihypertensive*** • *Pregnancy risk category C*

COMMON INDICATIONS AND DOSAGES	ADMINISTRATION	SPECIAL CONSIDERATIONS
Emergency treatment of hypertension. *Adults:* 10 to 20 mg initially, repeated and increased, p.r.n. *Children:* 0.1 to	Available in 1-ml ampules at 20 mg/ml. Store at room temperature; don't freeze or refrigerate. Avoid contact with metal syringe parts because discoloration and change in stability	• Check patient's vital signs q 5 to 10 minutes for 1 hr, q 1 hr for next 2 hr, then q 4 hr after injection. Monitor patient's ECG continuously.

0.2 mg/kg dose q 4 to 6 hr, p.r.n.
Pregnancy-induced hypertension. *Adults:* 5 mg, then 5 to 20 mg q 20 to 30 minutes, p.r.n. Consider another drug if patient doesn't respond after 20 mg.

may result. Prepare just before use. Discard unused portion.
Incompatibilities: Aminophylline, ampicillin sodium, chlorothiazide, dextrose 10% in 0.9% NaCl, D_5W, diazoxide, edetate calcium disodium, ethacrynate, furosemide, hydrocortisone sodium succinate, mephentermine, methohexital, nitroglycerin, phenobarbital sodium, and verapamil. Avoid mixing with other drugs in same container.
Direct injection: Inject undiluted drug at 10 mg/minute directly into vein or as close to I.V. insertion site as possible.

- Headache and tachycardia are common and can be minimized by starting with small dose and gradually increasing.
- Slow acetylation increases risk of adverse reactions.
- Withdraw drug gradually in patients with marked reduction in blood pressure to avoid rebound hypertension.
- Tell patient to change position slowly to minimize dizziness.

hydrocortisone sodium phosphate • Hydrocortone Phosphate
hydrocortisone sodium succinate • A-hydroCort, Solu-Cortef

Class: ***adrenocorticoid replacement*** • *Pregnancy risk category C*

Severe inflammation; adrenal insufficiency. *Adults:* 15 to 240 mg (phosphate) daily or 100 to 500 mg (succinate), repeated q 2 to 6 hr, p.r.n. *Children:* 0.16 to 1 mg/kg or 6 to 30 mg/m^2 (succinate) given 1 to 2 times daily. High-dose therapy should end within 72 hr.
Shock. *Adults:* 50 mg/kg (succinate), repeated in 4 hr or q 24 hr. Or, 0.5 to 2 g, repeated q 2 to 6 hr, p.r.n.

Hydrocortisone sodium phosphate is available in 2- and 10-ml multidose vials at 50 mg/ml. *Hydrocortisone sodium succinate* is available in 100-mg vials that require reconstitution with no more than 2 ml of bacteriostatic water for injection or bacteriostatic 0.9% NaCl for injection. Also supplied in 100-, 250-, and 500-mg and 1-g containers that require dilution with D_5W in water, 0.9% NaCl, or D_5W in 0.9% NaCl to yield 0.1 to 1 mg/ml. Store solutions at 77° F (25° C) or below for up to 3 days. Discard thereafter or if solutions aren't clear. Protect from light.
Incompatibilities: Amobarbital, ampicillin sodium, bleomycin, ciprofloxacin, colistimethate, cytarabine, diazepam, dimenhydrinate, diphenhydramine, doxapram, doxorubicin, ephedrine, ergotamine, furosemide, heparin sodium, hydralazine, idarubicin, kanamycin, metaraminol, methicillin, methylprednisolone sodium succinate, mitoxantrone, nafcillin, pentobarbital sodium, phenobarbital sodium, phenytoin, prochlorperazine edisylate, promethazine hydrochloride, sargramostim, secobarbital, and vitamin B complex with C.

- Hydrocortone sodium phosphate contains sulfites. A-hydroCort and Solu-Cortef contain benzyl alcohol.
- Avoid abrupt withdrawal after high-dose therapy.
- Because hydrocortisone has hyperglycemic effects, diabetic patients may need an adjustment in antidiabetic drug dosage.
- Tell patient to report signs of infection during therapy and for 12 months afterward.

(continued)

COMMON INDICATIONS AND DOSAGES	ADMINISTRATION	SPECIAL CONSIDERATIONS
hydrocortisone sodium phosphate hydrocortisone sodium succinate *(continued)*	***Direct injection:*** Inject 0.1 to 1 mg/ml directly into vein or I.V. tubing containing free-flowing, compatible solution over 30 seconds to several minutes. ***Intermittent infusion:*** Give diluted solution over prescribed duration. ***Continuous infusion:*** Infuse diluted solution over 24 hr.	

hydromorphone hydrochloride • Dilaudid◆, Dilaudid HP◆

Class: ***analgesic*** • *Pregnancy risk category C* • *Controlled substance schedule II*

COMMON INDICATIONS AND DOSAGES	ADMINISTRATION	SPECIAL CONSIDERATIONS
Moderate to severe pain. *Adults:* 1 to 4 mg q 4 to 6 hr p.r.n.	Available in preserved multidose vials and syringes at 1, 2, 3, 4, and 10 mg/ml. Also available in preservative-free ampules at 2 mg/ml. Dilution isn't needed, but most common I.V. solutions may be used as diluents. Store at 59° to 86° F (15° and 30° C). Protect from freezing and light. Don't refrigerate because precipitates or crystal may form. Yellowish tint doesn't mean loss of potency. ***Incompatibilities:*** Alkalies, ampicillin sodium, bromides, cefazolin, cloxacillin, dexamethasone, diazepam, gallium, iodides, minocycline, phenobarbital sodium, phenytoin sodium, prochlorperazine edisylate, sargramostim, sodium bicarbonate, sodium phosphate, and thiopental. ***Direct injection:*** Inject directly into a vein or I.V. line containing free-flowing, compatible solution over 2 to 5 minutes, especially if 10 mg/ml preparation is used. ***Intermittent infusion:*** Give diluted drug over prescribed duration. ***Continuous infusion:*** Using an infusion pump, give at the ordered dilution and rate.	• Rapid administration may lead to anaphylaxis, respiratory failure, or cardiac arrest. • Give smallest effective dose. High doses may be required for severe chronic or cancer pain. • Give drug with patient lying down to minimize hypotensive effects. • Monitor patient's respiratory status frequently for at least 1 hr after dose. Keep resuscitation equipment and naloxone readily available. • Duration of effects lengthens with repeated doses because drug accumulates. • Tell patient to avoid alcohol or other CNS depressants while taking drug.

ibutilide fumarate • Corvert

Class: ***supraventricular antiarrhythmic*** • *Pregnancy risk category C*

Rapid conversion of atrial fibrillation or flutter of recent onset to sinus rhythm. *Adults who weigh 132 lb (60 kg) or more:* 1 mg over 10 minutes. *Adults who weigh less than 132 lb:* 0.01 mg/kg over 10 minutes. Stop infusion if arrhythmia stops or if patient develops ventricular tachycardia or marked prolongation of QT or QTc interval. If arrhythmia continues 10 minutes after infusion ends, may repeat infusion.

Available as single-dose, 10-ml clear glass vials at 0.1 mg/ml. Store in original carton at controlled 68° to 77° F (20° to 25° C). Administer undiluted or add 50 ml of diluent to form admixture of about 0.017 mg/ml. May be diluted with 0.9% NaCl injection or 5% D_5W injection before infusion. May be used with polyvinyl chloride plastic bags or polyolefin bags. After dilution, product is stable 24 hr at 59° to 86° F (15° to 30° C) and 48 hr at 36° to 46° F (2° to 8° C). Inspect for particulates and discoloration before administration.
Incompatibilities: None reported.
Direct injection: Undiluted solution may be injected over 10 minutes.
Intermittent infusion: Give 50 ml infusion bag over 10 minutes.

- Patients with atrial arrhythmias of long duration are less likely to respond to drug.
- Correct hypokalemia and hypomagnesemia before therapy to reduce risk of proarrhythmia.
- Cardiac monitor, intracardiac pacing, cardioverter or defibrillator, and drugs for treating sustained ventricular tachycardia must be available.
- Monitor patient's ECG continuously during administration and for at least 4 hr afterward or until QTc interval returns to baseline. Drug can worsen ventricular arrhythmias. Longer monitoring is required if ECG shows arrhythmia.

idarubicin • Idamycin

Class: ***antineoplastic*** • *Pregnancy risk category D*

Combination therapy for acute myelogenous leukemia. *Adults:* 12 mg/m² for 3 days by slow (10 to 15 minutes) I.V. injection in combination with cytarabine, which may be given as a continuous infusion of 100 mg/m² daily for 7 days or as a 25 mg/m² bolus followed by continuous infusion of 200 mg/m² daily for 5 days. A second course may be administered.
Dosage adjustment. If patient experiences severe mucositis, delay administration until recovery is complete and reduce dose by 25%.

Follow facility protocol for handling chemotherapy drugs. Available as a powder for injection in 5-, 10- and 20-mg single-dose vials. Store at 59° to 86° F (15° to 30° C) and protect from light. Reconstitute with preservative-free 0.9% NaCl injection. Add 5 ml to 5-mg vial, 10 ml to 10-mg vial, or 20 ml to 20-mg vial to yield 1 mg/ml. Don't use bacteriostatic saline. Vial is under negative pressure; use care when inserting needle and avoid inhaling aerosol. Reconstituted solution stable for 72 hr at room temperature, 7 days if refrigerated.
Incompatibilities: Acyclovir sodium, allopurinol, ampicillin sodium, cefazolin, cefepime, ceftazidime, clindamycin phosphate, dexamethasone sodium phosphate, etoposide,

- Examine patient's mouth for ulceration before each dose.
- Check patient's CBC, liver function tests, BUN, and creatinine frequently.
- Give antiemetics to prevent or treat nausea and vomiting.
- Patient may develop hyperuricemia from lysis of leukemic cells.
- Patients over age 60, those who have heart disease, and those who have received anthracycline compounds have a higher risk of cardiotoxicity from drug.

(continued)

COMMON INDICATIONS AND DOSAGES	ADMINISTRATION	SPECIAL CONSIDERATIONS
idarubicin *(continued)*	furosemide, gentamycin, heparin, hydrocortisone sodium succinate, lorazepam, meperidine, methotrexate sodium, mezlocillin, piperacillin sodium, sulbactam, tazobactam, vancomycin, and vincristine. Don't mix with other drugs unless you have specific compatibility data. Drug degrades after prolonged contact with alkaline solutions. ***Direct injection:*** Administer over 10 to 15 minutes into tubing of free-flowing 5% dextrose injection or 0.9% NaCl. Use a winged-tip needle in a large vein.	• Tell patient to avoid vaccines and tell family members to avoid vaccination with oral polio vaccine.

ifosfamide • Ifex♦

Class: ***antineoplastic*** • *Pregnancy risk category D*

COMMON INDICATIONS AND DOSAGES	ADMINISTRATION	SPECIAL CONSIDERATIONS
Germ-cell testicular cancers. *Adults:* 1,200 mg/m^2 for 5 consecutive days. Repeat q 3 weeks or after recovery from hematologic toxicity. Give with mesna to prevent hemorrhagic cystitis.	Follow facility protocol for handling chemotherapy drugs. Available as an off-white powder in 1- and 3-g vials; in Canada, also available in 2-g vials. Store intact vials at room temperature and protect from temperatures above 104° F (40° C). May liquefy at temperatures above 95° F (35° C). Reconstitute with sterile water for injection or bacteriostatic water for injection. Add 20 ml diluent per gram of drug to yield 50 mg/ml. For intermittent infusion, drug may be added to D_5W, dextrose 2.5% in water, 0.45% NaCl injection, 0.9% NaCl injection, or lactated Ringer's injection. ***Incompatibilities:*** Cefepime. ***Intermittent infusion:*** Using 23G or 25G winged-tip needle, infuse over at least 30 minutes. Use new I.V. site for each infusion, if possible.	• Use cautiously if patient has renal impairment, previous radiation therapy, severely depressed bone marrow, or hypersensitivity to drug. • Obtain urinalysis before giving each dose. • Maintain daily fluid intake of at least 2 liters during therapy and for at least 3 days afterward to reduce risk of toxic urologic effects. Along with increased fluids, use of oral ascorbic acid further reduces toxicity risk. • Tell patient to report bloody urine, painful urination, and burning on urination right away. • Remind patient to void frequently to minimize contact between bladder mucosa and drug and its metabolites.

imipenem and cilastatin • Primaxin IV

Class: ***antibiotic*** • *Pregnancy risk category C*

Respiratory, urinary, intra-abdominal, gynecologic, bone, joint, skin, and skin-structure infections; bacterial septicemia; endocarditis; and polymicrobic infections with susceptible organisms. *Adults and children over age 12 with normal renal function:* 250 to 500 mg q 6 hr for mild infections; 500 mg or 1 g q 6 to 8 hr for severe infections. Maximum 4 g or 50 mg/kg daily, whichever is lower. **Dosage adjustment.** Adjust dosage based on creatinine clearance if patient has renal impairment.

Available as white or yellow powder in 13-ml vials or 120-ml infusion bottles that contain either 250 mg imipenem and 250 mg cilastatin or 500 mg imipenem and 500 mg cilastatin. Reconstitute 13-ml vial with 10 ml of compatible solution, such as 0.9% NaCl, dextrose 5% or 10% in water, D_5W in 0.9% NaCl, or D_5W with potassium chloride 0.15%. Shake until dissolved. Using a new needle, transfer reconstituted solution into container of remaining 90 ml of solution. Reconstitute 120-ml vial with 100 ml of compatible diluent. Most solutions stable for 4 hr at room temperature, 24 hr when refrigerated. Solutions prepared in 0.9% NaCl at no more than 5 mg/ml stay stable for 10 hr at room temperature, 48 hr when refrigerated. Solutions may turn deep yellow; discard any that turn brown.
Incompatibilities: D_5W in lactated Ringer's injection. Don't mix drug with other antibiotics. Manufacturer recommends against mixing in same solution or tubing with other drugs.
Intermittent infusion: Give diluted solution into I.V. line containing a free-flowing, compatible solution. Infuse 125-, 250-, or 500-mg doses over 20 to 30 minutes and 750-mg or 1-g doses over 40 to 60 minutes.

- Check for previous penicillin or cephalosporin hypersensitivity before giving first dose.
- Reduce rate if patient develops nausea, vomiting, hypotension, dizziness, or sweating.
- When giving with aminoglycosides, you can infuse through same I.V. line, but use separate solution containers. Avoid giving to patients receiving beta-lactams because of increased risk of serious hypersensitivity reactions.
- Monitor patient's BUN and serum creatinine levels to assess renal function.
- If patient has hemodialysis, give supplemental dose after treatment unless next dose is scheduled within 4 hr.
- If diarrhea persists during therapy, discontinue drug and collect stool specimens for culture to rule out pseudomembranous colitis.

immune globulin intravenous • Gamimune N, Gammagard S/D, Gammar-P I.V., Iveegam, Polygam S/D, Sandoglobulin, Venoglobulin-I, Venoglobulin-S

Class: ***antibody production stimulant*** • *Pregnancy risk category C*

Immunodeficiency diseases; B-cell chronic lymphocytic leukemia, Kawasaki syndrome, bone marrow transplantation, pediatric HIV infections.

Each immune globulin is produced by different isolation and purification methods, thus has a different constitution. See manufacturer's guidelines for reconstitution information. Use reconstituted solutions promptly. Don't administer turbid solutions. Discard unused drug.

- Giving corticosteroids before infusion may prevent adverse reactions. If they develop, reduce rate.
- Monitor patient's vital signs continuously during infusion.

(continued)

◆ Also available in Canada. ◇ Available in Canada only.

COMMON INDICATIONS AND DOSAGES	ADMINISTRATION	SPECIAL CONSIDERATIONS
immune globulin intravenous *(continued)* Dosages vary among brands. See manufacturer's guidelines. **Dosage adjustment.** Dosage must be adjusted to ensure adequate serum IgG levels. **Idiopathic thrombocytopenic purpura.** Dosages vary among brands. See manufacturer's guidelines.	***Incompatibilities:*** Don't mix with other drugs or fluids. Give in separate infusion line. ***Intermittent infusion:*** Infusion rates and techniques vary by brand. See manufacturer's guidelines.	• Signs of an allergic reaction may occur 30 to 60 minutes after start of infusion. If so, stop infusion immediately. • Don't give live-virus measles-mumps-rubella vaccine for 2 weeks before or 3 months after giving immune globulin.

indomethacin sodium trihydrate • Indocid PDA◇, Indocin I.V.

Class: ***adjunct for closure of patent ductus arteriosus*** • *Pregnancy risk category B (D in last trimester)*

COMMON INDICATIONS AND DOSAGES	ADMINISTRATION	SPECIAL CONSIDERATIONS
Patent ductus arteriosus. *Infants under 2 days old:* 0.2 mg/kg, then one to two doses of 0.1 mg/kg q 12 to 24 hr p.r.n. *Infants 2 to 7 days old:* 0.2 mg/kg, then one to two doses of 0.2 mg/kg q 12 to 24 hr if needed. *Infants over 7 days old:* 0.2 mg/kg, then one or two doses of 0.25 mg/kg q 12 to 24 p.r.n. **Dosage adjustment.** If patient has urine output below 0.6 ml/kg/hr at time of second or third dose, don't give additional doses until laboratory tests show normal renal function.	Available as white or yellow powder in single-dose vials containing equivalent of 1 mg of indomethacin. Protect from sunlight and store below 86° F (30° C). Reconstitute with 1 ml preservative-free sterile 0.9% NaCl or preservative-free sterile water for injection to yield 1 mg/ml. Or reconstitute with 2 ml to yield 0.5 mg/ml. Although drug concentrations of 1 mg/ml remain stable for 16 days, prepare them just before use because diluent is preservative-free. Don't dilute drug. Discard unused portion. ***Incompatibilities:*** Amino acid injection, calcium gluconate, cimetidine, dextrose injection, dobutamine, dopamine, gentamicin, solutions with pH of less than 6, tobramycin sulfate, and tolazoline. ***Direct injection:*** Give drug over 5 to 10 seconds through tubing of compatible I.V. solution. Avoid extravasation because drug irritates tissues.	• Give lowest dose that relieves symptoms. • Carefully monitor patient's hemodynamic indicators. • Monitor patient's intake and output, coagulation studies, and BUN and serum creatinine levels. • If renal function declines, next dose may need to be held temporarily. • Stop drug if severe hepatic reactions occur. • Ductus may reopen, possibly requiring additional indomethacin or surgery. However, spontaneous reclosure is common. Surgery may be indicated if infant doesn't respond to two courses of therapy (three doses per course).

infliximab • Remicade

Class: ***adjunct for Crohn's disease*** • *Pregnancy risk category C*

Reduction of signs and symptoms in patients with moderate to severe Crohn's disease and inadequate response to conventional therapy. *Adults:* 5 mg/kg as single infusion.
Reduction in the number of draining enterocutaneous fistulas in patients with fistulizing Crohn's disease. *Adults:* 5 mg/kg. Repeat at 2 and 6 weeks after initial infusion.

Available in single-use, preservative-free vials of 100 mg. Store at 36° to 46° F (2° to 8° C). Reconstitute with 10 ml sterile water for injection using a syringe with 21G or smaller needle. Gently swirl to dissolve powder. Solution should be colorless to light yellow and opalescent and may develop a few translucent particles. Do not use if other particles or discoloration are present. Dilute total volume of reconstituted dose to 250 ml with 0.9% NaCl injection. Prepare only in glass infusion bottles or polypropylene or polyolefin infusion bags. Infusion concentration range is 0.4 to 4 mg/ml. Infuse within 3 hr of preparation. Discard any unused portion.
Incompatibilities: Plasticized polyvinyl chloride equipment or devices. Don't infuse in same I.V. line with other drugs.
Intermittent infusion: Administer over at least 2 hr through polyethylene-lined administration sets with an in-line, sterile, nonpyrogenic, low-protein-binding filter (pore size 1.2 microns or less).

- Use cautiously in the elderly patients.
- If an infusion reaction develops, stop drug, notify doctor, and be prepared to give acetaminophen, antihistamines, corticosteroids, and epinephrine, as ordered.
- Monitor patient for development of lymphomas and infection.
- Drug may affect normal immune responses. If patient develops autoimmune antibodies and lupus-like syndrome, stop drug therapy and symptoms will most likely resolve.

insulin, regular • Humulin-R, Novolin R, Velosulin Human BR

Class: ***antidiabetic*** • *Pregnancy risk category B*

Diabetic ketoacidosis. *Adults:* 6 to 10 U, then 6 to 10 U/hr by infusion. Or 10 to 20 U regular insulin followed by 5 to 10 U/hr IM. Early in treatment, give at least 0.1 U/kg/hr but no more than 0.2 U/kg/hr. *Children:* 0.1 U/kg/hr initially. Maintenance dosage based on blood glucose levels.
Growth hormone secretion test. *Adults:* 0.05 to 0.15 U/kg.

Available in 10-ml vials at 100 U/ml. Can be added to most I.V. and hyperalimentation solutions. Store at 36° to 46° F (2° to 8° C); avoid freezing. Don't use cloudy, discolored, or unusually viscous preparations. Use only syringes calibrated for insulin concentration being given. Adding regular insulin to infusion solution may result in absorption of insulin by container and tubing. Amount lost is highly variable.
Incompatibilities: Aminophylline, amobarbital, chlorothiazide, cytarabine, dobutamine, methylprednisolone sodium succinate, pentobarbital sodium, phenobarbital sodium,

- Increased dosages may be required in high fever, hyperthyroidism, severe infections, trauma, or surgery. Reduced dosages may be required in diarrhea, hepatic or renal impairment, hypothyroidism, or nausea and vomiting.
- Assess patient for signs of hypoglycemia and dehydration.
- For overdose, give orange juice, sugar, or candy to conscious patient. In severe hypoglycemia or coma,

(continued)

◆ Also available in Canada. ◇ Available in Canada only.

COMMON INDICATIONS AND DOSAGES	ADMINISTRATION	SPECIAL CONSIDERATIONS
insulin, regular *(continued)*	phenytoin sodium, secobarbital, sodium bicarbonate, and thiopental. ***Direct injection:*** Inject directly into vein, through an intermittent infusion device, or into a port close to I.V. access site at ordered rate. ***Continuous infusion:*** Infuse drug diluted in 0.9% NaCl at a rate sufficient to reverse ketoacidosis.	give 10 to 30 ml of dextrose 50% or 1 U glucagon if hepatic glycogen stores are adequate. • Regular insulin added to dextrose infusion may promote intracellular potassium shift in hyperkalemia.

interferon alfa-2b, recombinant (IFN-alpha 2) • Intron-A

Class: ***antineoplastic*** • *Pregnancy risk category C*

COMMON INDICATIONS AND DOSAGES	ADMINISTRATION	SPECIAL CONSIDERATIONS
Adjuvant to surgery in patients with malignant melanoma who are free of disease postsurgery but at high risk for systemic recurrence for up to 8 weeks after surgery. *Adults:* 20 million IU/m² infusion 5 consecutive days weekly for 4 weeks, then 10 million IU/m² S.C. three times weekly for 48 weeks.	Reconstitute according to manufacturer's instructions. Dilute with 100 ml 0.9% NaCl injection to yield not less than 100,000 IU/ml. Store at 35.6° to 46.4° F (2° and 8° C) before and after reconstitution; stable for 30 days. Also available as solution for injection that's stable for up to 7 days at 45° F (7° C), up to 14 days at 86° F (30° C). ***Incompatibilities:*** None reported. ***Intermittent infusion:*** Infuse diluted dose over 20 minutes.	• Premedicate with acetaminophen to minimize flu-like symptoms. Fever is common; check temperature frequently. Report sudden temperature change. • Keep patient well hydrated during therapy. • Monitor patient's liver function tests. • Observe for adverse CNS reactions, especially in the elderly. • If patient has heart disease, monitor his ECG, especially early in therapy. • Monitor patient's hemodynamic status closely if he has underlying massive hemangiomas.

irinotecan hydrochloride • Camptosar

Class: ***antineoplastic*** • *Pregnancy risk category D*

COMMON INDICATIONS AND DOSAGES	ADMINISTRATION	SPECIAL CONSIDERATIONS
Metastatic carcinoma of the colon or rectum that has recurred or progressed after fluorouracil therapy. *Adults:* 125 mg/m² once weekly for 4 weeks, followed by 2-week rest period. May be re-	Follow facility protocol for handling chemotherapy drugs. Available in 5-ml vial that contains 20 mg/ml. Store at 59° to 86° F (15° to 30° C), protect from light, and leave in original packaging and carton. Dilute with D_5W injection or 0.9% NaCl injection to yield 0.12 to 1.1 mg/ml. Usually administered in	• Premedicate patient with antiemetic drug on day of treatment, starting at least 30 minutes before giving drug. • Monitor patient's WBC count with differential, hemoglobin, and platelet count before giving each dose.

peated q 6 weeks. Subsequent doses adjusted to patient tolerance.

500 ml of D_5W. If protected from light and stored at 36° to 46° F (2° to 8° C), D_5W solution is stable for 48 hr. However, because of possible contamination during dilution, manufacturer recommends using within 24 hr if refrigerated, 6 hr at room temperature. Don't freeze.
Incompatibilities: Other drugs should not be added to irinotecan infusion.
Intermittent infusion: Infuse appropriate dose over 90 minutes.

- Assess site for inflammation; avoid extravasation.
- Drug can induce severe diarrhea.

iron dextran • DexFerrum, InFeD, Infufer◇

Class: ***hematinic*** • *Pregnancy risk category C*

Iron-deficiency anemias. *Adults and children who weigh more than 33 lb (15 kg):* See manufacturer's dosage table or calculate total dose with this formula: Dose (ml) = 0.0442 (desired hemoglobin – observed hemoglobin) × lean body weight (kg) + (0.26 × lean body weight).
Iron replacement after blood loss. *Adults and children:* Replacement iron (mg) = blood loss (ml) × hematocrit.

Available as dark brown, slightly viscous liquid in 2-ml ampules that contain 50 mg/ml. Store at 59° to 86° F (15° to 30° C). Administer undiluted.
Incompatibilities: Don't mix with other drugs or add to parenteral nutrition solutions for I.V. infusion.
Direct injection: After initial test dose, give 2 ml or less, undiluted, over at least 2 minutes.

- Keep emergency equipment available in case of anaphylaxis.
- Because of risk of anaphylaxis, inject test dose of 0.5 ml (25 mg) over 5 minutes and observe patient for 1 hr. If no adverse reactions occur, proceed with full dose.
- Delayed reactions (1 to 2 days) are more common with parenteral administration. They cause fever, chills, aches, dizziness, headache, nausea, and vomiting.
- Because toxic reaction may not cause acute signs, monitor patient's serum ferritin and hemoglobin levels, hematocrit, and reticulocyte count. Late signs of toxic reaction are bluish lips, fingernails, and palms; drowsiness; pale, clammy skin; tachycardia; and unusual weakness.

COMMON INDICATIONS AND DOSAGES	ADMINISTRATION	SPECIAL CONSIDERATIONS

isoproterenol hydrochloride • Isuprel♦

Classes: ***bronchodilator, antiarrhythmic, cardiac stimulant*** • *Pregnancy risk category C*

COMMON INDICATIONS AND DOSAGES	ADMINISTRATION	SPECIAL CONSIDERATIONS
Acute asthma unresponsive to inhalation therapy. *Adults:* 0.01 to 0.02 mg (0.5 to 1 ml of a 1:50,000 dilution). Repeat p.r.n. **Bronchospasm during anesthesia.** *Adults:* 0.01 to 0.02 mg (0.5 to 1 ml of a 1:50,000 dilution). *Children:* individualized. **Arrhythmias.** *Adults:* bolus of 0.02 to 0.06 mg (1 to 3 ml of a 1:50,000 dilution), then 0.01 to 0.2 mg (0.5 to 10 ml of a 1:50,000 dilution). Or infuse 2 mg diluted in 500 ml of D_5W at 5 mcg/minute. Titrate to response. *Children:* 2.5 mcg/minute, titrated to response. **Shock.** *Adults:* 0.5 to 5 mcg/minute. In advanced shock, 5 to 30 mcg/minute.	Available in 1:5,000 dilution in 1-ml (0.2-mg) and 5-ml (1-mg) ampules and in 5-ml (1-mg) and 10-ml (2-mg) vials. For direct injection, add 1 ml of drug to 10 ml of 0.9% NaCl or D_5W to yield a 1:50,000 dilution (20 mcg/ml). For infusion, dilute 10 ml of drug with 500 ml of D_5W to yield a 1:250,000 dilution (2 mg in 500 ml). Drug is also compatible with lactated Ringer's and D_5W in lactated Ringer's. Store in a cool place, protect from light, and keep in an opaque container until used. Discard if solution turns pink or brown or if precipitate forms. ***Incompatibilities:*** Alkalies, aminophylline, furosemide, metals, and sodium bicarbonate. ***Direct injection:*** Inject diluted solution (1:50,000) directly into vein or into I.V. line that contains free-flowing, compatible solution. ***Continuous infusion:*** Using an infusion pump, give appropriate dose and dilution (1:250,000) at ordered rate.	• Adjust infusion rate according to heart rate and blood pressure. For heart rate above 110, lower or temporarily stop infusion. • In cardiac arrest, arrhythmias, shock, and heart block, observe patient's ECG closely to help adjust dosage. • Drug may aggravate ventilation-perfusion abnormalities.

ketamine hydrochloride • Ketalar♦

Class: ***anesthetic*** • *Pregnancy risk category C*

COMMON INDICATIONS AND DOSAGES	ADMINISTRATION	SPECIAL CONSIDERATIONS
Induction of anesthesia. Can be used as sole anesthetic for procedures that don't require skeletal muscle relaxation, as a preanesthetic, or as an adjunct to low-potency anesthetics. *Adults and children:* 1 to 4.5 mg/kg, then maintenance infusion of 0.1 to 0.5 mg/minute, augmented with diazepam. Adjust dosage based on patient's response.	Available in multidose vials of 10, 50, and 100 mg/ml. For direct injection, dilute 100 mg/ml concentration with equal volume of sterile water for injection, 0.9% NaCl, or D_5W. For continuous infusion, prepare a 1 mg/ml solution by adding 10 ml from 50-mg/ml vial or 5 ml from 100-mg/ml vial to 500 ml of D_5W in water or 0.9% NaCl. If patient must restrict fluids, prepare a 2 mg/ml solution by adding 10 ml of 50 mg/ml or 5 ml of 100 mg/ml solution to 250 ml of diluent. Store at room temperature and protect from light and heat.	• Only staff specially trained in administering anesthetics and managing their adverse effects should administer. • Monitor patient's ECG during administration, especially if patient has hypertension or cardiac decompensation. • Emergent reactions occur in about 12% of patients, least often in the young and elderly. If severe, give a small dose of short-acting sedative. Reduce risk by

Incompatibilities: Barbiturates and diazepam.
Direct injection: Over 1 minute, inject initial dose directly into vein or into I.V. tubing that contains free-flowing, compatible solution.
Continuous infusion: Infuse diluted drug at 0.5 mg/kg/minute (for induction) to 0.1 to 0.5 mg/minute (for maintenance) with diazepam.

lowering ketamine dose and giving with I.V. diazepam and by reducing postoperative sensory stimulation.

- Warn patient not to drive or perform other tasks that require alertness for 24 hr because of risk of psychomotor impairment.

ketorolac tromethamine • Toradol

Class: ***analgesic*** • *Pregnancy risk category C*

Short-term management of moderately severe, acute pain (single-dose treatment). *Adults under age 65:* 30 mg. *Adults age 65 or older, renally impaired patients, or those who weigh less than 110 lb (50 kg):* 15 mg.
Short-term management of moderately severe, acute pain (multiple-dose treatment). *Adults under age 65:* 30 mg q 6 hr, up to 120 mg/day. *Adults age 65 or older, renally impaired patients, or those who weigh less than 110 lb:* 15 mg q 6 hr, up to 60 mg/day.

Ketorolac tromethamine injection is a solution of the drug in alcohol and sterile water for injection, containing 15 or 30 mg/ml. Store at 59° to 86° F (15° to 30° C) and protect from light.
Incompatibilities: Solutions of drugs that result in a relatively low pH, such as opiate agonists (meperidine hydrochloride, morphine sulfate), because precipitation can occur.
Direct injection: Administer over at least 15 seconds.

- Drug contraindicated in patients with active peptic ulcer, recent GI bleeding, or renal impairment.
- Maximum combined duration of therapy should be limited to 5 days.
- Monitor patient's serum creatinine and BUN closely.
- Monitor patient's bleeding time and closely observe patients with coagulopathies or those who receive anticoagulants.
- Drug can mask signs and symptoms of infection.

labetalol hydrochloride • Normodyne, Trandate

Class: ***antihypertensive*** • *Pregnancy risk category C*

Severe hypertension and hypertensive crisis. *Adults:* 20 mg as direct injection, then 20 to 80 mg q 10 minutes, up to 300 mg. Or continuous infusion starting

Available as a clear, colorless to light-yellow solution in 20-, 40-, and 60-ml multidose vials at 5 mg/ml. Store at room temperature. For infusion, add two 20-ml ampules to 160 ml of D_5W, 0.9% NaCl, dextrose 2.5% in 0.45% NaCl, dextrose

- Check patient's blood pressure frequently.
- Drug masks common signs of shock and hypoglycemia.

(continued)

COMMON INDICATIONS AND DOSAGES	ADMINISTRATION	SPECIAL CONSIDERATIONS
labetalol hydrochloride *(continued)* at 2 mg/minute and titrated to blood pressure response. **Hypotension control during halothane anesthesia**. *Adults:* 10 to 25 mg after induction of anesthesia. Hypotension then controlled by halothane. **Hypotension control with use of other anesthetics.** *Adults:* 30 mg, then 5 to 10 mg if needed.	5% in lactated Ringer's, or lactated Ringer's to yield 1 mg/ml. To obtain 2 mg/3 ml, add two 20-ml ampules to 250 ml of diluent. Solutions remain stable for at least 24 hr at room temperature or when refrigerated. ***Incompatibilities:*** Cefoperazone, nafcillin, and sodium bicarbonate. ***Direct injection:*** Over 2 minutes, inject directly into vein or into I.V. line that contains free-flowing, compatible solution. ***Continuous infusion:*** Give 2 mg/minute until satisfactory response occurs, then stop infusion. May repeat in 6 to 8 hr.	• Give epinephrine or atropine for excessive bradycardia. • Tell patient to remain supine for 3 hr after administration to prevent severe orthostatic hypotension.

leucovorin calcium (citrovorum factor, folinic acid) • Wellcovorin

Classes: ***vitamin, antidote*** • *Pregnancy risk category C*

COMMON INDICATIONS AND DOSAGES	ADMINISTRATION	SPECIAL CONSIDERATIONS
Methotrexate overdose. *Adults:* up to 75 mg within 12 hr or an amount sufficient to produce serum levels at least equal to serum methotrexate levels. **Hematologic toxicity caused by other folic acid antagonists, such as trimethoprim.** *Adults and children:* 5 to 15 mg/day. **Neutralization of methotrexate's toxic effects (leucovorin rescue).** Used in various regimens. Dosage depends on extent of systemic toxicity. *Adults and children:* 10 mg/m^2 given q 6 hr for 10 doses starting 24 hr after methotrexate infusion starts. **Palliative treatment of advanced colorectal carcinoma.** *Adults:* 20 mg/m^2 followed by 425 mg/m^2 of fluorouracil, or	Available as yellow-white solution in 3-, 100-, and 350-ml ampules and as powder in 50-mg vials. Store at room temperature. Reconstitute powder for injection by adding 5 ml sterile or bacteriostatic water to 50-mg vial to yield 10 mg/ml. For intermittent infusion, add 15 to 50 mg of reconstituted drug to 50 ml of compatible solution, such as lactated Ringer's, D_5W, or dextrose 10% in water. For continuous infusion, add up to 200 mg reconstituted drug to 1 liter of compatible solution. If solution contains sterile water, use immediately. If it contains bacteriostatic water, refrigerate and use within 1 week. ***Incompatibilities:*** Droperidol and foscarnet. ***Direct injection:*** Inject into vein or I.V. tubing that contains free-flowing, compatible solution over 5 minutes. ***Intermittent infusion:*** Infuse over 15 minutes. ***Continuous infusion:*** Infuse over 24 hr at rate of about 40 ml/hr.	• Begin leucovorin rescue within 24 hr of high-dose methotrexate regimen. • Leucovorin infusion shouldn't exceed 16 ml/minute because of calcium concentration in the solution. • Don't give drug simultaneously with methotrexate. • Monitor patient's serum methotrexate and serum creatinine levels, creatinine clearance, and urine pH every 6 to 24 hr during leucovorin rescue.

200 mg/m^2 followed by 370 mg/m^2 of fluorouracil daily for 5 consecutive days. Repeat at 4-week intervals for two more courses; then repeat at 4- to 5-week intervals if tolerated.

levofloxacin • Levaquin

Class: ***antibiotic*** • *Pregnancy risk category C*

Mild, moderate, and severe infections, such as those listed below, caused by susceptible microorganisms in adults age 18 and older.
Acute maxillary sinusitis. *Adults:* 500 mg daily for 10 to 14 days.
Acute bacterial exacerbation of chronic bronchitis. *Adults:* 500 mg daily for 7 days.
Community-acquired pneumonia. *Adults:* 500 mg daily for 7 to 14 days.
Mild to moderate skin and skin-structure infections. *Adults:* 500 mg daily for 7 to 10 days.
Mild to moderate UTI. *Adults:* 250 mg daily for 10 days.
Mild to moderate acute pyelonephritis. *Adults:* 250 mg daily for 10 days.
Dosage adjustment. Dosage must be adjusted if patient has renal impairment.

Available in single-use, 20-ml vial that contains 500 mg of drug (25 mg/ml). Must be diluted to 5 mg/ml before I.V. use. Compatible with 0.9% NaCl, D_5W, 5% dextrose in 0.9% NaCl, 5% dextrose in lactated Ringer's solution, Plasma-Lyte 56/5% dextrose, and sodium lactate (1/6 M). Diluted solution is stable for 72 hr when stored below 77° F (25° C), 14 days when stored at 41° F (5° C) in plastic I.V. containers. If frozen in glass bottle or plastic I.V. container, stable for 6 months at –4° F (–20° C). Must be thawed at room temperature; don't refreeze. Discard unused portion. If preparing a 250-mg dose, withdraw entire amount and prepare a second dose for storage.
Incompatibilities: Don't give through same I.V. line with solutions that contain multivalent cations (such as magnesium).
Intermittent infusion: Infuse diluted dose (5 mg/ml) slowly over at least 60 minutes.

- Avoid rapid or bolus I.V. infusion because hypotension may result.
- Use cautiously if patient has history of seizures or other CNS diseases.
- If patient experiences increased CNS stimulation, stop drug and institute seizure precautions.

COMMON INDICATIONS AND DOSAGES	ADMINISTRATION	SPECIAL CONSIDERATIONS

levothyroxine sodium (L-thyroxine sodium, T_4) • Levothroid, Levoxine, Synthroid

Class: ***thyroid hormone replacement*** • *Pregnancy risk category A*

COMMON INDICATIONS AND DOSAGES	ADMINISTRATION	SPECIAL CONSIDERATIONS
Hypothyroidism. *Adults:* 50 to 100 mcg daily as a single dose. *Children ages 6 to 12:* 100 to 150 mcg or 4 to 5 mcg/kg daily. *Children ages 1 to 5:* 75 to 100 mcg or 5 to 6 mcg/kg daily. *Infants ages 6 to 12 months:* 50 to 75 mcg or 6 to 8 mcg/kg daily. *Healthy infants up to age 6 months:* 25 to 50 mcg or 10 to 15 mcg/kg daily. *Premature infants who weigh less than 4.4 lb (2 kg) and infants at risk for heart failure:* 25 mcg daily, increased to 37.5 mcg daily after 4 to 6 weeks. **Myxedema coma.** *Adults:* 200 to 500 mcg followed by 100 to 300 mcg on next day. *Children:* See schedule for hypothyroidism.	Available as a buff-colored, odorless powder in 6-ml vials of 200 or 500 mcg. Stable at room temperature. Store in light-resistant container; otherwise, powder may turn light pink. Reconstitute Levothroid powder by adding 2 to 5 ml of preservative-free 0.9% NaCl injection to the 200- or 500-mg vial respectively to yield 100 mcg/ml. Shake until clear. To reconstitute Synthroid powder, add 5 ml of 0.9% NaCl injection or (except in infants) bacteriostatic NaCl injection with benzyl alcohol to the 200- or 500-mcg vial to yield 40 or 100 mcg/ml. Shake to dissolve. Reconstitute drug immediately before use and discard unused portions. ***Incompatibilities:*** Don't mix with other solutions for I.V. infusion. ***Direct injection:*** Inject each 100 mcg over 1 to 2 minutes.	• Don't use diluent that contains benzyl alcohol for an infant. • Monitor patient's vital signs and thyroid function tests. • Monitor patient's ECG for ventricular arrhythmias, tachyarrhythmias, and signs of ischemia. • In myxedema coma, give levothyroxine with hydrocortisone to prevent adrenal crisis. • If symptoms of overdose or hyperthyroidism occur, stop drug for 2 to 6 days. Resume at a lower dose.

lidocaine hydrochloride • LidoPen Auto-Injector, Xylocaine, Xylocard◆

Classes: ***ventricular antiarrhythmic, anesthetic*** • *Pregnancy risk category B*

COMMON INDICATIONS AND DOSAGES	ADMINISTRATION	SPECIAL CONSIDERATIONS
Acute ventricular arrhythmias (PVCs, ventricular tachycardia) from acute MI, cardiac glycoside toxicity, cardioversion, cardiac manipulation from trauma or surgery, or adverse drug effects. *Adults:* 50 to 100 mg initial bolus, repeated after 5 minutes if arrhythmia continues. For maintenance, infuse 20 to 50 mcg/kg/minute (1 to 4 mg/minute in 154-lb [70-kg] adult). Don't exceed	Available for injection in 5-ml ampules and prefilled syringes at 10 and 20 mg/ml. Available for continuous infusion in 40-mg, 1-g, and 2-g, single-use, 25- or 50-ml vials and in 5- and 10-ml syringes that require mixing with D_5W in water. Dilute 1 g drug in 250 ml D_5W to obtain a 0.4% solution (4 mg/ml). Drug also comes in premixed 250-ml bottles of 0.4% or 0.8% solution or 500 ml bottles of 0.2%, 0.4%, or 0.8% solution. Store at room temperature. Use only solutions marked for treating arrhythmias. ***Incompatibilities:*** Amphotericin B, ampicillin sodium, ce-	• Monitor patient's ECG continuously during administration. Keep resuscitation equipment nearby. • Use smallest dose possible to control arrhythmia. Therapeutic level is 1.5 to 5 mcg/ml; toxic level is above 5 mcg/ml. • Assess often for signs of toxic effects. • In case of overdose, stop infusion immediately and notify doctor. Ensure an adequate airway and oxygenation. Monitor patient's vital signs and ECG closely. A different drug may be needed.

300 mg within 1 hr. Keep rate below 30 mcg/kg/minute if patient has heart failure or liver disease. *Children:* 0.5 to 1 mg/kg initial bolus, repeated as necessary. For maintenance, infuse 10 to 50 mcg/kg/minute. Maximum 5 mg/kg.
Status epilepticus unresponsive to all other measures. *Adults and children:* 1 mg/kg initial bolus. If seizure doesn't stop after 2 minutes, give 0.5-mg/kg bolus. For maintenance, infuse 30 mcg/kg/minute.

fazolin, hydromorphone, methohexital, and phenytoin.
Direct injection: Inject undiluted drug into large vein or cannula at 25 to 50 mg/minute.
Continuous infusion: Using an infusion pump and microdrip tubing, titrate dose according to suppression of ventricular ectopy.

lorazepam • Ativan

Classes: ***antianxiety, sedative-hypnotic*** • *Pregnancy risk category D* • *Controlled substance schedule IV*

Short-term relief of anxiety symptoms in patients who can't take oral drugs. *Adults:* 0.044 mg/kg or 2 mg total, whichever is smaller.
Preoperative sedation. *Adults:* 2 mg total dose or 0.044 mg/kg, whichever is smaller, given 15 to 20 minutes before surgery. In patients age 50 and younger, doses up to 0.05 mg/kg (up to 4 mg total) may be given.
Prevention of nausea and vomiting from chemotherapy. *Adults:* 2 mg 30 minutes before chemotherapy, then 2 mg q 4 hr, p.r.n.

Available in 1- and 10-ml vials and single-dose prefilled syringes at 2 and 4 mg/ml. Refrigerate drug (but don't freeze) and protect from light. Discard if drug becomes discolored or contains precipitate. Just before administration, dilute with an equal volume of sterile water for injection, 0.9% NaCl, or D_5W in water. Rotate syringe gently to ensure complete mixing.
Incompatibilities: Idarubicin.
Direct injection: Inject into vein or into I.V. line that contains a free-flowing, compatible solution at maximum of 2 mg/minute.

- Keep emergency resuscitation equipment nearby.
- Monitor patient's vital signs.
- Overly rapid infusion can cause apnea, hypotension, bradycardia, or cardiac arrest.
- If necessary, use flumazenil (Romazicon), a benzodiazepine antagonist, to reverse lorazepam's sedative and respiratory depressant effects.

magnesium sulfate

Classes: ***anticonvulsant, antiarrhythmic*** • *Pregnancy risk category A*

COMMON INDICATIONS AND DOSAGES

Preeclampsia or eclampsia. *Adults:* 4 g, then 1 to 2 g/hr by continuous infusion. Dosage over next 24 hr depends on serum magnesium levels and urine output. Maximum is 30 to 40 g/24 hr; in renal disease, 20 g q 48 hr.

Prevention and control of seizures in severe preeclampsia or eclampsia, epilepsy, glomerulonephritis, or hypothyroidism. *Adults:* 1 to 4 g (8 to 32 mEq of magnesium) of 10% to 20% solution.

Severe hypertension, encephalopathy, and seizures caused by nephritis. *Children:* 100 to 200 mg/kg of 1% to 3% solution. Give total dose within 1 hr, half in the first 15 to 20 minutes.

Severe magnesium deficiency. *Adults:* 5 g.

Magnesium supplement in total parenteral nutrition. *Adults:* 0.5 to 3 g daily (4 to 24 mEq of magnesium). *Infants:* 0.25 to 1.25 g daily (2 to 10 mEq of magnesium).

Barium poisoning. *Adults*: 1 to 2 g.

Paroxysmal atrial tachycardia. *Adults:* 3 to 4 g.

ADMINISTRATION

Available as 10% concentration in 10- and 20-ml ampules (100 mg/ml) and in 20- and 50-ml vials; as 12.5% concentration in 20-ml vials (125 mg/ml); and as 50% concentration in 2-ml ampules (500 mg/ml), 2-, 5-, 10-, 30-, and 50-ml vials, and 10-ml syringes. Store at room temperature and avoid freezing. For seizures, dilute dose in 250 ml D_5W. For magnesium deficiency, dilute dose in 1 liter D_5W or dextrose 5% in 0.9% NaCl. For all indications, don't use concentrations over 20% (200 mg/ml).

Incompatibilities: Alcohol, alkali carbonates and bicarbonates, calcium gluceptate, calcium gluconate, cefepime, ciprofloxacin, dobutamine, hydrocortisone sodium succinate, 10% I.V. fat emulsion, polymyxin B, procaine, sodium bicarbonate, and soluble phosphates.

Direct injection: Inject directly into vein at 150 mg/minute or less.

Intermittent infusion: Administer diluted drug over 1 to 3 hr.

Continuous infusion: Give by infusion pump at 150 mg/minute (1.2 mEq/minute) or less.

SPECIAL CONSIDERATIONS

- Keep I.V. calcium gluconate available, but use cautiously in patients undergoing digitalization because arrhythmias may develop.
- Monitor patient's vital signs and intake and output every 15 minutes. Watch for respiratory depression and signs of heart block.
- Disappearance of patellar reflexes signals onset of toxic effects. Treat with 5 to 10 mEq of calcium (10 to 20 ml of 10% calcium gluconate), as ordered. In severe overdose, patient may need peritoneal dialysis or hemodialysis.

mannitol • Osmitrol◆

Class: ***diuretic*** • *Pregnancy risk category C*

Prevention of oliguric phase in acute renal failure. *Adults:* 50 to 100 g, followed by infusion of 5% or 10% solution.
Test dose for marked oliguria or suspected inadequate renal function. *Adults and children over age 12:* 200 mg/kg, or 12.5 g as a 15% or 20% solution given over 3 to 5 minutes. *Children age 12 and under:* 0.2 g/kg given over 3 to 5 minutes, then 2 g/kg.
Treatment of oliguria. *Adults:* 100 g of a 15% to 20% solution given over 90 minutes to several hr.
Reduction of intracranial and intraocular pressure. *Adults:* 1.5 to 2 g/kg of a 15%, 20%, or 25% solution given over 30 to 60 minutes. *Children age 12 and under:* 1 to 2 g/kg of a 15% or 20% solution given over 30 to 60 minutes.
Reduction of nephrotoxic effects of amphotericin B. *Adults:* 12.5 g given just before and after each dose of amphotericin B.
Promotion of diuresis in drug intoxication (adjunct). *Adults:* 50 to 200 g of 5% to 25% solution, followed by infusion to maintain urine output at 100 to 500 ml/hr.
Adjunctive treatment of edema and ascites. *Adults:* 100 g of a 10% to 20% solution given over 2 to 6 hr. *Children age 12 and under:* 2 g/kg of a 15% or 20% solution given over 2 to 6 hr.

Available in strengths of 5%, 10%, 15%, 20%, and 25% in 150-, 250-, 500-, and 1,000-ml glass and plastic I.V. containers. Store at room temperature; avoid freezing. Drug may crystallize, especially if chilled. If crystals form, dissolve according to manufacturer's directions. Don't use solution that contains undissolved crystals.When giving mannitol solutions of 15% or above, make sure the administration set includes a filter.
Incompatibilities: Imipenem-cilastatin and blood products. If blood must be given with mannitol, add 20 mEq of NaCl to each liter of mannitol.
Intermittent infusion: Infuse appropriate dose and concentration at ordered rate.
Continuous infusion: Infuse appropriate dose and concentration at ordered rate.

- Avoid extravasation to prevent edema and necrosis.
- Rebound increase in intracranial and intraocular pressure may occur about 12 hr after giving mannitol.
- Rapid administration of large doses may lead to drug accumulation and circulatory overload.
- Large doses may cross the blood-brain barrier and cause CNS damage or death.
- Monitor patient's vital signs frequently during first hr of infusion and each hr thereafter, or as needed. Also monitor patient's intake and output, BUN, and serum electrolytes, especially sodium and potassium.
- Tell patient to change positions slowly to avoid dizziness from orthostatic hypotension.

◆ Also available in Canada. ◇ Available in Canada only.

COMMON INDICATIONS AND DOSAGES	ADMINISTRATION	SPECIAL CONSIDERATIONS

mechlorethamine hydrochloride (nitrogen mustard) • Mustargen ◆

Class: ***antineoplastic*** • *Pregnancy risk category D*

COMMON INDICATIONS AND DOSAGES	ADMINISTRATION	SPECIAL CONSIDERATIONS
Hodgkin's disease. *Adults and children:* 6 mg/m^2 daily on days 1 and 8 of 28-day cycle in combination with other antineoplastics. Repeat for six cycles. Subsequent doses reduced by 50% in MOPP regimen when WBC count is between 3,000 and 3,999/mm^3, by 75% when WBC count is between 1,000 and 2,999/mm^3, or by 75% if platelet count is between 50,000 and 100,000/mm^3. **Other neoplastic disorders.** *Adults and children:* 0.4 mg/kg as single dose or 0.1 to 0.2 mg/kg divided in two or four successive daily doses during each course of therapy. **Dosage adjustment.** Dosage is based on patient response and degree of toxicity.	Follow facility protocol for handling chemotherapy drugs. Available in 10-mg vials. Store at room temperature. Reconstitute with 10 ml sterile water for injection or 0.9% NaCl to yield 1 mg/ml. Shake vial several times to dissolve. Administer within 15 minutes. Highly unstable, the solution decomposes while standing. Don't use if drug is discolored or if water droplets appear in vial. Discard unused drug. ***Incompatibilities:*** Methohexital. ***Direct injection:*** Use one sterile needle to aspirate reconstituted drug from vial and another for direct injection. Inject reconstituted solution directly into vein or, preferably, into free-flowing I.V. solution over a few minutes or according to protocol. After administration, flush tubing and vein with I.V. solution for 2 to 5 minutes.	• Administer with hydrocortisone, as ordered, to reduce risk of phlebitis or pain. • If infiltration occurs, aspirate as much drug as possible from tissues. Then inject area with sterile isotonic sodium thiosulfate and apply ice compresses for 6 to 12 hr. • Expect some evidence of toxic effects with a therapeutic response. • Give antiemetics to reduce severity of nausea and vomiting, which usually begin 1 to 3 hr after administration. • Monitor patient's WBC, platelet count, BUN, hematocrit, ALT, AST, bilirubin, creatinine, lactic dehydrogenase, and uric acid levels.

melphalan hydrochloride • Alkeran

Class: ***antineoplastic*** • *Pregnancy risk category D*

COMMON INDICATIONS AND DOSAGES	ADMINISTRATION	SPECIAL CONSIDERATIONS
Palliative treatment of multiple myeloma. *Adults:* 16 mg/m^2 as a single infusion over 15 to 20 minutes at 2-week intervals for four doses, then at 4-week intervals after adequate recovery from toxicity. **Dosage adjustment.** Adjust dose based on blood cell counts at nadir and on day of treatment. Reduce dose by up to half if patient has renal insufficiency.	Follow facility protocol for handling chemotherapy drugs. Available as a 50-mg powder for injection in a single-use vial with a 10-ml vial of sterile diluent (water for injection). Protect from light and dispense in glass. To prepare, reconstitute with 10 ml of diluent supplied to yield 5 mg/ml. Shake vigorously until solution is clear. Immediately dilute calculated dose in 0.9% NaCl injection. Final concentration shouldn't exceed 0.45 mg/ml. Complete administration within 60 minutes of reconstitution because reconstituted and diluted solutions	• Obtain CBC before starting therapy and before each subsequent dose. If WBC falls below 3,000/mm^3, temporarily stop drug or decrease dosage. If platelet count falls below 100,000/mm^3, don't give IM injections. • Therapeutic effects are often accompanied by toxic effects. • Anticoagulants and aspirin products should be used cautiously. Watch for signs of bleeding and infection

are unstable. Don't refrigerate because precipitate will form.
Incompatibilities: amphotericin B, chlorpromazine, D_5W, and lactated Ringer's injection. Compatibility with 0.9% NaCl injection is concentration-dependent; don't prepare solutions exceeding 0.45 mg/ml.
Intermittent infusion: Administer diluted drug over 15 to 20 minutes and within 60 minutes of reconstitution and dilution.

meperidine hydrochloride (pethidine hydrochloride) • Demerol◆

Classes: ***narcotic analgesic, anesthesia adjunct*** • *Pregnancy risk category B (D for prolonged use or high doses at term)* • *Controlled substance schedule II*

Moderate to severe pain. *Adults:* 10 to 50 mg q 2 to 4 hr or 15 to 35 mg/hr by infusion. Dosage reflects patient response and severity of pain.
Adjunct in anesthesia. *Adults:* Fractional doses of a 10-mg/ml solution, repeated p.r.n., or 1 mg/ml by infusion.

Available in preservative-free ampules and vials and in preservative-containing syringes at strengths of 10, 25, 50, 75, and 100 mg/ml. Store vials and ampules at room temperature. Single doses in syringes remain stable at room temperature for 24 hr. For direct injection, dilute dose with compatible solution to yield 10 mg/ml. For infusion, dilute with compatible solution to yield 1 mg/ml.
Incompatibilities: Aminophylline, amobarbital, ephedrine, heparin, methicillin, morphine, phenobarbital sodium, phenytoin, sodium bicarbonate, sodium iodide, sulfadiazine, and thiopental.
Direct injection: Inject diluted dose over 3 to 5 minutes. Rapid injection increases risk of severe adverse reactions.
Continuous infusion: Give at 15 to 35 mg/hr using an infusion control device. Avoid rapid infusion.

- For improved analgesia, give before patient has intense pain.
- Give drug with patient in supine position to minimize hypotension.
- Monitor respirations frequently during infusion and every 15 minutes for 1 hr after infusion. Keep resuscitation equipment and naloxone nearby.
- Monitor for neurotoxic effects.
- During I.V. administration, tachycardia may occur.

COMMON INDICATIONS AND DOSAGES	ADMINISTRATION	SPECIAL CONSIDERATIONS
meropenem • Merrem I.V.		
Class: ***antibiotic*** • *Pregnancy risk category B*		
Complicated appendicitis and peritonitis; bacterial meningitis (pediatric only) caused by susceptible organisms. *Adults:* 1 g q 8 hr. *Children age 3 months and older:* 20 mg/kg for intra-abdominal infection or 40 mg/kg for bacterial meningitis every 8 hr; maximum 2 g q 8 hr. *Children who weigh more than 110 lb (50 kg):* 1 g q 8 hr for intra-abdominal infections or 2 g q 8 hr for meningitis. **Dosage adjustment.** Dosage must be adjusted for elderly patients and patients with renal impairment or creatinine clearance below 51 ml/minute.	Available in 20- and 30-ml injection vials containing 500 mg and 1 g, respectively. Also supplied in 100-ml infusion vials. ADD-Vantage vials contain 500 mg or 1 g. Store powder at controlled 68° to 77° F (20° to 25° C). For I.V. bolus, add 10 ml sterile water for injection to 500 mg/20-ml vial or add 20 ml to 1 g/30-ml vial. Shake to dissolve and let stand until clear. For I.V. infusion, reconstitute infusion vials (500 mg or 1 g/100 ml) directly with compatible infusion fluid. Or reconstitute injection vial and add resulting solution to I.V. container for further dilution with appropriate infusion fluid. Don't use ADD-Vantage vial for this purpose. For ADD-Vantage vials, follow manufacturer's guidelines closely. Use solutions immediately if possible. Stability varies with type of drug and type of solution. Consult manufacturer's literature for details. ***Incompatibilities:*** Compatibility with other drugs has not been established. Don't mix with or physically add to solutions containing other drugs. ***Direct injection:*** Administer over 3 to 5 minutes. ***Intermittent infusion:*** Infuse diluted drug over 15 to 30 minutes.	• To minimize risk of seizures, closely adhere to dosage regimen, especially in patients at risk of seizures. • Serious, occasionally fatal hypersensitivity reactions have been reported in patients receiving beta-lactams. Obtain thorough history and be prepared to treat reactions. • Monitor patient for signs and symptoms of superinfection. • Periodically monitor patient's renal, hepatic, and hematopoietic function. • Monitor patient for seizures and other CNS adverse reactions and report immediately.
mesna • Mesnex		
Class: ***uroprotectant*** • *Pregnancy risk category B*		
Prevention of ifosfamide-induced hemorrhagic cystitis. *Adults:* 60% of ifosfamide dose given in three bolus doses (each 20% of ifosfamide dose), the first given with ifosfamide dose and subsequent ones given 4 and 8 hr later.	Available in 2-, 4-, and 10-ml ampules at 100 mg/ml. Store at room temperature. Dilute the appropriate dose in D_5W, 0.9% NaCl injection, or Ringer's lactate to yield 20 mg/ml. Diluted solutions are stable for 24 hr at 77° F (25° C), but you should use within 6 hr. Because drug becomes oxidized in the presence of oxygen, discard unused drug from open ampules and	• Mesna doesn't prevent or alleviate other adverse reactions to ifosfamide. • Drug has been used to prevent cyclophosphamide-induced hemorrhagic cystitis.

prepare a new ampule for each administration.
Incompatibilities: Cisplatin.
Direct injection: Inject into vein or I.V. tubing that contains free-flowing, compatible solution.
Intermittent infusion: Infuse over 15 to 30 minutes.

methocarbamol • Robaxin◆

Class: ***skeletal muscle relaxant*** • *Pregnancy risk category NR*

Adjunct in severe musculoskeletal pain. *Adults:* 1 g q 8 hr. Maximum 3 g daily for 3 days.
Tetanus. *Adults:* 1 to 2 g by direct injection, followed by 1 to 2 g by infusion q 6 hr. Repeat until nasogastric tube can be inserted. *Children:* 15 mg/kg q 6 hr.

Available in 10-ml vials at 100 mg/ml. Dilute single-dose vial in up to 250 ml of 0.9% NaCl or D_5W for infusion. Store drug and diluted solution at room temperature.
Incompatibilities: None reported.
Direct injection: Inject drug into vein or I.V. tubing of free-flowing solution at maximum of 300 mg/minute. Slow injection helps minimize adverse effects.
Intermittent infusion: Infuse diluted solution through I.V. tubing that contains free-flowing solution at ordered rate.

- Keep patient in supine position during administration and for 10 to 15 minutes afterward.
- Monitor patient's blood pressure and observe for orthostatic hypotension.
- Monitor patient's I.V. sites carefully.
- Avoid extravasation because solution is hypertonic and may cause thrombophlebitis.
- Administer drug for no longer than 3 consecutive days.

methotrexate sodium • Folex, Folex PFS, Mexate, Mexate-AQ

Class: ***antineoplastic*** • *Pregnancy risk category D*

Induction of remission in lymphoblastic leukemia. *Adults:* 2.5 mg/kg q 14 days. Dosage varies widely.
Psoriasis. *Adults:* 10 to 25 mg once weekly. Up to 100 mg may be required, but manufacturer recommends maximum of 50 mg weekly.
Adjuvant therapy for osteosarcoma. *Adults:* 12 g/m^2. May be increased to 15 g/m^2 if lower dose can't provide 1×10^{-3} M blood level at end of infusion.

Follow facility protocol for handling chemotherapy drugs. Available in 20-, 50-, 100-, and 250-mg single-dose vials of lyophilized sterile powder and in 2-, 4-, 8-, and 10-ml vials containing 25 mg/ml solution. Reconstitute with 2 to 10 ml of sterile water for injection, 0.9% NaCl, or D_5W to yield 2 to 50 mg/ml. Dilute for injection with 0.9% NaCl or D_5W. Store drug preparations at room temperature and protect from light.
Incompatibilities: Bleomycin, chlorpromazine, droperidol, fluorouracil, metoclopramide, prednisolone, promethazine, and sodium phosphate.

- Generic preparations may contain benzyl alcohol.
- Monitor patient's CBC. If blood cell counts decrease, discontinue drug, as ordered.
- Monitor patient's serum creatinine and BUN levels daily during high-dose therapy.
- Monitor patient's serum methotrexate levels daily during therapy and until serum level falls below 5×10^{-8} M.
- Expect toxic reactions to accompany therapeutic doses. Drug is highly toxic and has a low therapeutic index.

(continued)

COMMON INDICATIONS AND DOSAGES	ADMINISTRATION	SPECIAL CONSIDERATIONS
methotrexate sodium *(continued)*	***Direct injection:*** Inject directly into vein or into side port of free-flowing I.V. line over prescribed duration. ***Intermittent infusion:*** May be given as a 4-hr infusion.	• For overdose, give leucovorin calcium as soon as possible, preferably in first hr of overdose. In massive overdose, urine alkalinization and hydration help prevent precipitation of methotrexate or its metabolites in renal tubules.

methyldopate hydrochloride • Aldomet♦

Class: ***antihypertensive*** • *Pregnancy risk category B*

Sustained mild to severe hypertension and, in combination therapy, acute hypertensive emergencies. *Adults:* 250 to 500 mg q 6 hr, as necessary. Maximum 1 g q 6 hr. *Children:* 20 to 40 mg/kg q 24 hr or 0.15 to 0.3 g/m^2 q 6 hr. Maximum 65 mg/kg, 2 g/m^2, or 3 g daily, whichever is smallest. **Dosage adjustment.** Dosage must be adjusted if patient has renal impairment.	Available at 50 mg/ml. For infusion, add required dose to 100 ml D_5W to yield 100 mg/10 ml. Drug stable for 24 hr in most I.V. solutions; however, exposure to air may accelerate decomposition. Protect from light and store at room temperature; avoid freezing. ***Incompatibilities:*** Amphotericin B, methohexital, and some total parenteral nutrition solutions. Mix cautiously with drugs that have poor solubility in acidic media, such as barbiturates and sulfonamides. ***Intermittent infusion:*** Infuse diluted dose through patent I.V. line over 30 to 60 minutes.	• Perform Coombs' test before therapy. • Monitor patient's CBC before and during therapy. If hemolytic anemia develops, stop drug. • Monitor patient's heart rate, blood pressure, cardiac output, blood volume, electrolyte balance, GI motility, renal function, and cerebral activity. To reverse hypotension, administer I.V. fluids. • Watch for signs of drug-induced depression.

methylene blue

Class: ***antidote*** • *Pregnancy risk category C*

Methemoglobin and cyanide poisoning. *Adults and children:* 1 to 2 mg/kg of 1% solution. May be repeated in 1 hr.	Available in 1- and 10-ml ampules at 10 mg/ml. No need to dilute before injection. ***Incompatibilities:*** Dichromates, iodides, and oxidizing and reducing substances. ***Direct injection:*** Administer over several minutes directly into vein or I.V. tubing that contains free-flowing, compatible solution. Overly rapid injection causes additional methemoglobin production. Don't exceed recommended dosage.	• S.C. injection may cause necrotic abscesses. • In prolonged therapy, monitor patient for signs of anemia. • Monitor patient's I.V. site carefully to avoid extravasation. • Tell patient that drug discolors urine and stools and stains skin. Stains can be removed with hypochlorite solution.

methylergonovine maleate • Methergine

Class: ***oxytocic*** • *Pregnancy risk category C*

Emergency treatment of severe postpartum and postabortion hemorrhage caused by uterine atony or subinvolution. *Adults:* 0.2 mg in single dose, repeated q 2 to 4 hr for up to five doses, if necessary.

Available in 1-ml ampules at 0.2 mg/ml. Store below 46° F (8° C) in a light-resistant container. Don't freeze. Ready-to-use injections are normally clear and colorless. Discard if solution is discolored or contains a precipitate. Dilute with 5 ml of 0.9% NaCl, if appropriate.

Incompatibilities: None reported.

Direct injection: Administer directly into vein or into I.V. tubing that contains free-flowing, compatible solution over at least 60 seconds. Can use diluted dosage to facilitate slow injection.

- Overly rapid administration can cause severe CV effects.
- Closely monitor patient's blood pressure and pulse. Give hydralazine or chlorpromazine I.V., as ordered, for hypertension.
- After administration, closely monitor patient's uterine activity. (Contractions are sustained and uterine tone is high.) If appropriate, give analgesics for discomfort.
- Tell patient to report shortness of breath, headache, numb or cold extremities, or severe abdominal cramps.

methylprednisolone sodium succinate • A-methaPred, Solu-Medrol◆

Classes: ***anti-inflammatory, immunosuppressant*** • *Pregnancy risk category C*

Severe inflammation or immunosuppression. *Adults:* 10 mg to 1.5 g daily. Usual dosage, 10 to 250 mg up to q 4 hr.
Severe shock. *Adults:* 30 mg/kg initially and repeated q 4 to 6 hr p.r.n. or 100 to 250 mg initially and repeated q 2 to 6 hr p.r.n. Initial dose may be followed by 30 mg/kg infusion q 12 hr for 24 to 48 hr.
Severe lupus nephritis. *Adults:* 1 g (intermittent infusion) for 3 days followed by oral prednisolone or prednisone.
Children: 30 mg/kg on alternate days for six doses followed by oral prednisolone or prednisone.

Available as drug and diluent in these strengths: 40 mg (1 ml), 125 mg (2 ml), 500 mg (8 ml), 1 g (16 ml), and 2 g (32 ml). Reconstitute with diluent provided and store at room temperature. Don't freeze. Don't use cloudy solution, and discard unused portion after 48 hr. Dilute for infusion with D_5W, 0.9% NaCl, or dextrose 5% in 0.9% NaCl.

Incompatibilities: Calcium gluconate, cephalothin, cytarabine, filgrastim, glycopyrrolate, metaraminol, nafcillin, and penicillin G sodium.

Direct injection: Inject diluted drug into vein or I.V. tubing that contains free-flowing, compatible solution over at least 1 minute. In life-threatening situations, give initial massive dose over 3 to 15 minutes.

- In all preparations, diluent contains benzyl alcohol.
- Because of risk of anaphylaxis, keep resuscitation equipment nearby.
- Adjust dosage as needed for patients taking insulin, antithyroid drugs, or thyroid hormones.

(continued)

COMMON INDICATIONS AND DOSAGES	ADMINISTRATION	SPECIAL CONSIDERATIONS
methylprednisolone sodium succinate *(continued)* **To decrease residual damage following spinal cord trauma.** *Adults:* 30 mg/kg as a bolus injection within 8 hr of injury followed by cautious infusion of 5.4 mg/kg/hr for next 23 hr. **Adjunctive treatment of *Pneumocystis carinii* pneumonia.** *Adults:* 30 mg b.i.d. for 5 days, then 30 mg daily for 5 days. Finally, 15 mg daily for 11 days or until anti-infective therapy is discontinued.	***Intermittent infusion:*** Using appropriately diluted dose, adjust flow rate, depending on disorder and patient's response. ***Continuous infusion:*** Using appropriately diluted dose, adjust flow rate, depending on disorder and patient's response.	

metoclopramide hydrochloride • Maxeran♦, Octamide PFS, Reglan♦

Classes: ***antiemetic, GI stimulant*** • *Pregnancy risk category B*

COMMON INDICATIONS AND DOSAGES	ADMINISTRATION	SPECIAL CONSIDERATIONS
Nausea and vomiting during chemotherapy. *Adults:* 2 mg/kg q 2 hr for three doses, beginning 30 minutes before chemotherapy; then 1 mg/kg q 3 hr for three doses. For less emetogenic regimens, 1 mg/kg/dose may be adequate. **Severely delayed gastric emptying in diabetic gastroparesis (in patients who can't take oral dose).** *Adults:* 10 mg q.i.d. 30 minutes before meals and h.s. **Passage of intestinal tubes for diagnostic tests.** *Adults:* 10 mg. *Children ages 6 to 14:* 2.5 to 5 mg. *Children under age 6:* 0.1 mg/kg. **Radiologic examination of GI tract (in delayed gastric emptying that interferes with exam).** *Adults:* 10 mg. *Children*	Available at 5 mg/ml in 2-, 10-, 30-, 50-, and 100-ml vials and in 2- and 10-ml ampules. For infusion, dilute with 50 ml of D_5W, 0.9% NaCl, dextrose 5% in 0.45% NaCl, Ringer's injection, or lactated Ringer's solution. Solution stable for 48 hr when stored at 39° to 86° F (4° to 30° C) and protected from light. If diluted with 0.9% NaCl, solution may be frozen in polyvinyl chloride bags for up to 4 weeks. Don't use dextrose 5% diluent with polyvinyl chloride bags if solution will be frozen. ***Incompatibilities:*** Allopurinol, ampicillin, calcium gluconate, cefepime, cephalothin, chloramphenicol sodium succinate, cisplatin, erythromycin lactobionate, furosemide, methotrexate sodium, penicillin G potassium, and sodium bicarbonate. ***Direct injection:*** Inject over 1 to 2 minutes directly into vein or into I.V. tubing that contains free-flowing, compatible solution. Each 10 mg of drug should be given slowly over 1 to 2 minutes.	• Slow infusion prevents anxiety and restlessness. • Contact doctor if patient has involuntary movements of face, eyes, or limbs. • Adjust insulin dosage, as ordered, if patient has diabetic gastroparesis. Drug affects intestinal food absorption. • For overdose, to control extrapyramidal symptoms, give antimuscarinic-antiparkinsonian drugs or antihistamines with antimuscarinic properties.

ages 6 to 14: 2.5 to 5 mg. *Children under age 6:* 0.1 mg/kg.
Dosage adjustment. Adjust dosage in renal impairment. For adults, decrease dose by half if creatinine clearance less than 40 ml/minute.

Intermittent infusion: Cover solution with a brown paper bag to prevent exposure to light. Infuse over at least 15 minutes.

metoprolol tartrate • Betaloc◆, Lopresor◆, Lopressor

Class: ***antihypertensive*** • *Pregnancy risk category C*

Early treatment in suspected or definitive acute MI. *Adults:* Three injections of 5 mg each q 2 minutes, followed by oral maintenance doses if patient tolerates I.V. doses.
Dosage adjustment. Patients with hepatic dysfunction may need reduced dosage.

Available in 5-ml ampules or prefilled syringes at 1 mg/ml. Store at room temperature and protect from light. Discard solution if discolored or if precipitate forms.
Incompatibilities: None reported.
Direct injection: Rapidly inject bolus into I.V. line of free-flowing solution.

- If bradycardia or hypotension develops before complete dosage is given, notify doctor. Injections may be stopped or changed to oral form.
- Don't withdraw drug abruptly; it could worsen angina, the MI, or ventricular arrhythmias, or it could cause death.
- Continuously monitor patient's hemodynamic status, blood pressure, heart rate, and ECG during infusion.

metronidazole • Flagyl 500 Injection◇, Flagyl IV RTU, Metro I.V.
metronidazole hydrochloride • Flagyl IV

Classes: ***antibacterial, amebicide, antiprotozoal*** • *Pregnancy risk category B*

Severe infections caused by susceptible bacteria. *Adults:* 15 mg/kg initially, then 7.5 mg/kg q 6 hr beginning 6 hr after loading dose. Maximum 4 g daily.
Surgical prophylaxis. *Adults:* 15 mg/kg, completed 1 hr before surgery, then 7.5 mg/kg q 6 hr for two doses at 6 and 12 hr after initial dose.

Flagyl IV available as sterile, off-white, lyophilized powder in single-dose vials containing 500 mg of metronidazole and 415 mg of mannitol. Before reconstitution, store below 86° F (30° C) and protect from light. Drug requires reconstitution, dilution, and neutralization. Order of mixing is important. Reconstitute drug with 4.4 ml of sterile water for injection, bacteriostatic water for injection, 0.9% NaCl injection, or bacteriostatic 0.9% NaCl injection. Mix thoroughly. Resulting so-

- Flagyl IV RTU contains 14 mEq (322 mg) of sodium. Neutralized I.V. solution contains 5 mEq (115 mg) of sodium.
- Obtain patient's CBC before and after therapy.
- Symptoms of known or previously undiagnosed candidiasis may become more prominent during therapy, requiring treatment with an antifungal agent.

(continued)

◆ Also available in Canada. ◇ Available in Canada only.

COMMON INDICATIONS AND DOSAGES	ADMINISTRATION	SPECIAL CONSIDERATIONS
metronidazole **metronidazole hydrochloride** *(continued)* **Dosage adjustment.** If patient has severe hepatic dysfunction, dosage may need to be reduced.	lution provides 5 ml (100 mg/ml). Reconstituted vials stable for 96 hr in room light if stored below 86° F. Using glass or plastic container, dilute further with 0.9% NaCl injection, dextrose 5% injection, or lactated Ringer's injection. Concentration should not exceed 8 mg/ml. Neutralize final dilution with 5 mEq sodium bicarbonate injection for each 500 mg of drug. Because this produces carbon dioxide, the container may need venting. Don't refrigerate when neutralized because precipitate may form. Use diluted and neutralized solutions within 24 hr. Flagyl IV RTU and Metro I.V. supplied in 100-ml single-dose plastic containers containing 500 mg of drug. They need no dilution or neutralization. Don't dilute, change pH, or mix any additive with these solutions. Also avoid using aluminum equipment that would come in contact with drug. Although drug may cause opacity of plastic containers, needle hubs, or cannulae, this reaction does not affect solution. Store at a controlled 59° to 86° F (15° to 30° C) and protect drug from light. Don't refrigerate or freeze. ***Incompatibilities:*** Aluminum, 10% amino acid, and dopamine. Manufacturer recommends mixing no other drugs with metronidazole. ***Intermittent infusion:*** Give by slow infusion only, over 1 hr (30 to 60 minutes when used for surgical prophylaxis). Discontinue primary solution during administration. ***Continuous infusion:*** Rarely used. Infuse diluted drug over ordered amount of time.	• If diarrhea persists during therapy, collect stool specimens for culture to rule out pseudomembranous colitis.

mezlocillin sodium • Mezlin

Class: ***antibiotic*** • *Pregnancy risk category B*

Severe infections caused by susceptible organisms. *Adults:* 200 to 300 mg/kg daily in four to six divided doses; 3 g q 4	Available as sterile powder in vials containing 1, 2, 3, or 4 g of drug or in infusion bottles containing 2, 3, or 4 g of drug. Store at or below 86° F (30° C). Reconstitute each gram of	• Institute seizure precautions in patients who receive high doses. • When giving drug with an aminoglycoside, adminis-

hr; or 4 g q 6 hr. *Children ages 1 month to 12 years:* 50 mg/kg q 4 hr. *Neonates age 8 days or older, weighing more than 4.4 lb (2 kg):* 75 mg/kg q 6 hr. *Neonates age 8 days or older, weighing 4.4 lb or less:* 75 mg/kg q 8 hr. *Neonates age 7 days or younger:* 75 mg/kg q 12 hr.

Life-threatening infections caused by susceptible organisms. *Adults:* 350 mg/kg daily or 4 g q 4 hr. Maximum 24 g daily. *Children and neonates:* Same as for severe infections above.

Uncomplicated UTI. *Adults:* 100 to 125 mg/kg daily in divided doses q 6 hr or 1.5 to 2 g q 6 hr. *Children and neonates:* Same as for severe infections above.

Complicated UTI. *Adults:* 150 to 200 mg/kg daily in six divided doses or 3 g q 6 hr. *Children and neonates:* Same as for severe infections above.

Acute, uncomplicated gonococcal urethritis caused by susceptible strains of *Neisseria gonorrhoeae*. *Adults:* 1 to 2 g plus 1 g probenecid at time of dosing or up to 30 minutes before. *Children and neonates:* Same as for severe infections above.

Dosage adjustment. Dosage may be reduced or administration interval lengthened if patient has renal or hepatic impairment.

sterile powder with at least 10 ml of sterile water for injection, dextrose 5% injection, or 0.9% NaCl injection. Shake vigorously to dissolve drug. After reconstitution in up to 100 mg/ml, solution may be frozen, remaining stable for 28 days. For infusion, dilute further with 50 to 100 ml sterile water for injection, 0.9% NaCl injection, dextrose 5% injection, dextrose 5% in 0.25% NaCl injection, lactated Ringer's injection, dextrose 5% in 0.45% NaCl injection, or Ringer's injection. Add daily dose of mezlocillin to amount of appropriate fluid to be administered within 24 hr. At room temperature, solutions of 10 to 100 mg/ml are stable for 24 hr when diluted in lactated Ringer's solution or Ringer's injection; for 48 hr when diluted in sterile water for injection, 0.9% NaCl, D_5W, or dextrose 5% in 0.45% NaCl; and for 72 hr when diluted in dextrose 5% in 0.25% NaCl. Refrigerated solutions of 10 to 100 mg/ml are stable for 24 hr when diluted in Ringer's injection; for 48 hr when diluted in dextrose 5% in 0.45% NaCl; and for 7 days when diluted in sterile water for injection, 0.9% NaCl, D_5W, dextrose 5% in 0.25% NaCl, or lactated Ringer's solution.

Incompatibilities: Amiodarone, aminoglycosides, filgrastim, meperidine, and idarubicin.

Direct injection: Inject reconstituted drug directly into vein or into I.V. tubing that contains free-flowing, compatible solution over 3 to 5 minutes.

Intermittent infusion: Infuse diluted drug over 30 minutes. If infused by piggyback, temporarily stop the primary solution while drug infuses.

Continuous infusion: Adjust rate according to infusion volume.

ter at separate sites and times.

- Therapy for group A beta-hemolytic streptococcal infections lasts for at least 10 days to reduce risk of rheumatic fever or glomerulonephritis. Other regimens last for 10 to 14 days or for at least 48 hr after infection is confirmed eradicated.
- Mezlocillin contains 43 mg of sodium per gram of drug.
- Check patient's CBC frequently and monitor serum potassium levels, especially in high-dose therapy or in fluid and electrolyte imbalance. Potassium supplements may be needed in hypokalemia.
- Watch bleeding time and platelet count, especially in patients with renal impairment who receive maximum doses.
- Monitor patient's hepatic and renal function.

midazolam hydrochloride • Versed♦

Classes: ***sedative-hypnotic, amnesic, anesthesia adjunct*** • *Pregnancy risk category D* • *Controlled substance schedule IV*

COMMON INDICATIONS AND DOSAGES

Dosages are highly individualized.

Conscious sedation. *Adults:* Maximum of 2.5 mg given over 2 to 3 minutes (some patients may respond to 1 mg), then increased in small increments at intervals of at least 2 minutes to assess drug effect until reaching desired effect. *Elderly or debilitated patients:* 1 to 1.5 mg initially, given over a longer duration.

Induction of general anesthesia without premedication. *Adults age 55 and over:* 300 mcg/kg. *Adults under age 55:* 300 to 350 mcg/kg given over 20 to 30 seconds. Increments of 25% of initial dose may be needed to complete induction. *Adults with debilitation or severe systemic disease:* 150 to 250 mcg/kg. Total dose shouldn't exceed 600 mcg/kg.

Induction of anesthesia following premedication with an opioid drug. *Adults age 55 and over:* 200 mcg/kg. *Adults under age 55:* 250 mcg/kg. *Adults with debilitation or severe systemic disease:* 150 mcg/kg.

ADMINISTRATION

Available in 1- and 5-mg/ml vials. Drug may be given undiluted or diluted with D_5W, 0.9% NaCl, or lactated Ringer's solution. Mixtures with D_5W or 0.9% NaCl are stable for 24 hr; those with lactated Ringer's solution, for 4 hr. Store undiluted solution at room temperature and protect from light. Once diluted, solution no longer requires protection from light.

Incompatibilities: Dimenhydrinate, pentobarbital sodium, perphenazine, prochlorperazine edisylate, and ranitidine hydrochloride.

Direct injection: Inject directly into vein or established I.V. line that contains compatible solution over 2 to 3 minutes for conscious sedation or over 20 to 30 seconds for anesthesia induction.

SPECIAL CONSIDERATIONS

- Only staff specially trained in administering anesthetics and managing their adverse reactions should give drug. Keep equipment for respiratory and CV support readily available.
- Monitor patient's vital signs during administration.
- Give slowly and in divided doses to titrate effect. Rapid administration can lead to severe apnea, respiratory arrest, and hypotension, especially in elderly or debilitated patients.
- Clinical experience has shown Versed to be three to four times as potent per milligram as diazepam.
- Give flumazenil 0.2 mg I.V. to reverse sedative effects.

milrinone lactate • Primacor

Class: ***inotropic vasodilator*** • *Pregnancy risk category C*

Heart failure. *Adults:* 50 mcg/kg over 10 minutes, then continuous infusion of 0.375 to 0.75 mcg/kg/minute. Adjust dosage to hemodynamic and clinical response. Maximum 1.13 mg/kg/day.
Dosage adjustment. If patient has renal impairment, dosage is based on creatinine clearance.

Available in 10- and 20-ml vials (1 mg/ml) and premixed 200 mcg/ml in 5% dextrose (100 ml). Dilute with 0.45% or 0.9% NaCl or D_5W only. Store at 59° to 86° F (15° to 30° C). Discard if drug discolors or contains particles.
Incompatibilities: Furosemide added to a line that contains this drug will form a precipitate.
Direct injection: Loading dose may be given undiluted, but diluting to a total volume of 10 to 20 ml helps visualize the injection rate.
Continuous infusion: Adjust maintenance dosage according to increase in cardiac output and decrease in pulmonary artery wedge pressure.

- Correct hypokalemia with potassium supplements before or during administration.
- Monitor patient's renal function and fluid and electrolyte changes.
- Monitor patient's blood pressure, heart rate, and clinical symptoms.

minocycline hydrochloride • Minocin ◆

Class: ***antibiotic*** • *Pregnancy risk category D*

Severe infections caused by susceptible organisms. *Adults:* 200 mg, then 100 mg q 12 hr. Maximum 400 mg/day. *Children over age 8:* 4 mg/kg, then 2 mg/kg q 12 hr.

Available in 100-mg vials. Reconstitute with 5 ml sterile water for injection. Then dilute each 100 mg in 500 to 1,000 ml of compatible I.V. solution for infusion, such as dextrose 5% in 0.9% NaCl, D_5W, Ringer's injection, lactated Ringer's, and 0.9% NaCl. Store vials below 104° F (40° C) in light-resistant containers. Reconstituted solution stable for 24 hr at room temperature. Once mixed with compatible I.V. solution, give diluted solution right away.
Incompatibilities: Calcium-containing solutions.
Intermittent infusion: Infuse over 6 hr; avoid rapid infusion.

- Observe I.V. site for signs of thrombophlebitis. Rotate I.V. site every 48 to 72 hr.
- Inform patient that tetracyclines may cause permanent tooth discoloration, enamel hypoplasia, and decreased bone growth in children age 8 or younger and when used during pregnancy.
- If diarrhea persists, collect stool specimen for culture to rule out pseudomembranous colitis.
- Switch to oral therapy as soon as possible.

◆ Also available in Canada. ◇ Available in Canada only.

COMMON INDICATIONS AND DOSAGES | **ADMINISTRATION** | **SPECIAL CONSIDERATIONS**

mitomycin • Mutamycin ◆

Class: ***antineoplastic*** • *Pregnancy risk category NR*

Neoplasms, including adenocarcinomas of the stomach, pancreas, and colon; head and neck cancers; chronic myelogenous leukemia; advanced biliary, ovarian, and lung cancers; cervical squamous cell carcinomas; and transitional cell carcinoma of the urinary bladder. *Adults:* dosage based on clinical and hematologic response and on concurrent myelosuppressant therapy. 20 mg/m² can be given in single dose and repeated q 6 to 8 weeks.

Follow facility protocol for handling chemotherapy drugs. Supplied in 5-, 20-, and 40-mg vials. Before reconstitution, store at room temperature. Reconstitute 5-mg vial with 10 ml (20 mg vial with 40 ml, 40 mg vial with 80 ml) of sterile water for injection. Shake to dissolve; don't use until completely dissolved. Reconstituted solutions stable 7 days at room temperature, 14 days if refrigerated. Solutions further diluted in D_5W stable 3 hr at room temperature; 12 hr in 0.9% NaCl; and 24 hr in sodium lactate. If not used within 24 hr, protect from light.

Incompatibilities: Bleomycin.

Direct injection: Administer through a new I.V. site, preferably with 23G or 25G winged-tip needle or an I.V. catheter. Use distal rather than major veins to allow repeated venipunctures.

Intermittent infusion: Infuse diluted drug through a new I.V. line.

- Expect toxic effects with therapeutic doses. Evaluate patient before each course of therapy.
- Assess patient for renal dysfunction.
- Because of cumulative myelosuppression, monitor patient's hematologic studies weekly during treatment and for at least 8 weeks afterward.
- Monitor pulmonary function during therapy.

mitoxantrone hydrochloride • Novantrone ◆

Class: ***antineoplastic*** • *Pregnancy risk category D*

Combination therapy for acute nonlymphocytic leukemia. *Adults:* Initial therapy, 12 mg/m² on days 1, 2, and 3 (combined with continuous I.V. infusion of cytosine arabinoside on days 1 to 7); consolidation therapy, 12 mg/m² on days 1 and 2 and cytosine arabinoside given as continuous infusion on days 1 to 5.

Follow facility protocol for handling chemotherapy drugs. Available as aqueous solution of 2 mg/ml in volumes of 10, 12.5, and 15 ml. Store undiluted solution at room temperature. Avoid freezing. Dilute dose in at least 50 ml of 0.9% NaCl injection or dextrose 5% injection. May be further diluted in D_5W, 0.9% NaCl, or dextrose 5% and 0.9% NaCl. Use immediately and discard unused solution.

Incompatibilities: Heparin sodium. Manufacturer recommends not mixing with any other drugs because not all in-

- Monitor patient's hematology and chemistry laboratory parameters and liver function tests closely.
- Monitor left ventricular ejection fraction during administration.
- Monitor serum uric acid levels during therapy. Keeping patient well hydrated, alkalinizing urine, and administering allopurinol may prevent uric acid nephropathy.

compatibilities are known.

Intermittent infusion: Infuse diluted solution slowly into I.V. line of free-flowing 0.9% NaCl or D_5W over at least 3 minutes.

- Tell patient that urine may appear blue-green within 24 hr after administration. Some bluish discoloration of the sclera may also occur.

mivacurium chloride • Mivacron

Class: ***Skeletal muscle relaxant*** • *Pregnancy risk category C*

As an adjunct to anesthesia, to facilitate endotracheal intubation, and to relax skeletal muscles during surgery or mechanical ventilation. *Adults:* Dosage is individualized. 0.15 mg/kg by I.V. push over 5 to 15 seconds 2.5 minutes before intubation. Supplemental doses 0.1 mg/kg q 15 minutes. Continuous infusion of 4 mcg/kg/ minute started together with initial dose maintains neuromuscular blockade. Or, 9 to 10 mcg/kg/minute started after spontaneous recovery begins from initial dose. Dosage is reduced up to 40% when used with isoflurane or enflurane anesthesia. *Children ages 2 to 12:* 0.20 mg/kg by I.V. push administered over 5 to 15 seconds. Maintenance doses are usually required more frequently in children. Neuromuscular blockade can be maintained with infusion titrated to effect. Most children respond to 5 to 31 mcg/kg/minute (average, 14 mcg/kg/minute).

Available in 5-ml single-use and 10-ml multidose vials at 2 mg/ml, and as an infusion of 0.5 mg/ml in 50- and 100-ml D_5W. Protect from ultraviolet light and from freezing. Use within 24 hr.

Incompatibilities: Don't mix with other drugs.

Direct injection: Give rapid I.V. bolus over 5 to 15 seconds.

Continuous infusion: Titrate drip to peripheral nerve stimulation and clinical criteria.

- To avoid patient distress, don't administer until patient's consciousness is obtunded by general anesthetic because drug has no effect on consciousness or pain threshold.
- Dosage requirements for children are higher on a mg/kg basis than for adults. Onset and recovery occur more rapidly in children.
- Maintain airway and control ventilation until recovery of normal neuromuscular function is ensured.
- Monitor patient's respirations closely until patient is fully recovered, as evidenced by tests of muscle strength (hand grip, head lift, and ability to cough).

◆ Also available in Canada. ◇ Available in Canada only.

COMMON INDICATIONS AND DOSAGES	ADMINISTRATION	SPECIAL CONSIDERATIONS

morphine sulfate • Astramorph PF, Duramorph, Epimorph, Morphine H.P.

Class: ***narcotic analgesic*** • *Pregnancy risk category C* • *Controlled substance schedule II*

Severe pain. *Adults:* 2.5 to 15 mg q 4 hr p.r.n. *Children:* 50 to 100 mcg/kg. Maximum single dose, 10 mg.
Pain from MI. *Adults:* 2 to 15 mg, followed by smaller doses q 3 to 4 hr p.r.n.
Severe chronic pain. *Adults:* 1 to 10 mg/hr by continuous infusion. Maintenance dosage, 20 to 150 mg/hr. *Children:* 0.025 to 2.6 mg/kg/hr.

Available with preservative in concentrations of 1, 2, 4, 5, 8, 10, 15, 25, and 50 mg/ml. Available without preservatives in concentrations of 0.5, 1, and 15 mg/ml. For direct injection, dilute with 4 or 5 ml of D_5W. Dilute with larger volumes for slow infusion. Morphine is compatible with most common I.V. solutions. Store below 104° F (40° C) and protect from light and freezing.
Incompatibilities: Aminophylline, amobarbital, soluble barbiturates, cefepime, chlorothiazide, heparin sodium, meperidine, methicillin, phenobarbital sodium, phenytoin sodium, promethazine hydrochloride, sodium bicarbonate, sodium iodide, and thiopental.
Direct injection: Inject diluted drug over 4 to 5 minutes through I.V. tubing that contains free-flowing, compatible solution.
Continuous infusion: Infuse diluted drug at 1 to 10 mg/hr initially, increasing rate until reaching effective dosage.

- Generic preparations may contain sulfites.
- Keep a narcotic antagonist available.
- Monitor patient's vital signs and respiratory status for at least 1 hr after injection and every 15 minutes during and for 1 hr after infusion.
- Give drug with patient in supine position to minimize hypotension.
- Rapid infusion can cause life-threatening adverse reactions. Ambulatory patients and those not experiencing severe pain have more adverse reactions.
- Dose may need to be extended in patients with severe chronic pain who have become tolerant to analgesic effects of opioids.

multivitamins • M.V.I.-12◆, M.V.I. Pediatric

Class: ***dietary supplement*** • *Pregnancy risk category NR*

Maintenance of vitamins during parenteral nutrition or in patients who can't take vitamins orally. *Adults and children age 11 and over:* Dosage varies. Maintenance nutrition requires one dose of multivitamin concentrate in I.V. infusion q 24 hr. *Children under age 11:* 1 vial of M.V.I. Pediatric daily in I.V. infusion. *Neonates who weigh 2.2 to 6.6 lb*

M.V.I.-12 available in a three-vial container with 5 ml of liquid in first vial, 5 ml of liquid in second vial, and 10 ml lyophilized powder in third vial. Mix contents of first two vials by pressing down to force liquid from upper chamber into lower chamber. Or add 5 ml of sterile water for injection to the 10-ml vial of powder. M.V.I. Pediatric available in a 5-ml vial. Reconstitute by adding 5 ml of sterile water for injection, D_5W, or 0.9% NaCl. Reconstituted solution stable for 24 hr if refrigerated. Dilute all prepared solutions in 500 to 1,000 ml

- M.V.I.-12 doesn't provide vitamin K_1, so you'll need to give it separately. M.V.I. Pediatric does contain vitamin K_1.
- Folic acid doses exceeding 0.1 mg/day may mask signs of pernicious anemia.
- Fat-soluble vitamins (A, D, E, and K) accumulate in the body and hypervitaminosis of A, D, and E can occur.
- Multivitamins shouldn't be used in severe vitamin

(1 to 3 kg): 65% of M.V.I. Pediatric vial daily in I.V. infusion. *Neonates who weigh less than 2.2 lb:* 30% of M.V.I. Pediatric vial daily.

of a compatible solution.

Incompatibilities: Acetazolamide, moderately alkaline solutions, amino acids (5.5%, 8.5%, or 10%), chlorothiazide, dextrose 5% in Normosol-M. Folic acid may be unstable in presence of calcium salts. Some vitamins, particularly thiamine, may be incompatible with sodium bisulfite. Manufacturer recommends against mixing M.V.I.-12 with fat emulsions.

Intermittent infusion: Infuse diluted solution over ordered amount of time. Add to only one I.V. solution daily.

Continuous infusion: Infuse diluted solution over 24 hr.

deficiency.

- Monitor patient for adverse reactions.
- Inform pregnant patient that megadoses of vitamins may be hazardous to the fetus.

muromonab-CD3 • Orthoclone OKT3◆

Class: ***immunosuppressant*** • *Pregnancy risk category C*

Acute allograft rejection in heart, liver, or kidney transplant. *Adults:* 5 mg daily for 10 to 14 days.

Available in 1-mg/ml ampules. Refrigerate unless otherwise specified by the manufacturer. Protect from freezing. Don't shake ampule. Draw solution into syringe through a low-protein-binding, 0.2- or 0.22-micrometer filter, then discard filter and attach appropriate needle. Fine, translucent particles in solution doesn't indicate loss of potency.

Incompatibilities: None reported. Don't give with other drugs.

Direct injection: Give by I.V. push directly into vein over less than 1 minute. Don't give with I.V. fluids.

- Keep equipment and drugs for advanced life support readily available during first dose.
- Give an antipyretic and antihistamine before therapy to reduce expected pyrexia and chills.
- Drug usually used with azathioprine, corticosteroids, or both.
- Monitor patient's temperature, CBC, and tests for circulating T cells expressing the CD3 antigen.

nafcillin sodium • Nafcil, Nallpen, Unipen◆

Class: ***antibiotic*** • *Pregnancy risk category B*

Severe systemic infection caused by susceptible organisms. *Adults:* 0.5 to 1 g q 4 hr for 14 days. *Children over 1 month old:* 50 to 100 mg/kg/day in equally divided doses q 6 hr for 14 days. **Osteomyelitis and endocarditis.** *Adults:*

Available as white to yellow-white powder in 500-mg, 1-g, 2-g, and 10-g vials. Store at room temperature. To reconstitute, use sterile water for injection, bacteriostatic water for injection, or 0.9% NaCl. Add 1.7 ml to 500-mg vial, 3.4 ml to 1-g vial, or 6.8 ml to 2-g vial. For larger doses, follow manufacturer's directions. After reconstitution with sterile water or

- Before giving first dose, ask patient about previous allergic reactions to penicillins or cephalosporins. Negative history does not rule out future hypersensitivity reaction.

(continued)

◆ Also available in Canada. ◇ Available in Canada only.

COMMON INDICATIONS AND DOSAGES	ADMINISTRATION	SPECIAL CONSIDERATIONS
nafcillin sodium *(continued)* 1 to 2 g q 4 hr for 4 to 8 weeks. *Children over 1 month old:* 100 to 200 mg/kg/day in equally divided doses q 4 to 6 hr for 4 to 8 weeks. **Meningitis.** *Adults:* 100 to 200 mg/kg/day in equally divided doses q 4 to 6 hr for at least 14 days.	0.9% NaCl, solution of 250 mg/ml is stable for 3 days at 77° F (25° C), 7 days if refrigerated, or 3 months if frozen. At 10 to 40 mg/ml, drug begins to lose potency in 24 hr at room temperature, 4 days if refrigerated. Drug is compatible with D_5W, lactated Ringer's, or 0.9% NaCl. ***Incompatibilities:*** Aminoglycosides, aminophylline, ascorbic acid, aztreonam, bleomycin, cytarabine, droperidol, fentanyl, hydrocortisone sodium succinate, regular insulin, labetalol, meperidine, metaraminol, methylprednisolone sodium succinate, nalbuphine, pentazocine lactate, promazine, verapamil hydrochloride, and vitamin B complex with C. ***Direct injection:*** Dilute reconstituted solution with 15 to 30 ml sterile water for injection or 0.45% or 0.9% NaCl for injection. Administer over 5 to 10 minutes. ***Intermittent infusion:*** Dilute reconstituted solution to 2 to 40 mg/ml or according to manufacturer's directions (Nallpen). Infuse over at least 30 minutes. ***Continuous infusion:*** Add daily amount of nafcillin (only as 2 to 40 mg/ml) to solution to be administered over 24 hr.	• Obtain WBC count and differential before therapy and 1 to 3 times weekly during therapy. • If diarrhea persists during therapy, collect stool specimens for culture to rule out pseudomembranous colitis.

nalbuphine hydrochloride • Nubain ◆

Classes: ***analgesic, adjunct to anesthesia*** • *Pregnancy risk category B (D for prolonged use or high doses at term)*

COMMON INDICATIONS AND DOSAGES	ADMINISTRATION	SPECIAL CONSIDERATIONS
Moderate to severe pain and preoperative analgesia; supplement to obstetric analgesia. *Adults:* 10 mg (or 0.14 mg/kg) q 3 to 6 hr. Maximum single dose, 20 mg; maximum daily dose, 160 mg. **Supplement to balanced anesthesia.** *Adults:* 0.3 to 3 mg/kg over 10 to 15 minutes. Maintenance, 0.25 to 0.5 mg/kg p.r.n.	Available in 1-ml ampules, 10-ml vials, and 1-ml disposable syringes in 10-mg/ml or 20-mg/ml concentrations. Protect from freezing, excessive light, and heat. Store at room temperature. Drug is compatible with D_5W, lactated Ringer's, and 0.9% NaCl. ***Incompatibilities:*** Allopurinol, cefepime, diazepam, ketorolac, nafcillin, pentobarbital sodium, piperacillin sodium-tazobactam sodium, promethazine hydrochloride, sargramostim, thiethylperazine, and tromethamine. ***Direct injection:*** Inject over 2 minutes or more.	• Drug may contain sulfites. • Avoid rapid injection because it can cause anaphylaxis, peripheral circulatory collapse, or cardiac arrest. • Administer with patient in supine position to minimize hypotensive effects.

naloxone hydrochloride • Narcan ◆

Class: ***narcotic antagonist*** • *Pregnancy risk category B*

Opioid toxicity. *Adults:* 0.4 mg to 2 mg, repeated q 2 to 3 minutes p.r.n. Or 0.4 mg followed by continuous infusion of 0.4 mg/hr titrated to patient's response. *Children:* 0.01 mg/kg, then 0.1 mg/kg repeated q 2 to 3 minutes for up to two more doses. Or 0.4 mg/hr by continuous infusion titrated to patient's response. *Neonates:* 0.01 mg/kg, repeated q 2 to 3 minutes until desired response occurs.
Postoperative opioid depression. *Adults:* 0.1 to 0.2 mg q 2 to 3 minutes until ventilation is adequate. Repeat p.r.n. at 1- to 2-hr intervals. *Children:* 0.005 to 0.01 mg q 2 to 3 minutes until ventilation is adequate and child is alert. Repeat p.r.n. at 1- to 2-hr intervals.

Available as 0.02-, 0.4-, and 1-mg vials, ampules, and syringes. Store at 59° to 86° F (15° to 30° C) and protect from light. Avoid freezing. To yield 0.004 mg/ml, mix 2 mg of drug in 500 ml of D_5W or 0.9% NaCl. Solution is stable for 24 hr. Discard unused portion after 24 hr. To yield 0.02 mg/ml, dilute 0.5 ml of adult dose (0.4 mg/ml) with 9.5 ml of sterile water or 0.9% NaCl for injection.
Incompatibilities: Don't mix with any other drugs, especially those that contain bisulfite, metabisulfite, long-chain or high-molecular-weight anions, or alkaline solutions.
Direct injection: Inject directly into vein or into established I.V. line that contains free-flowing, compatible solution.
Continuous infusion: Titrate rate to patient's needs. Pediatric rate may range from 0.024 to 0.16 mg/kg/hr.

- In a detoxified opioid addict, give naloxone challenge test, as ordered, before starting therapy.
- Closely monitor patient's respiratory, cardiac, and hemodynamic status for at least 24 hr. Duration of action of some narcotics may be longer than that of naloxone. Also, respiratory rate may rise suddenly.
- Monitor for signs of withdrawal.
- Lack of response indicates that condition isn't caused by opioid CNS depressant.

neostigmine methylsulfate • Prostigmin ◆

Class: ***muscle stimulant*** • *Pregnancy risk category C*

Myasthenia gravis. Dosage varies with response. *Adults:* 0.5 to 2.5 mg p.r.n.
Antidote for nondepolarizing neuromuscular blockers. *Adults:* 0.5 to 2 mg, repeated p.r.n. to maximum total dose of 5 mg. *Children:* 0.025 to 0.08 mg/kg.

Available as 1-ml ampules of 1:2,000 (0.5 mg/ml) and 1:4,000 (0.25 mg/ml). Also available in multidose vials of 1:1,000 (1 mg/ml) and 1:2,000 (0.5 mg/ml). Protect solution from light and avoid freezing. Drug needs no further dilution.
Incompatibilities: None reported.

- Assess patient's baseline vital signs and maintain a patent airway. If heart rate is below 80 beats/minute, may give atropine before neostigmine. Some doctors give adults 0.6 to 1.2 mg atropine I.V. or 0.2 to 0.6 mg glycopyrrolate I.V. several minutes before giving high doses of neostigmine.
- When reversing the effects of nondepolarizing neuromuscular blockers, keep patient on assisted ventilation.

(continued)

◆ Also available in Canada. ◇ Available in Canada only.

COMMON INDICATIONS AND DOSAGES	ADMINISTRATION	SPECIAL CONSIDERATIONS
neostigmine methylsulfate *(continued)*	***Direct injection:*** Inject slowly into tubing of patent, free-flowing I.V. line that contains D_5W, 0.9% NaCl, or other compatible I.V. solution.	• I.V. dose will be much smaller than oral dose. In a critically ill patient, exact dose may be titrated with peripheral nerve stimulators. • Be alert for cholinergic crisis (versus myasthenia crisis) in patients with myasthenia gravis.

nitroglycerin • Nitro-Bid IV♦, Tridil♦

Classes: ***antianginal, vasodilator*** • *Pregnancy risk category C*

COMMON INDICATIONS AND DOSAGES	ADMINISTRATION	SPECIAL CONSIDERATIONS
Heart failure and chest pain from MI; acute angina pectoris; blood pressure reduction during surgery. *Adults:* 5 mcg/minute, increased by 5 mcg/minute q 3 to 5 minutes until response achieved. If response inadequate at 20 mcg/minute, increase by 10 to 20 mcg/minute and give q 3 to 5 minutes p.r.n. Once partial response occurs, reduce the size and lengthen the interval of increases in dosage increments. Maximum dosage not established.	Drug is available for I.V. injection in several preparations and concentrations. Each comes with diluent instruction and dosage. Nitro-Bid IV available as 1-, 5-, and 10-ml vials of 5 mg/ml. Mix 1 ml of drug in 100 ml D_5W or 0.9% NaCl to yield 50 mcg/ml; mix 1 ml with 50 ml to yield 100 mcg/ml or 2 ml with 50 ml to yield 200 mcg/ml. Tridil available as 5-, 10-, and 20-ml ampules and vials at 5 mg/ml, and as 10-ml ampules at 0.5-mg/ml. Mix 25-mg or 50-mg ampule with 500 ml of D_5W or 0.9% NaCl to yield 50 or 100 mcg/ml, respectively. Diluting 5 mg of drug in 100 ml of solution yields 50 mcg/ml. Store at room temperature; protect from light and freezing. After reconstitution, drug is stable for 48 hr at room temperature. Mix and store in glass bottle supplied with most products. Use only nonabsorbent tubing; PVC tubing may absorb up to 80% of diluted drug from solution. ***Incompatibilities:*** Alteplase, hydralazine, and phenytoin sodium. Don't mix with other drugs. ***Continuous infusion:*** Infuse diluted drug using a volume-control device and microdrip regulator at a rate that produces therapeutic effect.	• Monitor patient's blood pressure and heart rate and rhythm continuously during therapy because response to drug varies greatly. • Tell patient to report chest pain or angina. • Help patient sit up and stand up until he can tolerate orthostatic hypotension.

nitroprusside sodium • Nipride◇, Nitropress

Class: ***antihypertensive*** • *Pregnancy risk category C*

Rapid blood pressure reduction in hypertensive emergencies, control of hypertension during anesthesia, reduction of preload and afterload in cardiac pump failure or cardiogenic shock.
Adults and children receiving no other hypotensive drugs: Average dose, 3 mcg/kg/minute (range, 0.3 to 10 mcg/kg/minute, titrated to blood pressure response). Maximum 10 mcg/kg/minute.

Available as a powder in 50-mg vials. Reconstitute with 2 to 3 ml D_5W or sterile water for injection without preservatives. Then dilute in 250 to 1,000 ml D_5W to desired concentration. Store at room temperature and protect from light, heat, and moisture (not necessary to cover tubing or drip chamber). Reconstituted solution stable for 24 hr. Discard if discolored (blue, green, or dark red), because drug has reacted with another substance. After reconstitution, protect solution from light by covering with aluminum foil.
Incompatibilities: Bacteriostatic water for injection. Don't mix with any other drug or preservative.
Continuous infusion: Using an infusion pump, administer diluted solution at a rate that maintains desired hypotensive effect.

- Use only when patient's arterial blood pressure can be monitored adequately.
- Monitor patient's blood pressure frequently.
- Avoid extravasation.
- Assess patient's serum thiocyanate levels.
- If metabolic acidosis occurs, discontinue drug and expect to try alternative therapy.
- For overdose, give nitrites to promote methemoglobin formation. For massive overdose, stop drug and give amyl nitrate by inhalation for 15 to 30 seconds per minute until a 3% sodium nitrite solution can be prepared.

norepinephrine bitartrate • Levophed♦

Class: ***vasopressor*** • *Pregnancy risk category C*

Control of acute hypotension and as adjunct in treatment of cardiac arrest.
Adults: 8 to 12 mcg/minute, adjusted (usually by 2 to 4 mcg/minute) to maintain desired blood pressure range.
Children: 0.1 mcg/kg/minute, adjusted (usually by 2 mcg/minute) to maintain desired blood pressure range.

Available as 4-ml ampules at 1 mg/ml. Store ampules at room temperature. For infusion, mix one ampule in 1,000 ml D_5W or dextrose 5% in 0.9% NaCl to yield 4 mcg/ml. Adjust concentration as needed to reflect patient's drug and fluid volume requirements. Discard diluted solution after 24 hr or if it contains precipitate or turns brown, pink, or yellow.
Incompatibilities: Aminophylline, amobarbital, cephalothin, cephapirin, chlorothiazide, chlorpheniramine, lidocaine, pentobarbital sodium, phenobarbital sodium, phenytoin sodium, secobarbital, sodium bicarbonate, sodium iodide, streptomycin, thiopental, and whole blood. Manufacturer recommends not mixing drug with 0.9% NaCl.
Continuous infusion: Use an infusion pump to carefully

- Drug may contain sulfites.
- Use large vein to deliver drug; avoid those in hands and legs.
- During infusion, check patient's blood pressure every 2 minutes until stable, then every 5 to 15 minutes using intra-arterial monitoring.
- Monitor patient's mental status, skin temperature, and color of extremities, especially earlobes, lips, and nail beds.
- Avoid prolonged use, if possible, to prevent ischemia of vital organs.

(continued)

♦ Also available in Canada. ◇ Available in Canada only.

COMMON INDICATIONS AND DOSAGES	ADMINISTRATION	SPECIAL CONSIDERATIONS
norepinephrine bitartrate *(continued)*	regulate flow so it keeps a low-normal blood pressure, usually 80 to 100 mm Hg systolic. For previously hypertensive patient, maintain pressure that's 40 mm Hg below previous systolic pressure.	

octreotide acetate • Sandostatin

Class: ***somatropic hormone*** • *Pregnancy risk category B*

COMMON INDICATIONS AND DOSAGES	ADMINISTRATION	SPECIAL CONSIDERATIONS
Flushing and diarrhea from carcinoid tumors. *Adults:* 100 to 600 mcg daily in two to four divided doses for first 2 weeks (usual daily dosage, 300 mcg). Subsequent dosage based on response. **Watery diarrhea from vasoactive intestinal peptide-secreting tumors.** *Adults:* 200 to 300 mcg daily in two to four divided doses for first 2 weeks. Subsequent dosage based on response, but usually not more than 450 mcg daily. **Acromegaly.** *Adults:* 50 mcg t.i.d. initially. Subsequent dosage based on response: usually 100 mcg t.i.d. but some patients need up to 500 mcg t.i.d.	Available in 50-, 100-, and 500-mcg/ml ampules and 200- and 1,000-mcg/ml multidose vials. Refrigerate and protect from light. Stable at room temperature for 14 days if protected from light. Don't warm solution artificially. Dilute in volumes of 50 to 200 ml and give by I.V. push or intermittent infusion. Solution stable in sterile isotonic saline solution or D_5W for 24 hr. Discard unused portion of ampule. After initial use, discard multidose vial after 14 days. Also discard if particulates or discoloration develop. ***Incompatibilities:*** Total parenteral nutrition. ***Direct injection:*** Inject directly into vein or compatible I.V. solution over 3 minutes. ***Intermittent infusion:*** Administer diluted solution over 15 to 30 minutes.	• Perform baseline and periodic tests of patient's thyroid function because drug suppresses secretion of thyroid-stimulating hormone. • Monitor patient's fluid and electrolyte balance during therapy. • Transient, mild increases or decreases in blood sugar may occur during therapy. • Tell patient to notify doctor about abdominal discomfort because drug may cause gallstones.

ofloxacin • Floxin I.V.

Class: ***antibiotic*** • *Pregnancy risk category C*

COMMON INDICATIONS AND DOSAGES	ADMINISTRATION	SPECIAL CONSIDERATIONS
Acute bacterial exacerbations of bronchitis or pneumonia caused by susceptible organisms. *Adults:* 400 mg q 12 hr for 10 days. **Endocervical and urethral chlamydial in-**	Available premixed in 100-ml glass bottles or 50- and 100-ml plastic bags with 4 mg/ml of drug in dextrose 5% injection. Premixed solutions need no dilution. Also available as 10- and 20-ml single-use vials with 400 mg of drug in water for injection. Store below 86° F (30° C) and protect from freezing	• Avoid rapid infusion because hypotension may result. • If rash or other signs of hypersensitivity develop, stop drug and notify doctor. • Perform regular blood studies and hepatic and renal

fection with or without concurrent gonorrhea. *Adults:* 300 mg q 12 hr for 7 days.
Uncomplicated gonorrhea. *Adults:* 400 mg as single dose.
Prostatitis from *Escherichia coli*. *Adults:* 300 mg q 12 hr for 6 weeks (can switch to oral route after 10 days).
Skin and soft-tissue infections. *Adults:* 400 mg q 12 hr for 10 days.
Cystitis from *E. coli* or *Klebsiella pneumoniae*. *Adults:* 200 mg q 12 hr for 3 days.
UTI caused by susceptible organisms. *Adults:* 200 mg q 12 hr for 7 to 10 days.
Dosage adjustment. Adjust dosage if patient's creatinine clearance is 50 ml/minute or less.

and light. Use immediately after opening. Discard unused portions. To dilute, withdraw appropriate dose from vial and add to 50 or 100 ml of 0.9% NaCl, D_5W, or other compatible I.V. fluid to yield 4 mg/ml. Solution stable 72 hr when stored at or below 75° F (24° C), 14 days when refrigerated at 41° F (5° C) in glass bottle or plastic I.V. container. Diluted, frozen solution stable 6 months at –4° F (–20° C).
Incompatibilities: Don't mix with other drugs or infuse simultaneously through the same line.
Intermittent infusion: Infuse over 60 minutes.

function tests during prolonged therapy.

- Patient treated for gonorrhea should have a serologic test for syphilis. Drug is not effective against syphilis, and treatment of gonorrhea may mask or delay syphilis symptoms.

ondansetron hydrochloride • Zofran

Class: ***antiemetic*** • *Pregnancy risk category B*

Prevention of nausea and vomiting from chemotherapy. *Adults and children age 4 and over:* 0.15 mg/kg given 30 minutes before chemotherapy and 4 and 8 hr later. Or, adults and children age 12 and over may receive 32-mg infusion starting 30 minutes before chemotherapy.
Prevention of postoperative nausea and vomiting. *Adults:* 4 mg undiluted.

Available in 2-ml and 20-ml multidose vials of 2 mg/ml. Solution has pH of 3.3 to 4. Before infusion, dilute in 50 ml of compatible solution, such as D_5W for injection, 0.9% NaCl for injection, dextrose 5% in 0.9% NaCl for injection, dextrose 5% in 0.45% NaCl for injection, or 3% NaCl for injection. Drug is stable for up to 48 hr in polyvinyl chloride bags after dilution when refrigerated at 39° F (4° C) or kept at room temperature 77° F (25° C). Store at room temperature and protect from light. Not necessary to protect drug from light during administration.
Incompatibilities: Acyclovir, allopurinol, aminophylline, amphotericin B, ampicillin sodium, ampicillin sodium and sulbactam sodium, amsacrine, cefepime, cefoperazone, fluorouracil, furosemide, ganciclovir, lorazepam, methylpred-

- Tell patient to report immediately discomfort at I.V. site.
- Tell patient to report immediately difficulty in breathing after drug administration.
- Monitor liver function tests for hepatotoxicity.
- In clinical trials, ondansetron combined with dexamethasone controlled emesis significantly better than ondansetron alone.

(continued)

◆ Also available in Canada. ◇ Available in Canada only.

COMMON INDICATIONS AND DOSAGES	ADMINISTRATION	SPECIAL CONSIDERATIONS
ondansetron hydrochloride *(continued)*	nisolone sodium succinate, mezlocillin, piperacillin sodium, sargramostim, and sodium bicarbonate. ***Direct injection:*** Give undiluted over 2 to 5 minutes. (For postoperative nausea and vomiting only.) ***Intermittent infusion:*** Infuse over 15 minutes.	

orphenadrine citrate • Banflex, Flexoject, Norflex◆

Class: ***skeletal muscle relaxant*** • *Pregnancy risk category C*

COMMON INDICATIONS AND DOSAGES	ADMINISTRATION	SPECIAL CONSIDERATIONS
Acute pain in musculoskeletal disorders. *Adults:* 60 mg q 12 hr.	Available as 2-ml ampules and 10-ml vials at 30 mg/ml. Store at room temperature; protect ampules from light. Drug needs no further dilution for injection. ***Incompatibilities:*** None reported. ***Direct injection:*** Administer over 5 to 10 minutes with patient in supine position.	• Carefully check all dosages. Even a slight overdose can cause toxicity. • Keep patient recumbent for 5 to 10 minutes after injection, then help him sit up slowly. • Replace parenteral therapy with oral therapy as soon as possible. • Monitor patient's vital signs and input and output.

oxacillin sodium • Bactocill

Class: ***antibiotic*** • *Pregnancy risk category B*

COMMON INDICATIONS AND DOSAGES	ADMINISTRATION	SPECIAL CONSIDERATIONS
Severe infections caused by susceptible organisms. *Adults:* 1 g q 4 to 6 hr. *Children who weigh less than 88 lb (40 kg):* 100 to 200 mg/kg/day in equal doses q 4 to 6 hr. **Mild to moderate infections caused by susceptible organisms.** *Adults:* 250 to 500 mg q 4 to 6 hr. *Children who weigh less than 88 lb:* 50 mg/kg/day in equal doses q 6 hr. **Endocarditis or chronic osteomyelitis caused by susceptible organisms.**	Available as powder in 250- and 500-mg vials and in 1-, 2-, and 4-g vials. Reconstitute with sterile water for injection or 0.9% NaCl. Stable for 3 days at room temperature, 1 week if refrigerated. Compatible solutions include dextrose 5% in lactated Ringer's, dextrose 5% in 0.9% NaCl, D_5W or dextrose 10% in water, lactated Ringer's, and 0.9% NaCl. ***Incompatibilities:*** Acidic drugs, aminoglycosides, cytarabine, and verapamil hydrochloride. ***Direct injection:*** Add 5 ml sterile water for injection or 0.9% NaCl to 250- or 500-mg vial; 10 ml to 1-g vial, 20 ml to 2-g vial; or 40 ml to 4-g vial. Then inject over 10 minutes. ***Intermittent infusion:*** Mix 50 to 100 ml of diluent with 1-	• Drug contains about 3.1 mEq of sodium per gram. • Tell patient to expect some discomfort at injection site. • Monitor patient's WBC count before therapy and 1 to 3 times weekly during therapy. • Assess patient's renal and hepatic function before therapy and periodically during therapy. Closely monitor neonates for hepatotoxicity and nephrotoxicity. • Instruct patient to notify doctor if sore throat, fever, mucosal ulcers, rash, or unusual bleeding or bruising occurs.

Adults: 1.5 to 2 g q 4 hr.
Dosage adjustment. Adjust dosage in renal impairment.

or 2-g vial or mix 93 ml with 4-g vial. Then infuse over ordered duration.

oxymorphone hydrochloride • Numorphan◆

Class: ***analgesic*** • *Pregnancy risk category C* • *Controlled substance schedule II*

Moderate to severe pain. *Adults:* 0.5 mg q 3 to 4 hr initially, increased cautiously up to 1 mg in nondebilitated patients.

Available as 1- and 1.5-mg/ml ampules and 1.5-mg/ml vials. Protect from freezing and light. Store at 59° to 86° F (15° and 30° C). No further dilution needed for direct injection. Compatible solutions include D_5W, dextrose 5% in 0.9% NaCl, and lactated Ringer's.
Incompatibilities: None reported.
Direct injection: Inject directly into vein or I.V. line that contains free-flowing, compatible solution. Administer over 2 to 3 minutes.

- To minimize hypotension, keep patient supine when giving drug.
- Don't give drug if patient has less than 12 breaths/minute. Monitor his respirations for at least 1 hr after giving dose. Keep resuscitation equipment available.
- For improved analgesia, give before patient has intense pain.
- For overdose, give naloxone, repeating as needed to reverse respiratory depression.
- Reduce dosage gradually after prolonged use to avoid withdrawal symptoms.

oxytocin, synthetic injection • Pitocin

Class: ***oxytocic*** • *Pregnancy risk category NR*

Induction and stimulation of labor. *Adults:* Dosage determined by uterine response. Usually 0.5 to 2 milliunits/minute. May be increased 1 to 2 milliunits/minute q 30 to 60 minutes until contraction pattern simulates normal labor. Maximum 10 milliunits/minute.
Incomplete or inevitable abortion. *Adults:* 10 to 20 milliunits/minute. After abortion, 20 to 100 milliunits/minute.
Control of postpartum uterine bleeding.

Available as 10-ml vials, as 0.5- and 1-ml ampules, and as 1-ml disposable syringes at 10 U/ml. Store below 77° F (25° C). If stored correctly, drug reportedly remains stable for 5 years. *For infusion to start labor,* add 1 ml drug to 1,000 ml D_5W, 0.9% NaCl, or lactated Ringer's. *For infusion to control postpartum bleeding,* add 1 to 4 ml drug to 1,000 ml D_5W or 0.9% NaCl. *For use after abortion,* thoroughly mix 1 ml drug with 500 ml dextrose 5% in 0.9% NaCl or with 0.9% NaCl. *For evaluation of fetal distress,* dilute 0.5 to 1 ml in 1,000 ml D_5W.
Incompatibilities: Fibrinolysin or Normosol-M with dextrose 5%.

- Don't administer simultaneously by more than one route.
- Continuously monitor frequency, duration, and force of uterine contractions; resting uterine tone; fetal heart rate; maternal blood pressure; and intrauterine pressure.
- Stop infusion with signs of fetal distress or if contractions are less than 2 minutes apart, exceed 50 mm Hg, or last longer than 90 seconds. Turn patient on her side and notify doctor.

(continued)

◆ Also available in Canada. ◇ Available in Canada only.

COMMON INDICATIONS AND DOSAGES	ADMINISTRATION	SPECIAL CONSIDERATIONS
oxytocin, synthetic injection *(continued)* *Adults:* 20 to 40 milliunits/minute to total of 10 U. **Evaluation of fetal distress after 31 weeks.** *Adults:* 0.5 milliunits/minute, increased q 15 to 30 minutes to maximum of 20 milliunits/minute. Stop when three moderate contractions occur within 10 minutes.	***Continuous infusion:*** Use an infusion pump. Start I.V. line with 0.9% NaCl and add oxytocin solution as a secondary line to port as close to infusion needle as possible. Don't administer for more than 8 hr.	• Keep magnesium sulfate (20% solution) available to relax myometrium.

paclitaxel • Taxol

Class: ***antineoplastic*** • *Pregnancy risk category D*

COMMON INDICATIONS AND DOSAGES	ADMINISTRATION	SPECIAL CONSIDERATIONS
Ovarian cancer after failure of first-line or subsequent chemotherapy. *Adults:* 135 mg/m^2, repeated q 21 days (optimal dosages not established). **Breast cancer after failure of combination chemotherapy for metastatic disease.** *Adults:* 175 mg/m^2, repeated q 21 days (optimal dosages not established).	Follow facility protocol for handling chemotherapy drugs. Available as 5-ml single-dose vial containing 30 mg/5 ml. Unopened vial stable until expiration date when stored at 36° to 46° F (2° to 8° C). Keep in original package to protect from light. To prepare, calculate dose and dilute in 0.9% NaCl, D_5W, dextrose 5% in 0.9% NaCl, or dextrose 5% in lactated Ringer's solution to a final concentration of 0.3 to 1.2 mg/ml. Diluted solution stable up to 27 hr at room temperature and controlled lighting. May show haziness from formulation vehicle. Avoid contact of undiluted concentrate with polyvinyl chloride equipment. Store diluted solution in glass or polypropylene bottles or polypropylene, polyolefin bags. Administer through polyethylene-lined administration set. ***Incompatibilities:*** Amphotericin B, chlorpromazine, hydroxyzine hydrochloride, methylprednisolone sodium succinate, and mitoxantrone. ***Intermittent infusion:*** Infuse over 3 hr through a 0.22 micron in-line filter. Change filter every 12 hr to reduce clogging.	• To prevent hypersensitivity reactions, manufacturer suggests premedicating with corticosteroids (dexamethasone 20 mg P.O. or I.V.) about 12 and 6 hr before therapy, diphenhydramine 50 mg I.V. 30 to 60 minutes before therapy, and cimetidine 300 mg I.V. 30 to 60 minutes before therapy (or ranitidine 50 mg I.V. or famotidine 20 mg I.V.). • Monitor patient's vital signs frequently, especially during first hr. Keep emergency equipment readily available in case of anaphylaxis. • Monitor patient's CBC before and at intervals during treatment.

pamidronate disodium • Aredia

Class: ***antihypercalcemic*** • *Pregnancy risk category C*

Moderate to severe hypercalcemia from cancer (with or without bone metastases). *Adults:* For moderate hypercalcemia (corrected calcium of 12 to 13.5 mg/dl), 60 to 90 mg as a single dose infused over 4 and 24 hr, respectively. For severe hypercalcemia (corrected calcium above 13.5 mg/dl), 90 mg as a single dose infused over 24 hr. Wait at least 7 days before retreatment, if needed.
Osteolytic bone lesions from multiple myeloma. *Adults:* 90 mg over 4 hr on monthly basis.
Paget's disease. *Adults:* 30 mg daily over 4 hr for 3 consecutive days.

Available as 30-, 60-, and 90-mg lyophilized powder in single-dose vials. Store at 59° to 86° F (15° to 30° C). Don't freeze. To prepare, reconstitute with 10 ml sterile water for injection and let drug dissolve completely. Reconstituted solution stable up to 24 hr when kept at 36° to 46° F (2° to 8° C). Withdraw daily dose and dilute in 1,000 ml of 0.45% or 0.9% NaCl or D_5W. Diluted product stable for up to 24 hr. In Paget's disease and osteolytic bone lesions from multiple myeloma, dilute in 500 ml of 0.9% NaCl or D_5W.
Incompatibilities: Don't mix with calcium-containing infusion solutions, such as Ringer's injection or lactated Ringer's solution.
Continuous infusion: Infuse as directed for specific indication and dosage.

- Vigorously hydrate patient with saline before administration, if not contraindicated. If patient has mild to moderate hypercalcemia, hydration alone may be sufficient.
- Periodically monitor patient's alkaline phosphatase, a marker for Paget's disease, during therapy.
- Monitor patient's electrolytes (including serum calcium, potassium, magnesium, and phosphate), hemoglobin, hematocrit, CBC with differential, and serum creatinine periodically during therapy.
- Use of corticosteroids may be helpful in hypercalcemia from hematologic cancers.

pancuronium bromide • Pavulon◆

Class: ***skeletal muscle relaxant*** • *Pregnancy risk category C*

Adjunct to anesthesia. *Adults and children over 1 month old:* 0.04 to 0.1 mg/kg, with additional doses of 0.01 mg/kg given if needed at 25- to 60-minute intervals. *Neonates:* After giving a test dose of 0.02 mg/kg, individualize carefully.
To facilitate mechanical ventilation and endotracheal intubation. *Adults and children over 1 month old:* 0.015 mg/kg. *Neonates:* After giving a test dose of 0.02 mg/kg, individualize carefully.

Available as 2- and 5-ml ampules, as vials and syringes containing 2 mg/ml, and as 10-ml vials containing 1 mg/ml. Store at 36° to 46° F (2° to 8° C). Drug remains potent for 6 months at room temperature. Don't store in plastic containers, although drug may be given in plastic syringes. For infusion, dilute with ordered amount of D_5W, 0.9% NaCl, or lactated Ringer's.
Incompatibilities: Barbiturates and diazepam.
Direct injection: Slowly inject into established I.V. line that contains compatible, free-flowing solution.
Intermittent infusion: Infuse diluted drug at ordered rate.

- Drug may contain benzyl alcohol.
- Be prepared to give mechanical ventilation or airway support because apnea follows administration.
- Large doses may increase frequency and severity of tachycardia.
- Anesthesia is necessary because drug has no effect on consciousness, pain threshold, or cerebration.
- A nerve stimulator and train-of-four monitoring are recommended to assess recovery of muscle strength. Before attempting reversal with neostigmine, some evidence of spontaneous recovery should be present.

◆ Also available in Canada. ◇ Available in Canada only.

COMMON INDICATIONS AND DOSAGES	ADMINISTRATION	SPECIAL CONSIDERATIONS

paricalcitol • Zemplar

Class: ***antihyperparathyroid agent*** • *Pregnancy risk category C*

COMMON INDICATIONS AND DOSAGES

Prevention and treatment of secondary hyperparathyroidism from chronic renal failure. *Adults:* 0.04 to 0.1 mcg/kg (2.8 to 7 mcg) I.V. no more frequently than every other day during dialysis. Doses as high as 0.24 mcg/kg (16.8 mcg) have been given. If response inadequate, increase by 2 to 4 mcg at 2- to 4-week intervals.

ADMINISTRATION

Available as 1- and 2-ml single dose vials at 5 mcg/ml. Store at room temperature. Inspect for particulates and discoloration before use. Discard unused portion.

Incompatibilities: None reported.

Direct injection: Administer as an I.V. bolus.

SPECIAL CONSIDERATIONS

- Use cautiously in patients taking digitalis compounds; they have increased risk of digitalis toxicity during therapy secondary to potential for hypercalcemia.
- Watch for ECG abnormalities and symptoms of hypercalcemia.
- Monitor patient's serum calcium and phosphorus levels twice weekly when dose is being adjusted, then monitor monthly.
- Measure parathyroid hormone level every 3 months during therapy. If decreased, dose may need to be decreased as well.

pegaspargase • Oncaspar

Class: ***antineoplastic*** • *Pregnancy risk category C*

COMMON INDICATIONS AND DOSAGES

Acute lymphoblastic leukemia in patients who need L-asparaginase but are hypersensitive to native form. *Adults and children with body surface area of at least 0.6 m^2:* 2,500 IU/m^2 q 14 days. *Children with body surface area below 0.6 m^2:* 82.5 IU/kg q 14 days.

ADMINISTRATION

Follow facility protocol for handling chemotherapy drugs. Available as preservative-free, single-use, 5-ml vial containing 750 IU/ml. Don't shake vial. Keep refrigerated at 36° to 46° F (2° to 8° C); don't freeze or expose to excessive heat. Don't use if cloudy or precipitated. Drug stable at room temperature for 48 hr. Desired dose should be diluted in 100 ml 0.9% NaCl or dextrose 5%. Discard unused portions.

Incompatibilities: None reported, but don't mix with other drugs.

Intermittent infusion: Administer diluted solution into tubing of free-flowing, compatible I.V. solution over 1 to 2 hr.

SPECIAL CONSIDERATIONS

- Take preventive measures (including adequate hydration) before starting treatment. Allopurinol may be ordered.
- Monitor patient closely for hypersensitivity reactions and anaphylaxis for 1 hr. Keep emergency equipment available.
- Monitor patient's peripheral blood count and bone marrow, serum amylase, glucose, fibrinogen, PT, and PTT.
- Monitor patient for liver dysfunction when drug is used with hepatotoxic chemotherapy.

penicillin G potassium • Pfizerpen
penicillin G sodium

Class: ***antibiotic*** • *Pregnancy risk category B*

Moderate to severe systemic infection. *Adults:* 5 to 24 million units daily in divided doses q 4 hr. *Children:* 25,000 to 300,000 units/kg daily in divided doses q 4 hr.

Dosage adjustment. In adults with renal or hepatic impairment, dosage reflects degree of impairment, severity of infection, and causative organism.

Available in various vial sizes containing 200,000 or 500,000 U and 1, 5, 10, or 20 million U of penicillin G potassium; and 5 million U of penicillin G sodium. Reconstitute with sterile water for injection, 0.9% NaCl, or D_5W as manufacturer directs. For intermittent infusion, dilute in 50 to 100 ml of 0.9% NaCl or D_5W. For continuous infusion, dilute daily dose in 1 to 2 L of compatible I.V. solution. Diluted solution stable 24 hr at room temperature, 7 days at 36° to 46° F (2° to 8° C). Also available in premixed frozen I.V. bags containing 1, 2, and 3 million U in 50 ml dextrose 5%. Thaw frozen container at room temperature. Thawed solution stable 24 hr at room temperature, 14 days if refrigerated.

Incompatibilities: *Penicillin G potassium* incompatible with alcohol 5%, amikacin, aminophylline, amphotericin B, cephalothin, chlorpromazine, dextran, dopamine, heparin, hydroxyzine hydrochloride, lincomycin, metaraminol, metoclopramide, pentobarbital sodium, phenytoin, prochlorperazine mesylate, promazine, promethazine hydrochloride, sodium bicarbonate, thiopental, vancomycin, and vitamin B complex with C.

Penicillin G sodium incompatible with 10% fat emulsions, 10% invert sugar, amphotericin B, bleomycin, cephalothin, chlorpromazine, heparin, hydroxyzine hydrochloride, lincomycin, methylprednisolone sodium succinate, potassium chloride, prochlorperazine mesylate, and promethazine hydrochloride.

Intermittent infusion: Infuse diluted solution over 1 to 2 hr.

Continuous infusion: Infuse diluted solution over 24 hr.

- Ask patient about allergies to penicillin, cephalosporin, or imipenem before giving first dose.
- Anaphylaxis may occur within 30 minutes of infusion.
- Patients with poor renal function are at risk for seizures.
- Give penicillin and aminoglycosides separately at different sites.
- Take special care to prevent extravasation near major peripheral nerves or blood vessels; severe or permanent neurovascular damage may occur.
- Monitor patient's vital signs, CBC, PT, PTT, BUN, AST, and serum electrolyte and creatinine levels.
- Monitor patient's intake and output and give fluids.

COMMON INDICATIONS AND DOSAGES	ADMINISTRATION	SPECIAL CONSIDERATIONS
pentamidine isethionate • Pentam 300		
Class: ***antiprotozoal*** • *Pregnancy risk category C*		
***Pneumocystis carinii* pneumonia.** *Adults and children:* 3 to 4 mg/kg once daily for 14 to 21 days. *Alternative children's dosage:* 150 mg/m^2 once daily for 5 days, then 100 mg/m^2 once daily for 9 days. Adults and children with AIDS who don't respond in 14 days may receive drug for 7 more days. **Leishmaniasis (visceral) caused by *Leishmania donovani*.** *Adults and children:* 2 to 4 mg/kg once daily or every other day up to 15 doses, or 4 mg/kg three times weekly for 5 to 25 weeks or longer, based on response. **Trypanosomiasis.** *Adults and children:* 4 mg/kg once daily for 10 days, or 3 to 4 mg/kg once daily or every other day for 7 to 10 doses. **Dosage adjustment.** If creatinine clearance is less than 10 ml/minute, give usual dose q 48 hr.	Available as powder in 300-mg vials. Before reconstituting, store at 59° to 86° F (15° to 30° C). Protect both dry powder and reconstituted solution from light. Drug contains no preservatives. Reconstitute with 3 to 5 ml sterile water for injection or D_5W. For infusion, dilute further in 50 to 250 ml of D_5W. Solutions of 1 to 2.5 mg/ml prepared in dextrose 5% remain potent up to 24 hr at room temperature. Discard unused portion. ***Incompatibilities:*** Fluconazole and foscarnet. ***Intermittent infusion:*** Infuse diluted drug over 60 minutes.	• Because drug can cause severe hypotension, keep patient supine during administration and for several hr afterward. Monitor patient's blood pressure, and keep resuscitation equipment available. • Monitor patient's fluid status to ensure adequate hydration and minimize risk of nephrotoxicity. • Before, during, and after therapy, check ECG, CBC, platelets, AST, ALT, BUN, serum alkaline phosphatase, bilirubin, calcium, creatinine, and glucose levels.
pentazocine lactate • Talwin◆		
Classes: ***analgesic, adjunct to anesthesia*** • *Pregnancy risk category C (D with prolonged use or high doses at term)* • *Controlled substance schedule IV*		
Pain. *Adults and children over age 12:* 30 mg (maximum single dose) q 3 to 4 hr p.r.n. Maximum daily, 360 mg.	Available as 1-, 1.5-, and 2-ml ampules; 1-, 1.5-, and 2-ml disposable syringes; and 10-ml multidose vials at 30 mg/ml. Store below 104° F (40° C), preferably at room temperature.	• Drug may contain sulfites. • Rapid injection may lead to anaphylaxis, peripheral circulatory collapse, or cardiac arrest.

Obstetric pain. *Adults:* 20 mg when contractions regular, then 20 mg q 2 to 3 hr p.r.n. for 2 or 3 doses.

Protect from freezing. No dilution needed.
Incompatibilities: Aminophylline, amobarbital, glycopyrrolate, heparin, pentobarbital sodium, phenobarbital sodium, secobarbital, and sodium bicarbonate.
Direct injection: Inject drug slowly into I.V. tubing that contains compatible, free-flowing solution. Monitor patient's tolerance.

- Keep patient supine during administration to minimize hypotension. Closely monitor his respiratory status.
- Elderly patients may require lower doses.
- For patient receiving long-term therapy with other opioid agonist, give 25% of initial pentazocine dose and assess for withdrawal symptoms. If necessary, give dose slowly in small increments. If no adverse reactions occur, increase dose progressively to desired level of analgesia.

pentobarbital sodium • Nembutal◆

Classes: ***sedative-hypnotic, anticonvulsant*** • *Pregnancy risk category D* • *Controlled substance schedule II*

Insomnia, anesthesia (adjunct), and seizures. *Adults:* 100 mg initially, then smaller doses p.r.n. at 1-minute intervals to reach 200 to 500 (maximum) mg. Dose lower in elderly. *Children:* 50 mg initially, then smaller doses at 1-minute intervals until desired effect is reached.

Available as 2-ml vials; 1- and 2-ml prefilled syringes; and 20- and 50-ml multidose vials at 50 mg/ml. Store at room temperature. Drug is compatible with most common solutions, such as D_5W and 0.9% NaCl.
Incompatibilities: Acidic solutions (because precipitation may occur), benzquinamide, butorphanol, chlorpheniramine, chlorpromazine, cimetidine, codeine phosphate, dimenhydrinate, diphenhydramine, droperidol, ephedrine, fentanyl citrate, glycopyrrolate, hydrocortisone sodium succinate, hydroxyzine hydrochloride, regular insulin, meperidine, methadone, midazolam, morphine sulfate, nalbuphine, norepinephrine, opium alkaloids, penicillin G potassium, pentazocine lactate, perphenazine, phenytoin, prochlorperazine, promazine, promethazine, ranitidine, sodium bicarbonate, streptomycin, succinylcholine, triflupromazine, and vancomycin.
Direct injection: Inject drug into I.V. tubing of free-flowing, compatible solution at no more than 50 mg/minute.

- Keep emergency resuscitation equipment available.
- Monitor patient's vital signs, blood pressure, and cardiac function.
- Monitor patient's EEG and blood levels when used for barbiturate coma. Patient will require mechanical ventilation.
- Avoid extravasation because solution is alkaline and may cause local tissue damage and necrosis. Inadvertent arterial injection may cause arterial spasm, severe pain, and possibly gangrene.
- Tell patient to change positions and rise slowly; drug may alter equilibrium and cause hangover effect.

◆ Also available in Canada. ◇ Available in Canada only.

COMMON INDICATIONS AND DOSAGES	ADMINISTRATION	SPECIAL CONSIDERATIONS

pentostatin (2'-deoxycoformycin; DCF) • Nipent

Class: ***antineoplastic*** • *Pregnancy risk category D*

COMMON INDICATIONS AND DOSAGES	ADMINISTRATION	SPECIAL CONSIDERATIONS
Treatment of hairy cell leukemia refractory to alpha-interferon. *Adults with creatinine clearance of 60 ml/minute or more:* 4 mg/m^2 every other week by I.V. bolus or infusion until complete response achieved.	Follow facility protocol for handling chemotherapy drugs. Available as powder for injection in single-dose, 10-mg vial. Store at 36° to 46° F (2° to 8° C). To prepare, add 5 ml sterile water for injection and mix to dissolve completely. Resulting solution contains 2 mg/ml of pentostatin. Administer as I.V. bolus or dilute with 25 or 50 ml D_5W or 0.9% NaCl and infuse. Use reconstituted vials and diluted infusions within 8 hr if stored at room temperature (contains no preservatives). ***Incompatibilities:*** Don't mix with other drugs without specific compatibility data. ***Direct injection:*** Give by rapid I.V. bolus over 5 minutes. ***Intermittent infusion:*** Infuse diluted solution over 20 to 30 minutes.	• Hydrate patient with 500 to 1,000 ml of dextrose 5% in 0.45% NaCl before treatment and with 500 ml after treatment to minimize risk of adverse renal effects. • Monitor patient's creatinine level, CBC, and uric acid level. • Withhold or discontinue drug in patients with evidence of CNS toxicity, severe rash, or active infection. • Temporarily withhold drug, as ordered, if absolute neutrophil count falls below 200 $cells/mm^3$.

perphenazine • Trilafon◆

Class: ***antiemetic*** • *Pregnancy risk category C*

COMMON INDICATIONS AND DOSAGES	ADMINISTRATION	SPECIAL CONSIDERATIONS
Severe vomiting, intractable hiccups, violent retching during surgery. *Adults:* 1 mg at 1- to 2-minute intervals for 5 mg total, or maximum dose of 5 mg by infusion.	Available in 1-ml ampules at 5 mg/ml. Dilute to 0.5 mg/ml by adding 1 ml of drug to 9 ml of 0.9% NaCl for direct injection or to an ordered amount for infusion. Store at 59° to 86° F (15° to 30° C). Slight yellowing won't affect potency or efficacy, but discard if marked discoloration or precipitate forms. ***Incompatibilities:*** Aminophylline, cefoperazone, midazolam, opium alkaloids, oxytocin, pentobarbital sodium, and thiethylperazine. ***Direct injection:*** Inject at 1- to 2-minute intervals into I.V. line that contains free-flowing, compatible solution. ***Intermittent infusion:*** Infuse drug slowly into I.V. line that contains free-flowing, compatible solution.	• Prevent contact dermatitis by keeping drug away from skin and clothes. • Keep patient supine during and for 30 to 60 minutes after administration. Monitor his blood pressure before and after administration. • For severe hypotension that requires a vasopressor, use norepinephrine or phenylephrine—not epinephrine. • Tell patient that drug may cause drowsiness and to avoid activities that require mental alertness or coordination until CNS effects are clear. • Tell patient that drug may turn urine pink to red-brown.

phenobarbital sodium • Luminal◆

Classes: ***sedative-hypnotic, anticonvulsant*** • *Pregnancy risk category D* • *Controlled substance schedule IV*

Status epilepticus and acute seizure disorders. *Adults:* 200 to 600 mg, or 40 to 120 mg at 5- to 10-minute intervals. Total dosage, 20 mg/kg. *Children:* 100 to 400 mg, or 20 to 80 mg at 5- to 10-minute intervals. Total dosage, 20 mg/kg.

Available in single-dose vials, ampules, and prefilled syringes at 30, 60, 65, 120, and 130 mg/ml. Discard if precipitates visible. Drug compatible with commonly used I.V. solutions, such as 0.45% and 0.9% NaCl, dextrose 5% and lactated Ringer's.

Incompatibilities: Alcohol-dextrose solutions, cephalothin, chlorpromazine, codeine phosphate, ephedrine, hydralazine, hydrocortisone sodium succinate, regular insulin, levorphanol, meperidine, morphine, norepinephrine, pentazocine lactate, prochlorperazine mesylate, promazine, promethazine hydrochloride, ranitidine, streptomycin, and vancomycin.

Direct injection: Inject at no more than 60 mg/minute into vein or tubing of I.V. that contains free-flowing, compatible solution.

- Establish baseline blood pressure and respiratory rate, then monitor patient continuously.
- Observe injection site for signs of thrombophlebitis. If patient reports pain at site, stop injection and check cannula. High alkalinity of drug causes necrosis in extravasation.
- Stop drug immediately if a skin reaction occurs to avoid possible fatal reaction.
- For full anticonvulsant effect, wait 30 minutes after initial dose before giving additional doses. Maintain serum level at 15 to 40 mcg/ml. Halt injections when seizures stop or when total dosage reached.

phentolamine mesylate • Regitine, Rogitine◇

Classes: ***antihypertensive, vasodilator*** • *Pregnancy risk category C*

Diagnosis of pheochromocytoma. *Adults:* 5 mg. *Children:* 1 mg, 0.1 mg/kg, or 3 mg/m^2.

Hypertension in pheochromocytoma before surgical removal of tumor. *Adults:* 5 mg 1 to 2 hr before surgery. *Children:* 1 mg, 0.1 mg/kg, or 3 mg/m^2 1 to 2 hr before surgery, repeated if needed.

Left ventricular heart failure from acute MI. *Adults:* 0.17 to 0.4 mg/minute by continuous infusion.

Norepinephrine extravasation. *Adults:* 5 to 10 mg in 10 ml of 0.9% NaCl into af-

Available as powder in 5-mg vial with 1-ml ampule of sterile water for injection as diluent. Store at room temperature. Reconstitute with diluent to 5 mg/ml. Reconstituted product stable 48 hr at room temperature, 7 days at 36° to 46° F (2° to 8° C). Manufacturer recommends using immediately after reconstitution. For infusion, dilute 5 to 10 mg of drug in 500 ml of 0.9% NaCl.

Incompatibilities: None known.

Direct injection: Delay injection until venipuncture effect subsides, then rapidly inject desired dose.

Continuous infusion: Infuse at rate ordered for norepinephrine solution. To treat left-ventricular heart failure, infuse with an infusion pump at rate needed to control symptoms.

- Before performing pheochromocytoma test, make sure patient's blood pressure has returned to pretreatment level. Give drug rapidly, recording blood pressure immediately after injection, every 30 seconds for 3 minutes, then every 60 seconds for 7 more minutes. Severe hypotension after test dose indicates pheochromocytoma.
- For overdose with severe hypotension or other signs of shock, treat with norepinephrine and supportive measures. For arrhythmias, give cardiac glycosides. Don't use epinephrine.

(continued)

◆ Also available in Canada. ◇ Available in Canada only.

COMMON INDICATIONS AND DOSAGES	ADMINISTRATION	SPECIAL CONSIDERATIONS
phentolamine mesylate *(continued)* fected tissues within 12 hr of extravasation. **Prevention of severe tissue sloughing in norepinephrine infusion.** *Adults:* 10 mg added to each 1,000 ml norepinephrine infusion. **Hypertensive crisis from interaction between MAO inhibitor and sympathomimetic amine.** *Adults:* 5 to 10 mg.		• When treating left-ventricular heart failure, continuously monitor patient's ECG and left ventricular function.

phenylephrine hydrochloride • Neo-Synephrine

Class: ***vasopressor*** • *Pregnancy risk category C*

COMMON INDICATIONS AND DOSAGES	ADMINISTRATION	SPECIAL CONSIDERATIONS
Shock or severe hypotension. *Adults:* 0.1 to 0.18 mg/minute; after blood pressure stabilizes, 0.04 to 0.06 mg/minute. **Mild to moderate hypotension.** *Adults:* 0.1 to 0.5 mg (usually 0.2 mg). Later doses given at intervals of 10 to 15 minutes. **Paroxysmal supraventricular tachycardia.** *Adults:* Up to 0.5 mg, with later doses in 0.1- to 0.2-mg increments depending on blood pressure (systolic not to exceed 160 mm Hg), with no single dose over 1 mg. **Hypotensive emergencies during spinal anesthesia.** *Adults:* 0.2 mg, with later doses in 0.1- to 0.2-mg increments and no single dose over 0.5 mg.	Available as 1-ml ampules and 1- and 5-ml vials (10 mg/ml or 1% solution). Store at room temperature. Discard brown or precipitated solution. For infusion, dilute 10 mg in 500 ml D_5W or 0.9% NaCl. Discard diluted solution after 48 hr. Drug is compatible with most I.V. solutions. ***Incompatibilities:*** Alkaline solutions and iron salts. ***Direct injection:*** Inject over 1 minute for mild to moderate hypotension or hypotensive emergencies during spinal anesthesia. Inject over 20 to 30 seconds for paroxysmal supraventricular tachycardia. ***Continuous infusion:*** Infuse diluted drug at rate required to maintain adequate blood pressure and tissue perfusion. Regulate rate with microdrip tubing and infusion pump. Administer into large vein in antecubital fossa to prevent extravasation.	• Drug may contain sulfites. • Correct hypovolemia either before or during drug administration. • Rapid injection may cause short paroxysms of ventricular tachycardia, ventricular extra systoles, or a sensation of fullness in the head. • Closely monitor infusion site. If extravasation occurs, restart at another site and treat infiltrated area with phentolamine within 12 hr. • During infusion, check blood pressure q 2 minutes until stable, then q 5 to 15 minutes using intra-arterial monitoring. Taper slowly to avoid severe hypotension. • Continuously monitor patient's ECG and tell doctor about any arrhythmias.

phenytoin sodium • Dilantin ◆

Classes: ***anticonvulsant, antiarrhythmic*** • *Pregnancy risk category D*

Status epilepticus. *Adults:* 10 to 15 mg/kg by direct injection, then 100 to 150 mg after 30 minutes if necessary; or, 8 to 18 mg/kg at no more than 50 mg/minute. Maximum daily dose, 1.5 g. *Children:* 15 to 20 mg/kg at 0.5 to 1.5 mg/kg/minute. Maximum daily dose, 20 mg/kg.

Ventricular tachycardia, paroxysmal atrial tachycardia, or arrhythmias caused by digitalis toxicity. *Adults:* 50 to 100 mg at 5-minute intervals p.r.n. to terminate arrhythmia. Maximum daily dose, 15 mg/kg.

Available as 100- and 250-mg ampules and vials at 50 mg/ml. Store at room temperature, and avoid freezing. Solution should be clear. If refrigerated, discard if slight yellowing doesn't clear after slow warming. Manufacturer warns against using with other drugs or infusion solutions, but researchers have diluted drug for intermittent infusion with 0.9% NaCl injection. Add no more than 100 ml (preferably 25 or 50 ml) to 100 mg drug. Prepare immediately before use, always use an in-line filter, and infuse within 1 hr.

Incompatibilities: Amikacin, aminophylline, bretylium, cephapirin, clindamycin phosphate, codeine phosphate, D_5W, dobutamine, fat emulsions, regular insulin, levorphanol, lidocaine, lincomycin, meperidine, metaraminol, methadone, morphine sulfate, nitroglycerin, norepinephrine, pentobarbital sodium, procaine, secobarbital, and streptomycin.

Direct injection: Inject directly into vein (except dorsal hand vein, which may extravasate) using a 0.22-micron in-line filter. Or inject into I.V. line that contains compatible solution infusing at less than 50 mg/minute. In elderly or debilitated patient, give at 17 to 25 mg/minute.

Intermittent infusion: Infuse prescribed dose at ordered rate.

- Flush I.V. tubing with 0.9% NaCl before and after use to remove drug and reduce vein irritation.
- Monitor patient's ECG, blood pressure, respiratory status, and seizure activity.
- Frequently check I.V. site because extravasation causes severe tissue damage.
- If measleslike rash appears, immediately discontinue drug.
- Therapeutic serum level is 10 to 20 mcg/ml; more than 20 mcg/ml is toxic; 100 mcg/ml is lethal. No known antidote exists.

physostigmine salicylate • Antilirium ◆

Class: ***antimuscarinic antidote*** • *Pregnancy risk category C*

Reversal of anticholinergic drug effects (except atropine or scopolamine) or sedative effects of benzodiazepines. *Adults:* 0.5 to 2 mg, repeated q 20 min-

Available as 2-ml ampules at 1 mg/ml. Parenteral solution may be slightly red, blue, or brown; discard solution if discoloration is marked. Store in light-resistant container at room temperature. Avoid freezing.

- Draw physostigmine and atropine into separate syringes.

(continued)

◆ Also available in Canada. ◇ Available in Canada only.

COMMON INDICATIONS AND DOSAGES	ADMINISTRATION	SPECIAL CONSIDERATIONS
physostigmine salicylate *(continued)* utes to desired effect or until adverse cholinergic effects occur. If life-threatening signs recur, give 1 to 4 mg at 30- to 60-minute intervals p.r.n. *Children:* 0.02 mg/kg, repeated at 5- to 10-minute intervals to desired effect or until adverse cholinergic effects occur. Maximum total dose, 2 mg. Or, 0.03 mg/kg or 0.9 mg/m^2 as needed. **Reversal of anticholinergic effects of atropine sulfate or scopolamine hydrobromide as preanesthetics.** *Adults:* Dose is twice that of anticholinergic drug, depending on weight. For example, to reverse effects of 0.5 mg atropine, give 1 mg physostigmine. **Postoperative intestinal atony.** *Adults:* 0.5 to 2 mg.	***Incompatibilities:*** None reported. ***Direct injection:*** Don't exceed 1 mg/minute for adults or 0.5 mg/minute for children.	• Keep suction and cardiopulmonary resuscitation equipment and atropine available. • Establish baseline heart rate and blood pressure. Monitor closely. • Rapid injection can cause bradycardia, breathing difficulty, hypersalivation, and seizures. • Monitor patient for signs of cholinergic crisis. • Watch closely for changes in level of consciousness. Because drug's action lasts only 1 to 2 hr, patient may relapse into coma and need additional physostigmine.

phytonadione (vitamin K_1) • AquaMEPHYTON

Class: ***blood coagulation modifier*** • *Pregnancy risk category C*

Drug-induced hypoprothrombinemia with existing or imminent bleeding. *Adults:* 10 to 50 mg q 4 hr p.r.n. Dosage guided by coagulation studies.	Available as 0.5- and 1-ml ampules and 2.5- and 5-ml multidose vials containing 2 and 10 mg/ml. Protect from light, even after dilution. For direct injection, dilute with 10 ml preservative-free D_5W, 0.9% NaCl, or dextrose 5% in 0.9% NaCl. For infusion, dilute with 50 to 100 ml of any of these solutions. Administer immediately after dilution. Discard unused drug.	• Drug used in hypoprothrombinemia caused by vitamin K deficiency or in moderate to severe bleeding caused by Coumadin or indanedione derivatives. It doesn't antagonize the action of heparin. • Drug may contain benzyl alcohol. • Even dilution and slow infusion may not prevent severe reactions. To reverse vitamin K effects, admin-

Incompatibilities: Dobutamine and phenytoin sodium.
Direct injection: Inject diluted drug directly into vein or tubing of I.V. that contains free-flowing, compatible solution at no more than 1 mg/minute.
Intermittent infusion: Infuse diluted drug at no more than 1 mg/minute.

ister heparin or warfarin, as ordered.
- Monitor patient's coagulation studies 12 hr after administration and repeat as needed.

pipecuronium bromide • Arduan

Class: ***skeletal muscle relaxant*** • *Pregnancy risk category C*

Induction of skeletal muscle relaxation during surgery as an adjunct to general anesthesia. *Adults and children:* Dosage must be individualized. If patient has normal renal function and isn't obese, usually 70 to 85 mcg/kg used for intubation and to maintain paralysis for 1 to 2 hr. If succinylcholine used for intubation, initial dose of 50 mcg/kg will provide good relaxation for 45 minutes or more. Maintenance doses of 10 to 15 mcg/kg may be used to provide relaxation for about 50 minutes.

Available as vials containing 10 mg of powdered drug. Store powder at room temperature or refrigerate. Reconstitute with 10 ml solution before use to yield mg/ml. Don't use large volume of diluent or add drug to hanging I.V. solution. If refrigerated, drug stable 24 hr when reconstituted with sterile water for injection, 0.9% NaCl injection, D_5W, lactated Ringer's injection, or dextrose 5% in 0.9% NaCl. Discard unused portion. If reconstituted with bacteriostatic water for injection, drug stable 5 days at room temperature or in refrigerator. Bacteriostatic water contains benzyl alcohol and shouldn't be used in neonates.
Incompatibilities: Limited data available. Don't mix with other drugs or administer from a large-volume I.V.
Direct injection: Inject into tubing of a free-flowing I.V. solution.

- Because of prolonged duration of action, drug is recommended only for procedures that take 90 minutes or longer.
- Evaluate patient's renal function before drug administration.
- Adjust dosage to ideal body weight in obese patients.
- If succinylcholine used to facilitate intubation, administer drug afterward.
- Drug isn't recommended for use in children under 3 months old.
- A nerve stimulator and train-of-four monitoring are recommended to assess recovery of muscle strength. Before attempting reversal, some evidence of spontaneous recovery should appear.

piperacillin sodium • Pipracil◆

Class: ***antibiotic*** • *Pregnancy risk category B*

Severe systemic infections caused by susceptible organisms. *Adults:* 200 to 300 mg/kg or 12 to 18 g daily in divided doses q 4 to 6 hr.
Complicated UTI. *Adults:* 125 to 200 mg/kg or 8 to 16 g daily in divided

Available in powder form in 2-, 3-, 4-, and 40-g vials. Store at room temperature. Reconstitute each gram of drug with 5 ml of sterile bacteriostatic water for injection or bacteriostatic NaCl injection. Shake vigorously to dissolve. For infusion, dilute reconstituted solution with at least 50 ml D_5W, 0.9% NaCl, dextrose 5% in 0.9% NaCl, or lactated Ringer's. After

- Obtain specimens for culture and sensitivity tests before giving first dose.
- Before giving drug, ask patient if he has penicillin allergy.

(continued)

◆ Also available in Canada. ◇ Available in Canada only.

COMMON INDICATIONS AND DOSAGES	ADMINISTRATION	SPECIAL CONSIDERATIONS
piperacillin sodium *(continued)* doses q 6 to 8 hr. **Uncomplicated UTI.** *Adults:* 100 to 125 mg/kg or 6 to 8 g daily in divided doses q 6 to 12 hr. **Acute *Pseudomonas aeruginosa* infection in cystic fibrosis (with aminoglycosides).** *Adults:* 300 to 600 mg/kg daily. **Prophylaxis for abdominal surgery.** *Adults:* 2 g before surgery, during surgery, and q 6 hr after surgery for up to 24 hr. **Dosage adjustment.** Maximum daily adult dose for any indication, 24 g. Adjust dosage to reflect creatinine clearance in adults.	reconstitution, drug stable 24 hr at room temperature, 7 days 36° to 46° F (2° to 8° C). ***Incompatibilities:*** Fluconazole. ***Direct injection:*** Inject drug directly into vein over 3 to 5 minutes. ***Intermittent infusion:*** Infuse diluted solution over 30 minutes. ***Continuous infusion:*** Inject reconstituted 24-hr dose into required daily I.V. volume. Infuse at rate needed to deliver required fluid volume.	• Closely monitor patient for possible hypersensitivity for at least 30 minutes after administration. • Establish patient's baseline renal function, then periodically monitor his renal, hepatic, and CV status during prolonged therapy. • Check CBC frequently and serum potassium level, PT, and bleeding times. Assess for bleeding.

piperacillin sodium and tazobactam sodium • Zosyn

Class: ***antibiotic*** • *Pregnancy risk category B*

Complicated appendicitis, peritonitis, uncomplicated and complicated skin and skin-structure infections, postpartum endometritis, pelvic inflammatory disease, and community-acquired pneumonia caused by piperacillin-resistant organisms. *Adults:* 12 g piperacillin and 1.5 g tazobactam given as 3.375 g (3 g piperacillin and 0.375 g tazobactam) q 6 hr by I.V infusion. **Dosage adjustment.** Adjust dosage to reflect patient's creatinine clearance. If 20 to 40 ml/minute, give 8 g piperacillin and	Available as powder for injection in single-dose vials containing 2 g piperacillin and 0.25 g tazobactam, 3 g piperacillin and 0.375 g tazobactam, or 4 g piperacillin and 0.5 g tazobactam. Reconstitute with 5 ml of suitable diluent for each 1 g of piperacillin. Shake well until dissolved. May further dilute to desired volume (at least 50 ml). Drug is compatible with 0.9% NaCl, sterile water for injection, 6% dextrose in 0.9% NaCl, D_5W, potassium chloride 40 mEq, bacteriostatic saline with parabens, bacteriostatic water with parabens, bacteriostatic water with benzyl alcohol, or bacteriostatic saline with benzyl alcohol. Use reconstituted single-dose vial immediately. After reconstitution, product is stable in glass or plastic container up to	• Monitor patient's CBC, differential blood count, platelet count, and electrolytes (especially potassium). Assess for occult bleeding. • Monitor patient's neurologic status. • Tell patient to report sore throat, fever, rash, or easy bruising or bleeding.

1 g tazobactam daily in divided doses of 2.25 g q 6 hr. If below 20 ml/minute, give 6 g piperacillin and 0.75 g tazobactam daily in divided doses of 2.25 g q 8 hr.

24 hr at room temperature, 1 week if refrigerated. Stable 12 hr at room temperature in ambulatory I.V. infusion pump. Discard unused portion after 24 hr if stored at room temperature, 48 hr if refrigerated.

Incompatibilities: Acyclovir, amphotericin B, chlorpromazine, dacarbazine, daunorubicin, dobutamine, doxorubicin, doxycycline, droperidol, famotidine, ganciclovir, haloperidol, hydroxyzine hydrochloride, idarubicin, miconazole, minocycline, mitomycin, mitoxantrone, nalbuphine, prochlorperazine, promethazine, streptozocin, and vancomycin. Don't reconstitute with lactated Ringer's because drug degrades over 8 hr, losing potency.

Intermittent infusion: Infuse over 30 minutes.

plasma protein fraction 5% • Plasmanate, Plasma-Plex, Plasmatein, Protenate

Class: ***plasma volume expander*** • *Pregnancy risk category C*

Hypovolemic shock in hypoproteinemic patients (total protein below 5.2 g/dl). *Adults:* 250 to 500 ml. *Children:* 6.6 to 33 ml/kg. Rate and volume reflect patient's condition and response. Dose may be repeated after 15 to 30 minutes if response inadequate.

Hypoproteinemia in burn patients, after first 24 hr. *Adults:* 1,000 to 1,500 ml daily. Larger doses may be necessary in severe hypoproteinemia with continuing loss of plasma proteins. Maximum daily dose, 44 ml/kg.

Drug is ready for use. Solution varies from nearly colorless to straw-colored to dark brown. Store at room temperature, not above 86° F (30° C). Don't use if solution is cloudy, has been frozen, or contains sediment. Give within 4 hr after opening container. Use bottle only once; it contains no preservatives. Discard unused portion.

Incompatibilities: Alcohol-containing solutions, norepinephrine, and protein hydrolysates.

Intermittent infusion: Infuse undiluted or with other parenteral solutions, such as whole blood, plasma, 0.9% NaCl, glucose, or sodium lactate. Infusion rate depends on response but shouldn't exceed 10 ml/minute. As volume approaches normal, reduce to 5 to 8 ml/minute. In children, infuse at 5 to 10 ml/minute. Make sure administration set has adequate filter (provided by manufacturer).

- Solution is isotonic.
- Although product is a pooled human plasma derivative, cross-matching isn't needed.
- Don't give near site of infection or trauma.
- Rapid rates may result in sudden hypotension.
- Frequently monitor blood pressure in shock patients.
- Stop infusion if blood pressure suddenly falls. Correct with vasopressors.
- If allergic reaction occurs, discontinue and give antihistamines.
- Monitor patient's hemoglobin; increased blood volume may cause significant drop.

COMMON INDICATIONS AND DOSAGES	ADMINISTRATION	SPECIAL CONSIDERATIONS

plicamycin (mithramycin) • Mithracin

Class: ***antineoplastic, antihypercalcemic*** • *Pregnancy risk category X*

COMMON INDICATIONS AND DOSAGES	ADMINISTRATION	SPECIAL CONSIDERATIONS
Testicular cancer. *Adults:* 25 to 30 mcg/kg daily for 8 to 10 days or until toxicity develops. Maximum, 10 daily doses or 30 mcg/kg daily. May repeat monthly. **Cancer-related hypercalcemia and hypercalciuria.** *Adults:* 25 mcg/kg daily for 3 or 4 days. May repeat at intervals of 1 week or more.	Follow facility protocol for handling chemotherapy drugs. Available in 2,500-mcg vials. Refrigerate to store. Reconstitute with 4.9 ml sterile water for injection to yield 500 mcg/ml. For infusion, dilute appropriate dose in 1,000 ml D_5W or 0.9% NaCl. Reconstituted solution stable 24 hr at room temperature, 48 hr when refrigerated. Discard unused portion. ***Incompatibilities:*** None reported. However, drug may form a complex with metal ions, such as iron, and readily hydrolyzes in acidic solutions (pH below 4). ***Intermittent infusion:*** Infuse diluted drug over 4 to 6 hr.	• Give antiemetics before and during treatment to help reduce nausea. • Frequently obtain platelet counts, PT, and bleeding times during therapy and for several days afterward. • Monitor patient's liver and kidney function daily if he has preexisting impairment. • If extravasation occurs, stop infusion and restart in another area. Apply cold compress. If swelling develops, apply moderate heat. • Tell patient to report sore throat, fever, mucosal ulcer, easy bruising, or bleeding.

potassium chloride

Class: ***electrolyte supplement*** • *Pregnancy risk category C*

COMMON INDICATIONS AND DOSAGES	ADMINISTRATION	SPECIAL CONSIDERATIONS
Hypokalemia. Dosage reflects patient needs and response. *Adults:* If serum potassium exceeds 2.5 mEq/L, give up to 200 mEq daily at a concentration below 40 mEq/L. Don't exceed 10 mEq/hr. If serum potassium is below 2 mEq/L, give up to 400 mEq daily. Don't exceed 20 mEq/hr. *Children:* 2 to 3 mEq/kg or 40 mEq/m^2 daily. Maximum daily, 3 mEq/kg. Don't exceed 0.5 mEq/kg/hr.	Available as 5-, 10-, 15-, 20-, 30-, and 60-ml ampules and vials containing 10, 20, 30, 40, 60, 90, and 120 mEq potassium. Store at room temperature. Always dilute before use. Dilution varies widely, but potassium concentration usually shouldn't exceed 40 mEq/L. In emergencies, maximum concentration of 80 mEq/L may be temporarily exceeded. When adding potassium solutions, invert plastic container to avoid pooling of concentrated potassium at its base. Then knead the container to mix contents. ***Incompatibilities:*** Amikacin, amphotericin B, diazepam, ergotamine, fat emulsion (10%), mannitol (20% or 25%), penicillin G sodium, phenytoin sodium, promethazine hydrochloride, and streptomycin. ***Intermittent infusion:*** Infuse diluted solution slowly at no	• Never administer undiluted. • If patient is dehydrated, give 1 L of potassium-free fluid before potassium therapy begins. • Monitor patient's ECG, serum potassium, BUN, serum creatinine, pH, and intake and output. • For overdose, stop potassium-containing foods and drugs. Give insulin I.V., as ordered, in 10% to 25% dextrose solution (10 U insulin/20 g dextrose) at 300 to 500 ml/hr. Also give sodium bicarbonate by infusion to correct acidosis. Patient may receive exchange resins, hemodialysis, or peritoneal dialysis.

more than 20 mEq/hr. Rapid infusion can cause fatal hyperkalemia; don't exceed 1 mEq/minute for adult or 0.02 mEq/kg/minute for child.

Continuous infusion: Same as intermittent infusion.

potassium phosphate

Class: ***electrolyte supplement*** • *Pregnancy risk category C*

Electrolyte imbalance. *Adults:* Equivalent of 10 mmol (or 310 mg) of phosphorus daily. *Children:* Equivalent of 1.5 to 2 mmol (or 46.5 to 62 mg) of phosphorus daily. Dose must be individualized.

Available as 5- and 15-ml flip-top vials, 5-ml pin-top vial, and 50-ml bulk additive vial. Strength is equivalent to 3 mmol or 93 mg/ml of phosphorus. For infusion, dilute and mix thoroughly in a larger volume of compatible fluid. Store at room temperature.

Incompatibilities: Dobutamine and solutions that contain calcium and magnesium, such as lactated Ringer's, Ringer's injection, dextrose and Ringer's injection, dextrose 10% in 0.9% NaCl, and Ionosol solutions.

Intermittent infusion: Infuse diluted solution slowly over the ordered time to avoid phosphate intoxication and severe hyperkalemia. Rate must be individualized.

Continuous infusion: Same as intermittent infusion.

- Never administer undiluted.
- Don't give postoperatively until patient has urine flow.
- I.V. infusion of highly concentrated phosphates can cause hypocalcemia.
- Frequently monitor patient's serum electrolyte levels and renal function. Also watch ECG for signs of conduction disturbances.

pralidoxime chloride • Protopam Chloride◆

Class: ***antidote*** • *Pregnancy risk category C*

Poisoning by organophosphate cholinesterase inhibitors. *Adults:* 1 to 2 g. *Children:* 20 to 40 mg/kg. May repeat in 1 hr if weakness persists.

Overdose of anticholinesterase drugs (ambenonium, neostigmine, pyridostigmine) used in myasthenia gravis. *Adults:* 1 to 2 g, then 250 mg q 5 minutes.

Available as a 20-ml vial that contains 1 g of drug in white to off-white porous cake. Store vial at room temperature. Reconstitute with 20 ml sterile water for injection (without preservatives) to yield 50 mg/ml. For infusion, dilute reconstituted drug with 100 ml of 0.9% NaCl. Use solution within a few hr.

Incompatibilities: None reported.

Direct injection: Inject dose over at least 5 minutes directly into vein or tubing of I.V. that contains free-flowing, com-

- Monitor patient's vital signs and intake and output.
- Reduce administration rate or discontinue drug if hypertension develops. As ordered, give 5 mg of phentolamine I.V.
- Give drug with atropine to treat poisoning from organophosphate cholinesterase inhibitors. Watch closely for signs and symptoms of atropine toxicity, such as blurred vision, delirium, dry mouth, excite-

(continued)

◆ Also available in Canada. ◇ Available in Canada only.

COMMON INDICATIONS AND DOSAGES	ADMINISTRATION	SPECIAL CONSIDERATIONS
pralidoxime chloride *(continued)* **Dosage adjustment.** Reduce dosage if patient has renal impairment.	patible solution. Don't exceed 200 mg/minute. ***Intermittent infusion:*** Infuse diluted drug over 15 to 30 minutes.	ment, hallucinations, and tachycardia. Concurrent administration speeds onset of toxicity. • Watch for rapid weakening in patient with myasthenia gravis and carbamate anticholinesterase overdose. Patient can pass quickly from cholinergic crisis to myasthenic crisis.

prednisolone sodium phosphate • Hydeltrasol, Key-Pred-SP

Class: ***immunosuppressant*** • *Pregnancy risk category C*

Severe inflammation, immunosuppression. *Adults:* Depending on disorder, 4 to 60 mg, then 10 to 400 mg daily. *Children:* 0.04 to 0.25 mg/kg or 1.5 to 7.5 mg/m^2 daily in a single dose or b.i.d. Dosage reflects severity of disorder and response to drug.	Available as 2-, 5-, and 10-ml vials with 20 mg/ml. For infusion, dilute with D_5W, 0.9% NaCl, or dextrose 5% in 0.9% NaCl. Store at 59° to 86° F (15° to 30° C). Protect from freezing and light. ***Incompatibilities:*** Calcium gluceptate or gluconate, dimenhydrinate, metaraminol, methotrexate sodium, polymyxin B, prochlorperazine edisylate, promazine, and promethazine hydrochloride. ***Direct injection:*** Inject undiluted drug over 1 minute. ***Intermittent infusion:*** Infuse ordered dose over prescribed duration. ***Continuous infusion:*** Infuse ordered dose over prescribed duration.	• Drug may contain sulfites. • Keep emergency resuscitation equipment nearby in case of anaphylactoid reaction. • In acute adrenal insufficiency, expect to begin therapy by direct injection, then continue with slow I.V. infusion or I.M. administration. • Monitor patient's ECG for arrhythmias and watch for signs of infection, depression, or psychotic episodes, especially with high-dose therapy. • If patient has diabetes, monitor his glucose levels. • Assess drug's effect, gradually titrating to lowest effective dose and shortest possible time. Discontinue gradually.

procainamide hydrochloride • Pronestyl◆

Class: ***antiarrhythmic*** • *Pregnancy risk category C*

Arrhythmias, such as paroxysmal atrial tachycardia, PVCs, ventricular tachycardia, and sometimes atrial fibrillation. *Adults:* 50 to 100 mg at no more than 50 mg/minute, repeated q 5 minutes	Available as 10-ml (100 mg/ml) and 2-ml (500 mg/ml) vials. Store at room temperature. Protect from light and freezing. Discard if markedly discolored or precipitated. For injection or loading infusion, dilute 1 g with 50 ml D_5W to yield 20 mg/ml. For continuous infusion, dilute 1 g with 500 ml D_5W to	• Drug may contain benzyl alcohol and sulfites. • During administration, continuously monitor patient's blood pressure and cardiac function (including ECG). Place patient in a supine position for blood pressure monitoring.

until arrhythmia is controlled or you've given 500 mg. As needed, continue giving 100 mg slowly q 10 minutes until arrhythmia is controlled, adverse reactions occur, or you've given maximum loading dose of 1 g. Maintenance dose, 1 to 6 mg/minute. *Children:* Dosage not established. 2 to 5 mg/kg recommended (not to exceed 100 mg), repeated p.r.n. at 10- to 30-minute intervals (not to exceed 30 mg/kg in 24 hr), or 3 to 6 mg/kg over 5 minutes followed by maintenance infusion of 0.02 to 0.08 mg/kg/minute.
Malignant hyperthermia. *Adults:* 200 to 900 mg, then maintenance infusion of 0.02 to 0.08 mg/kg/minute.
Dosage adjustment. Reduced doses may be required if patient has heart failure or renal impairment.

yield 2 mg/ml. If patient has fluid restriction, dilute 1 g with 250 ml D_5W to yield 4 mg/ml. Note that drug may form a complex with dextrose, causing gradual loss of potency.
Incompatibilities: Bretylium, esmolol, ethacrynate, milrinone, and phenytoin sodium.
Direct injection: Inject dose over 2 minutes or longer.
Intermittent infusion: Give loading infusion at 1 ml/minute for 25 to 30 minutes. Therapeutic effects usually occur after infusion of 100 to 200 mg. If no effect occurs after infusing 500 mg, wait at least 10 minutes to allow drug distribution, then continue administration.
Continuous infusion: Using an infusion pump, give diluted solution at ordered rate, usually 2 to 6 mg/minute.

- Keep phenylephrine or norepinephrine available to treat severe hypotension.
- In ventricular tachycardia, stop infusion if ventricular rate declines significantly without attaining regular AV conduction.

prochlorperazine edisylate • Compazine

Class: ***antiemetic*** • *Pregnancy risk category C*

Severe nausea and vomiting from surgery or toxins, radiation, or cytotoxic drugs. *Adults:* 2.5 to 10 mg (0.5 to 2 ml). May repeat q 3 to 4 hr.
Prevention of nausea and vomiting during surgery. *Adults:* 5 to 10 mg by direct injection 15 to 30 minutes before induction of anesthesia. Repeat once before surgery, if necessary. Or 20 mg/L by infusion 15 to 30 minutes before induction of anesthesia. Maximum, 40 mg daily.

Available as 2-ml ampules, 10-ml vials, 2-ml disposable syringes, and 1- and 2-ml prefilled cartridges at 5 mg/ml. Store at room temperature and protect from light and freezing. Don't use if markedly discolored or if precipitate appears. Dilute for continuous infusion with at least 1 L of compatible isotonic solution, such as 0.9% NaCl, to yield 20 mg/L.
Incompatibilities: Aminophylline, amphotericin B, ampicillin sodium, calcium gluceptate and gluconate, cephalothin, chloramphenicol sodium succinate, chlorothiazide, dexamethasone sodium phosphate, dimenhydrinate, heparin, hydrocortisone sodium succinate, hydromorphone, methicillin, methotrexate, midazolam, penicillin G potassium and sodium,

- Monitor patient's blood pressure closely.
- Because of risk of hypotension, use I.V. route only when patient can be monitored closely.
- For elderly patient, start with low doses and increase gradually.
- Antiemetic effect may mask signs of drug toxicity or obscure diagnosis of conditions with nausea as primary symptom.
- Anticholinergic antiparkinson drugs may help control extrapyramidal reactions.

(continued)

◆ Also available in Canada. ◇ Available in Canada only.

COMMON INDICATIONS AND DOSAGES	ADMINISTRATION	SPECIAL CONSIDERATIONS
prochlorperazine edisylate *(continued)*	phenobarbital, phenytoin, prednisolone sodium phosphate, thiopental, and vitamin B complex with C. Also incompatible with solutions containing methylparaben or propylparaben. Don't mix in same syringe with other drugs. ***Direct injection:*** Slowly inject undiluted drug at 5 mg/minute. Never give as bolus injection. ***Continuous infusion:*** Infuse diluted drug at ordered rate and duration.	

promethazine hydrochloride • Phenergan◆

Classes: ***antiemetic, adjunct to analgesics*** *• Pregnancy risk category C*

COMMON INDICATIONS AND DOSAGES	ADMINISTRATION	SPECIAL CONSIDERATIONS
Allergic reaction. *Adults:* 25 mg, repeated in 2 hr p.r.n. **Nausea and vomiting.** *Adults:* 12.5 to 25 mg q 4 hr p.r.n. *Children:* 0.25 to 0.5 mg/kg 4 to 6 times daily. **Obstetric sedation.** *Adults:* 50 mg during early labor; then 25 to 75 mg in established labor (given with an opioid agonist). 25 to 50 mg may be repeated once or twice at 4-hr intervals. Maximum, 100 mg in 24 hr. **Sedation and relief of apprehension, postoperative pain (anesthesia and analgesia adjunct).** *Adults:* 25 to 50 mg p.r.n. Maximum, 150 mg daily.	Available as 1- and 10-ml ampules, 1- and 10-ml vials, and 1-ml prefilled cartridges at 25 mg/ml. Store at room temperature; protect from light and freezing. Discard if solution is discolored or precipitate appears. ***Incompatibilities:*** Aminophylline, chloramphenicol sodium succinate, chlorothiazide, diatrizoate meglumine and sodium (34.3%-35% and 52%-8%), diatrizoate sodium (75%), dimenhydrinate, heparin sodium, hydrocortisone sodium succinate, iodipamide meglumine (52%), iothalamate meglumine (60%), iothalamate sodium (80%), methicillin, methohexital, morphine, penicillin G potassium and sodium, pentobarbital sodium, phenobarbital, phenytoin, prednisolone sodium phosphate, thiopental, and vitamin B complex. ***Direct injection:*** Inject at no more than 25 mg/minute into tubing of I.V. line that contains free-flowing, compatible solution. Rapid administration may reduce blood pressure temporarily.	• Don't exceed 25 mg/ml. Make sure I.V. line is patent before injection. Avoid extravasation or inadvertent arterial injection because of possible gangrene or severe arteriospasm. • Monitor patient's blood pressure closely. • Watch for extrapyramidal reactions, especially in older adult. • Drug's antiemetic effect may obscure signs of intestinal obstruction, brain tumor, or promethazine overdose.

propofol • Diprivan

Class: ***general anesthetic*** • *Pregnancy risk category B*

Induction of anesthesia. *Adults:* Usually 40-mg bolus q 10 seconds until desired response occurs, individualized to patient's condition and age. Most patients with American Society of Anesthesiologists physical status I or II under age 55 need 2 to 2.5 mg/kg.
Maintenance of anesthesia. *Adults:* Usually 0.1 to 0.2 mg/kg/minute (6 to 12 mg/kg/hr) but may be given at variable rate, titrated to effect.
Sedation of intubated ICU patient. *Adults:* 5 mcg/kg/minute (0.3 mg/kg/hr) for 5 minutes. Increments of 5 to 10 mcg/kg/minute (0.3 to 0.6 mg/kg/hr) over 5 to 10 minutes may be used until desired sedation is achieved. Maintenance, 5 to 50 mcg/kg/minute (0.3 to 3 mg/kg/hr).
Dosage adjustment. Patients who are elderly, debilitated, hypovolemic, or assigned American Society of Anesthesiologists physical status III or IV receive half of usual doses for induction and maintenance of anesthesia.

Available as 20-ml ampules with 10 mg/ml. Use strict aseptic technique during handling. If diluting before infusion, use only D_5W and don't dilute to less than 2 mg/ml. Afterward, drug may be more stable in glass than in plastic container. When given into a running I.V. line, propofol emulsion is compatible with D_5W, lactated Ringer's injection, lactated Ringer's and 5% dextrose injection, 5% dextrose and 0.45% NaCl injection, and 5% dextrose and 0.2% NaCl injection.
Store unopened ampules above 40° F (4° C) and below 72° F (22° C). Don't refrigerate.
Incompatibilities: Don't mix with other drugs.
Direct injection: Varies with patient condition and response to drug.
Continuous infusion: Varies with indication, patient condition, and response to drug.

- Contraindicated if patient hypersensitive to drug or components, including soybean oil, egg lecithin, and glycerol.
- Use cautiously in elderly or debilitated patients.
- Apnea commonly occurs during induction and may persist more than 60 seconds. Ventilatory support may be required.
- Monitor patient's lipids daily.
- Don't stop drug abruptly to avoid sudden awakening with anxiety, agitation, and resistance to mechanical ventilation.

COMMON INDICATIONS AND DOSAGES	ADMINISTRATION	SPECIAL CONSIDERATIONS
propranolol hydrochloride • Inderal◆		
Classes: ***antiarrhythmic, antianginal, antihypertensive*** • *Pregnancy risk category C*		
Life-threatening arrhythmias or those occurring under anesthesia. *Adults:* 0.5 to 3 mg repeated after 2 minutes and again after 4 hr if needed. *Children:* 0.01 to 0.02 mg/kg. **Substitute for oral administration during surgery.** *Adults:* 10% of oral dose.	Available as 1-ml ampules with 1 mg/ml. Compatible with 0.9% NaCl and D_5W. Store at room temperature and protect from light and freezing. ***Incompatibilities:*** Diazoxide. ***Direct injection:*** Inject at no more than 1 mg/minute through an I.V. line that contains free-flowing, compatible solution. ***Intermittent infusion:*** In children, infuse over 10 minutes.	• Manufacturer doesn't recommend using drug for children. • Remember that I.V. doses are considerably smaller than oral ones. • Carefully monitor patient's ECG, blood pressure, and central venous pressure during administration. • Inform diabetic patient that signs of hypoglycemia may be masked.
protamine sulfate		
Class: ***antidote*** • *Pregnancy risk category C*		
Severe heparin overdose. *Adults:* 1 to 1.5 mg/100 U heparin when given a few minutes after I.V. heparin injection; 0.5 to 0.75 mg/100 U heparin when given 30 to 60 minutes after I.V. heparin injection; 0.25 to 0.375 mg/100 U heparin when given more than 2 hr after I.V. heparin injection; 25 to 50 mg after continuous infusion of heparin; 1 to 1.5 mg/100 U heparin after deep S.C. heparin injection. Or 25 to 50 mg by slow I.V. injection and remaining calculated dose by continuous I.V. infusion over 8 to 16 hr or expected duration of heparin absorption. **Neutralization of heparin given during extracorporeal circulation in arterial and cardiac surgery or dialysis.** *Adults and children:* Usually 1.5 mg/100 U heparin.	Available as liquid (10 mg/ml) in 5- and 25-ml vials or as powder in 50- and 250-mg vials. Refrigerate liquid; store powder at room temperature. Avoid freezing. Reconstitute powder with sterile water for injection or bacteriostatic water for injection containing 0.9% benzyl alcohol (5 ml for 50 mg vial or 25 ml for 250 mg vial) to yield 10 mg/ml. Shake vigorously. If reconstituted with sterile water, use immediately and discard unused portions. If reconstituted with bacteriostatic water and benzyl alcohol, solution stable 72 hr at room temperature. Reconstituted solutions need no further dilution but may be diluted in D_5W or 0.9% NaCl. Don't store diluted solutions; they contain no preservatives. ***Incompatibilities:*** Cephalosporins, diatrizoate meglumine, diatrizoate sodium, ioxaglate meglumine, ioxaglate sodium, and penicillins. ***Direct injection:*** Inject reconstituted drug slowly over 1 to 3 minutes. Don't give more than 50 mg in 10 minutes.	• Drug is used to treat severe overdose; mild overdose corrected by stopping heparin. • Typically, 1 mg of drug neutralizes about 90 U heparin sodium from bovine lung tissue, 100 U of heparin calcium from porcine intestinal mucosa, or 115 U of heparin sodium from porcine intestinal mucosa. • Overly rapid administration can cause severe hypotension and anaphylactoid reactions. • Carefully titrate drug dose, especially if patient received large heparin dose. • Check patient's vital signs frequently. • Perform coagulation studies 5 to 15 minutes after therapy; repeat as needed. • Don't give more than 100 mg over 2 hr (drug's duration of action) unless coagulation studies indicate need for higher dosage.

pyridostigmine bromide • Mestinon, Regonol

Class: ***muscle stimulant*** • *Pregnancy risk category C*

Myasthenia gravis. *Adults:* 2 mg q 2 to 3 hr or about one-thirtieth (1/30) of oral maintenance dose. Dosage varies widely.
Antidote for nondepolarizing neuromuscular blocker. *Adults:* 10 to 20 mg or 0.1 to 0.25 mg/kg, given with or shortly after 0.6 to 1.2 mg atropine sulfate I.V. or 0.2 to 0.6 mg glycopyrrolate I.V. (about 0.2 mg glycopyrrolate for each 5 mg pyridostigmine bromide).

Available as 2-ml ampules and 5-ml vials with 5 mg/ml. Store at room temperature. Protect from light and freezing.
Incompatibilities: Unstable in alkaline solutions.
Direct injection: Inject undiluted drug very slowly into I.V. line that contains compatible, free-flowing solution. Watch for thrombophlebitis at I.V. site.

- Establish baseline respiratory rate, heart rate, and blood pressure. Maintain patent airway.
- Keep atropine sulfate available in separate syringe. Give 0.6 to 1.2 mg, as ordered, before or with high doses of pyridostigmine.
- If patient's heart rate is below 80 beats/minute, expect to give atropine before pyridostigmine.
- Stop all other cholinergic drugs during pyridostigmine therapy to avoid toxicity.
- While reversing effects of nondepolarizing neuromuscular blockers, keep patient on ventilator. Wait 15 to 30 minutes for full effects. Observe closely for recurrence of respiratory depression.
- Stay alert for cholinergic crisis, which can occur with overdose.

pyridoxine hydrochloride (vitamin B_6)

Class: ***nutritional supplement*** • *Pregnancy risk category A (C if greater than RDA)*

Vitamin B_6 deficiency. *Adults:* 4.0 to 6.3 mg daily.
Pyridoxine dependency syndrome. *Adults:* 30 to 600 mg daily. *Infants with seizures:* 10 to 100 mg during seizure.
Drug-induced pyridoxine deficiency. *Adults:* 50 to 200 mg daily for 3 weeks, then 25 to 100 mg daily p.r.n.
Cycloserine poisoning. *Adults:* 300 mg or more daily.
Isoniazid poisoning. *Adults:* Dose equal to amount of isoniazid ingested, usually 1

Available as 1-, 10-, and 30-ml vials with 100 mg/ml. Store at room temperature; protect from light and freezing. For intermittent infusion, dilute with recommended solutions to ordered concentrations.
Incompatibilities: Alkaline solutions, erythromycin estolate, iron salts, kanamycin, oxidizing agents, riboflavin, sodium phosphate, and streptomycin.
Direct injection: Inject undiluted drug into I.V. line that contains free-flowing, compatible solution.
Intermittent infusion: Infuse diluted drug over prescribed duration.

- Give I.V. when oral route is unsuitable or impossible.
- Increase dosage, as ordered, in hemodialysis patients.
- Dosages of 200 mg daily for more than 30 days may cause pyridoxine dependency syndrome.
- Infants with hereditary pyridoxine dependency syndrome require high doses in first week after birth to prevent seizures and mental retardation. Drug usually stops seizures within 3 minutes.

(continued)

COMMON INDICATIONS AND DOSAGES	ADMINISTRATION	SPECIAL CONSIDERATIONS
pyridoxine hydrochloride *(continued)* to 4 g, followed by 1 g I.M. q 30 minutes until entire dose is given. Usually given with anticonvulsants p.r.n. **Hydrazine poisoning.** *Adults:* 25 mg/kg; one-third given I.M. and remainder by I.V infusion over 3 hr. **Mushroom poisoning (genus *Gyromitra*).** *Adults:* 25 mg/kg infused over 15 to 30 minutes and repeated p.r.n. Maximum, 15 to 20 g daily.		• Stay alert for symptoms of overdose (ataxia and severe neuropathy) in patient receiving high doses for several weeks or months.

quinidine gluconate

Class: ***antiarrhythmic*** *• Pregnancy risk category C*

COMMON INDICATIONS AND DOSAGES	ADMINISTRATION	SPECIAL CONSIDERATIONS
Arrhythmias. *Adults:* up to 0.25 mg/kg/minute, then adjusted as needed. Usual dose needed to control ventricular arrhythmias is 300 mg or less. Maximum, 4 g daily. *Children:* 30 mg/kg daily or 900 mg/m^2 daily in five divided doses. **Severe malaria caused by *Plasmodium falciparum* (when I.V. quinine dihydrochloride unavailable).** *Adults:* 10 mg/kg diluted in 250 ml 0.9% NaCl given over 1 to 2 hr, followed by continuous infusion of 0.02 mg/kg/minute for 72 hr or until parasitemia is reduced to less than 1%. **Dosage adjustment.** Dosage may need adjustment in patient with heart failure, hepatic disease, or need for hemodialysis.	Available as 10-ml vials with 80 mg/ml. Store at room temperature; protect from light and freezing. For intermittent infusion, dilute with D_5W to ordered concentration. For continuous infusion, dilute 800 mg (one vial) with 40 ml D_5W to yield 16 mg/ml. Discard diluted solution after 24 hr or if solution turns brown. ***Incompatibilities:*** Alkalies, amiodarone, furosemide, heparin sodium, and iodides. ***Intermittent infusion:*** Infuse solution through I.V. line over prescribed duration. ***Continuous infusion:*** Start infusing solution through I.V. line at prescribed rate, then adjust rate to control arrhythmias.	• Use cautiously in older adults. • During infusion, continuously monitor patient's blood pressure and cardiac function (including ECG). • Check serum quinidine and potassium levels; quinidine levels above 8 mcg/ml are toxic. • Adverse GI effects, especially diarrhea, indicate toxicity.

ranitidine • Zantac

Class: ***antiulcer agent*** • *Pregnancy risk category B*

Active duodenal or gastric ulcer and pathologic hypersecretory conditions in hospitalized patients who can't take drug orally. *Adults:* 50 mg q 6 to 8 hr. Maximum, 400 mg daily.
Dosage adjustment. Adjust dosage if patient has renal impairment.

Available as 2- and 10-ml vials with 25 mg/ml. Store at room temperature; protect from light and freezing. For direct injection, dilute 50-mg dose with compatible I.V. solution (such as 0.9% NaCl, D_5W, dextrose 10% in water, lactated Ringer's, or sodium bicarbonate 5%) to a total volume of 20 ml. For intermittent infusion, dilute 50-mg dose with 100 ml of a compatible I.V. solution. For continuous infusion, dilute 150 mg in 1,000 ml of compatible solution. Solutions stable 48 hr at room temperature. Discard if drug discolors or precipitate forms.
Incompatibilities: Amphotericin B, chlorpromazine, clindamycin phosphate, methotrimeprazine, midazolam, opium alkaloids hydrochloride, and pentobarbital sodium.
Direct injection: Inject diluted drug into patent I.V. line over at least 5 minutes.
Intermittent infusion: Infuse diluted drug into patent I.V. line through piggyback set over 15 to 20 minutes.
Continuous infusion: Infuse over 24 hr at 6.25 mg/hr. No loading dose required.

- Monitor AST levels if patient receives 400 mg daily for 5 days or longer. Begin on day 5 of therapy and check daily until discontinuation.
- Tell patient to report rash, sore throat, fever, easy bruising, or bleeding.
- Drug can be removed by hemodialysis.

remifentanil hydrochloride • Ultiva

Classes: ***analgesic, anesthetic*** • *Pregnancy risk category C* • *Controlled substance schedule II*

Analgesic during induction or maintenance of general anesthesia; use during monitored anesthesia care and immediate postoperative period, and as an analgesic component under the direct supervision of anesthesia practitioner; induction of anesthesia through intubation. *Adults:* 0.5 to 1 mcg/kg/minute with

Available as preservative-free 1-, 2-, and 5-mg lyophilized powder vials. Store at room temperature. Reconstitute with 1 ml diluent per 1 mg of each drug and shake well to make clear, colorless liquid. Dilute to final concentration of 25, 50, or 250 mcg/ml. Final product stable 24 hr at room temperature when diluted with sterile water, D_5W, dextrose 5% in 0.9% NaCl, 0.45% and 0.9% NaCl, or D_5W and lactated Ringer's. Don't give undiluted.

- Monitor patient's vital signs and oxygenation continually during administration.
- Stopping infusion will cause rapid offset.
- Before stopping drug, establish adequate postoperative analgesia.
- If patient is breathing spontaneously but has respiratory depression, decrease infusion rate by 50% or temporarily stop it.

(continued)

COMMON INDICATIONS AND DOSAGES	ADMINISTRATION	SPECIAL CONSIDERATIONS
remifentanil hydrochloride *(continued)* hypnotic or volatile agent; may load with 1 mcg/kg over 30 to 60 seconds if endotracheal intubation occurring less than 8 minutes after start of infusion. **Maintenance of anesthesia.** *Adults:* 0.25 to 0.4 mcg/kg/minute, depending on concurrent anesthesia. Increase doses by 25% to 100% and decrease by 25% to 50% q 2 to 5 minutes p.r.n. If rate exceeds 1 mcg/kg/minute consider increases in concomitant anesthetics. May supplement with 1 mcg/kg boluses over 30 to 60 seconds q 2 to 5 minutes p.r.n. **Continuation as analgesic in immediate postoperative period.** *Adults:* 0.1 mcg/kg/minute followed by infusion of 0.025 to 0.2 mcg/kg/minute. Adjust by 0.025 mcg/kg/minute q 5 minutes. Rates above 0.2 mcg/kg/minute can cause respiratory depression (less than 8 breaths/minute).	***Incompatibilities:*** Blood products. Don't mix with lactated Ringer's. ***Direct injection:*** Inject directly into vein over 30 to 60 seconds. ***Continuous infusion:*** Use an I.V. infusion device and injection site that's close to venous cannula. Clear site when infusion discontinued.	• Can administer with propofol into a running I.V. administration set. • Skeletal muscle rigidity may occur and is treated by stopping or decreasing rate of infusion if patient is breathing spontaneously. If rigidity occurs during anesthesia, give neuromuscular blocker and induction drugs.

respiratory syncytial virus immune globulin intravenous, human (RSV-IGIV) • RespiGam

Class: ***immune serum*** • *Pregnancy risk category C*

COMMON INDICATIONS AND DOSAGES	ADMINISTRATION	SPECIAL CONSIDERATIONS
Prevention of serious lower respiratory tract infections from respiratory syncytial virus. *Premature infants and children under age 2, especially those with bronchopulmonary dysplasia:* Give monthly as single infusion starting at 1.5 ml/kg/hr for 15 minutes; then, if condi-	Available as single-use vial containing 2,500 mg. Store at 35.6° to 46.4° F (2° to 8° C). Don't freeze. Don't shake vial; avoid foaming. Discard after use. Compatible with 2.5%, 5%, 10%, and 20% dextrose in water (with or without NaCl). Don't dilute more than 1:2 with any of these solutions. ***Incompatibilities:*** Give separately from other drugs. ***Intermittent infusion:*** Begin infusion within 6 hr and	• Give first dose before infection season begins and subsequent doses monthly during the season to maintain protection. Children with respiratory syncytial virus should receive monthly doses for duration of season. • Assess patient's cardiopulmonary status and vital signs before starting infusion, before each rate in-

tion allows, 3 ml/kg/hr for 15 minutes; then 6 ml/kg/hr (the maximum) until infusion complete. Maximum recommended total dose for each infusion is 750 mg/kg.

complete it within 12 hr after vial has been entered. Don't predilute drug. Administer with constant infusion pump. Use separate I.V. line, if possible, although drug may be piggybacked into compatible solution. Filter unnecessary, but in-line filter with pore size larger than 15 micrometers may be used.

crease, and every 30 minutes thereafter until 30 minutes after infusion completed.
- Monitor patient closely for signs of fluid overload, especially if he has bronchopulmonary dysplasia.
- If patient develops hypotension, anaphylaxis, or severe allergic reaction, stop infusion and give epinephrine (1:1,000), as ordered.

reteplase, recombinant • Retavase

Class: ***thrombolytic*** • *Pregnancy risk category C*

Management of acute MI. *Adults:* Double-bolus injection of 10 + 10 U. If first bolus doesn't cause complications (such as serious bleeding or anaphylactoid reaction), give second bolus 30 minutes after start of first bolus.

Available as sterile, preservative-free lyophilized powder in 10.8-U (18.8-mg) vials. Reconstitute only with materials (10 ml sterile water for injection) provided by manufacturer to yield 1 U/ml. Solution should be colorless. If foaming occurs, allow vial to stand for several minutes. Use within 4 hr of reconstitution if stored at 36° to 86° F (2° to 30° C). Protect from light. Discard if drug discolors or precipitates.
Incompatibilities: Add no other drug to injection solution that contains reteplase.
Direct injection: Give each bolus by I.V. infusion over 2 minutes.

- Potency is expressed in units specific to reteplase that aren't comparable to other thrombolytics.
- Carefully monitor patient's ECG for reperfusion arrhythmias during treatment.
- Monitor patient for bleeding and avoid use of noncompressible puncture sites.

Rh_o(D) immune globulin intravenous, human • WinRho SD

Class: ***anti-Rh_o(D)-positive prophylaxis*** • *Pregnancy risk category C*

After abortion, amniocentesis (after 34 weeks' gestation), or other manipulation (after 34 weeks' gestation) linked to increased risk of Rh isoimmunization. *Adults:* 120 mcg given within 72 hr after delivery, miscarriage, or manipulation.
Pregnancy. *Adults:* 300 mcg at 28 weeks' gestation. If given early in pregnancy, give

Available in kits containing either 120- or 300-mcg single-dose vials of anti-Rh_o(D) IGIV, a single-dose vial of 2.5 ml 0.9% NaCl injection, and a package insert. Reconstitute only with 0.9% NaCl. Store at 35° to 46° F (2° to 8° C). Don't freeze or shake vials. If reconstituted product isn't used immediately, store at room temperature for no more than 4 hr; don't freeze. Discard unused portion.
Incompatibilities: Give separately from other drugs.

- Obtain history of patient's allergies and reactions to vaccination. Keep epinephrine 1:1,000 available in case of anaphylaxis.
- Immediately after delivery, send a sample of neonate's cord blood to laboratory for typing and crossmatching. Confirm if mother is Rh_o(D)-negative and D^u-negative. As ordered, give drug to

(continued)

COMMON INDICATIONS AND DOSAGES	ADMINISTRATION	SPECIAL CONSIDERATIONS
Rh_o(D) immune globulin intravenous, human *(continued)* additional doses at 12-week intervals to maintain levels of passively acquired anti-Rh antibodies. Then give 120 mcg within 72 hr of delivery or up to 28 days later, if necessary. **Transfusion accident.** *Adults:* 600 mcg q 8 hr until total dose given. Total dose varies with volume of packed RBCs or whole blood transfused. **Idiopathic thrombocytopenic purpura in Rh_o(D)-antigen-positive patient.** *Adults:* 50 mcg/kg as single dose or divided into two doses given on separate days. Reduce initial dose to 25 to 40 mcg/kg if hemoglobin below 10 g/dl. Then, 25 to 60 mcg/kg (individualized) may be given p.r.n. to raise platelet counts.	***Direct injection:*** Inject directly into vein or free-flowing compatible I.V. solution over 3 to 5 minutes.	mother only if infant is Rh_o(D)-positive or D^u-positive. • Mini-dose preparations are recommended for every patient undergoing abortion or miscarriage up to 12 weeks' gestation unless she's Rh_o(D)-positive or D^u-positive or has Rh antibodies, or unless the father or fetus is Rh-negative.

rifampin • Rifadin

Class: ***antituberculotic*** • *Pregnancy risk category C*

COMMON INDICATIONS AND DOSAGES	ADMINISTRATION	SPECIAL CONSIDERATIONS
***Neisseria meningitidis* carrier state.** *Adults:* 600 mg b.i.d. for 2 days. *Children ages 1 month to 12 years:* 10 mg/kg q 12 hr for 2 days. *Infants under 1 month old:* 5 mg/kg q 12 hr for 2 days. **Primary treatment of pulmonary tuberculosis.** *Adults:* 10 mg/kg up to 600 mg daily as a single dose. *Children over age 5:* 10 to 20 mg/kg daily as a single dose. Maximum, 600 mg daily.	Available as lyophilized powder in 600-mg vial. Store at room temperature, protect from light, and avoid temperatures above 104° F (40° C). Reconstitute with 10 ml sterile water to yield 60 mg/ml. Solution stable at room temperature for 24 hr. Immediately before use, withdraw calculated amount and add to 500 ml D_5W; if patient's condition permits, add to 100 ml of D_5W. Use either solution within 4 hr to avoid precipitation. Use 0.9% NaCl solution when dextrose is contraindicated; stability is reduced slightly.	• Avoid extravasation. • Monitor patient's liver function tests, bilirubin, and blood counts. Watch closely for signs of hepatic impairment. • Tell patient that urine, feces, saliva, sputum, sweat, and tears may turn red or orange, and that soft contact lenses can be permanently stained. • Tell patient to report sore throat, fever, malaise, easy bruising, or bleeding.

Incompatibilities: Minocycline.
Intermittent infusion: Infuse 100 ml over 30 minutes; 500 ml over 3 hr.

Ringer's injection

Class: ***fluid and electrolyte supplement*** • *Pregnancy risk category C*

Replacement of extracellular fluid and electrolytes. *Adults and children:* Usually 1.5 to 3 L (2% to 6% of body weight) daily, but dosage highly individualized.

Available in 500- and 1,000-ml containers. Store at room temperature. Avoid excessive exposure to high temperatures (up to 104° F [40° C]). Protect from freezing. Before administration, inspect for precipitates and discoloration. Don't use unless solution is clear and container undamaged.
Incompatibilities: Ampicillin sodium, cefamandole, chlordiazepoxide, diazepam, erythromycin lactobionate, methicillin, potassium phosphate, sodium bicarbonate, and thiopental.
Continuous infusion: Infuse through central or peripheral I.V. line over ordered duration.

- Solution may be given with dextrose, other carbohydrates, or sodium lactate.
- I.V. administration of Ringer's injection can cause fluid or solute overload.
- Electrolyte content is insufficient for treating severe electrolyte deficiencies.
- Assess changes in fluid and electrolyte balance during prolonged therapy.
- Tell patient to promptly report difficulty in breathing.

Ringer's injection, lactated (Ringer's lactate solution)

Class: ***fluid and electrolyte supplement*** • *Pregnancy risk category C*

Replacement of extracellular fluid and electrolytes. *Adults and children:* Usually 1.5 to 3 L (2% to 6% of body weight) daily, but dosage highly individualized.

Available in 250-, 500-, and 1,000-ml containers. Store at room temperature. Avoid excessive exposure to high temperatures (up to 104° F [40° C]).
Incompatibilities: Amphotericin B, ampicillin sodium, cefamandole, chlordiazepoxide, diazepam, erythromycin lactobionate, methicillin, methylprednisolone sodium succinate, phenytoin sodium, potassium phosphate, sodium bicarbonate, thiopental, and whole blood.
Continuous infusion: Infuse ordered amount through peripheral or central I.V. line over ordered duration.

- Monitor patient's fluid and electrolyte balance during long-term therapy.
- Tell patient to report pain or swelling at infusion site.

COMMON INDICATIONS AND DOSAGES	ADMINISTRATION	SPECIAL CONSIDERATIONS

ritodrine hydrochloride • Yutopar♦

Class: ***tocolytic*** • *Pregnancy risk category B*

COMMON INDICATIONS AND DOSAGES	ADMINISTRATION	SPECIAL CONSIDERATIONS
Management of uncomplicated preterm labor after gestation of 20 or more weeks, but less than 36 weeks. *Adults:* 50 mcg/minute, gradually increasing q 10 minutes in 50-mcg increments until contractions cease. (Usual effective dosage, 150 to 350 mcg/minute.) Maintenance, 150 to 350 mcg/minute for 12 to 24 hr after contractions stop. Maximum, 350 mcg/minute.	Available as 5- and 10-ml ampules, vials, and syringes at 10 and 15 mg/ml. Store at room temperature. For infusion, add 150 mg drug to 500 ml D_5W to yield 300 mcg/ml. If patient has fluid restriction, make a higher concentration, as ordered. Drug also may be diluted with 10% Dextran 40 in NaCl or 10% invert sugar solution. Avoid diluting with Ringer's injection, 0.9% NaCl, or lactated Ringer's. Also avoid diluting in NaCl solutions except when mother has diabetes, because of increased risk of pulmonary edema. Use within 48 hr; discard if discolored or precipitated. ***Incompatibilities:*** None reported. ***Continuous infusion:*** Using a pump to control rate, infuse by I.V. piggyback into patent primary I.V. line at port closest to infusion needle. Adjust delivery as above until contractions or dilation stops, adverse maternal or fetal effects occur, or maximum of 350 mcg/minute is reached. At recommended dilution, maximum fluid volume after 12 hr is about 840 ml.	• Contraindicated if patient hypersensitive to sulfites, ritodrine, or other $beta_2$-adrenergic receptor agonists. • Place patient in left lateral position to minimize hypotension. • Closely monitor patient's intake and output. Check fetal and maternal heart rates and maternal blood pressure, breath sounds, respirations, and uterine activity. • If preterm labor recurs, I.V. infusion may be repeated. If contractions don't recur after about 36 hr, patient may gradually resume ambulation. • Sinus bradycardia may follow drug withdrawal.

rituximab • Rituxan

Class: ***antineoplastic*** • *Pregnancy risk category C*

COMMON INDICATIONS AND DOSAGES	ADMINISTRATION	SPECIAL CONSIDERATIONS
B-cell malignant lymphoma with relapsed or refractory low-grade or follicular, CD20 positive disease. *Adults:* 375 mg/m^2 once weekly for four doses (days 1, 8, 15, 22). Start first infusion at 50 mg/hr. If no hypersensitivity or adverse events occur, increase by 50 mg/hr q 30 minutes to maximum of 400 mg/hr. Later	Follow facility protocol for handling chemotherapy drugs. Available as 10- and 50-ml single-use, sterile vials at 10 mg/ml. Protect vials from direct sunlight. Dilute in D_5W or 0.9% NaCl to final concentration of 1 to 4 mg/ml. Gently invert bag to mix. Discard unused portion left in vial. ***Incompatibilities:*** Don't mix or dilute with any other drugs.	• Monitor patient closely for signs and symptoms of hypersensitivity. • Monitor patient's blood pressure closely during infusion. If hypotension, bronchospasm, or angioedema occurs, stop infusion, wait for symptoms to resolve, and restart infusion at half previous rate. • Obtain CBC at regular intervals, more frequently if patient develops cytopenia.

infusions can start at 100 mg/hr and increase by 100 mg/hr at 30-minute intervals to 400 mg/hr as tolerated.

Intermittent infusion: Give by I.V. infusion at prescribed rate according to patient tolerance; don't give by I.V. push or bolus.

- Stop infusion if serious or life-threatening arrhythmias occur. Patients will undergo cardiac monitoring during and after subsequent infusions.

rocuronium bromide • Zemuron

Class: ***skeletal muscle relaxant*** • *Pregnancy risk category B*

Adjunct to general anesthesia to facilitate intubation or relax skeletal muscles during surgery or mechanical ventilation. *Adults and children over 3 months old:* Dosage varies with anesthetic and patient's individual needs and response. 0.6 mg/kg by I.V. bolus allows intubation in most patients within 2 minutes and causes paralysis for about 31 minutes. Maintenance of 0.1 mg/kg gives another 12 minutes of relaxation; 0.15 mg/kg another 17 minutes; 0.2 mg/kg another 24 minutes. Maintenance of 0.075 to 0.125 mg/kg provides relaxation for 7 to 10 minutes in children. Continuous infusion may be used to maintain neuromuscular blockade. Infusion for adults may start after early evidence of spontaneous recovery from intubating dose; start at 0.01 to 0.012 mg/kg/minute. Infusion for children may start at 0.012 mg/kg/minute after one twitch is present in train-of-four. Dosages adjusted to patient's twitch response.

Available in vials containing 10 mg/ml. Refrigerated at 36° to 46° F (2° to 8° C); don't freeze. Use vial within 30 days after removal to room temperature. If given by continuous infusion, dilute with D_5W, 0.9% NaCl injection, dextrose 5% in 0.9% NaCl injection, sterile water for injection, or lactated Ringer's. Refrigerate reconstituted solution and discard after 24 hr or if precipitates develop.

Incompatibilities: Alkaline solutions. Don't mix with other drugs.

Direct injection: Give undiluted drug by rapid injection.

Continuous infusion: Give diluted drug by infusion pump. Rates are highly individualized but range from 0.004 to 0.016 mg/kg/minute.

- Keep emergency respiratory support materials readily available.
- Remember that neuromuscular blockers don't alter consciousness or pain threshold.
- A nerve stimulator and train-of-four monitoring are recommended to confirm antagonism of neuromuscular blockade and recovery of muscle strength.
- Monitor respirations until patient recovers fully from neuromuscular blockade, as evidenced by tests of muscle strength (hand grip, head lift, and ability to cough).

sargramostim • Leukine

Class: ***colony-stimulating factor*** • *Pregnancy risk category C*

COMMON INDICATIONS AND DOSAGES

Acceleration of myeloid reconstitution after autologous bone marrow transplant in patients with malignant lymphoma or acute lymphoblastic leukemia; or during autologous bone marrow transplant in patients with Hodgkin's disease. *Adults:* 250 mcg/m^2 over 2 hr daily for 21 days, beginning 2 to 4 hr after transplant. In clinical studies, doses of 60 to 1,000 mcg/m^2/day have been used.

Failure of bone marrow transplant or delay of engraftment. *Adults:* 250 mcg/m^2/day over 2 hr for 14 days. May be repeated after 7 days without therapy if engraftment has not occurred. A third course at 500 mcg/m^2/day for 14 days may be tried after 7 days without therapy.

Neutrophil recovery after chemotherapy in acute myelogenous leukemia. *Adults:* 250 mcg/m^2/day over 4 hr on about day 11 (or 4 days after induction chemotherapy complete) if bone marrow at day 10 is hypoplastic with fewer than 5% blasts. If patient needs second cycle of induction chemotherapy, give about 4 days after completion of chemotherapy if bone marrow is hypoplastic with fewer than 5% blasts. Continue until absolute neutrophil count exceeds 1,500/mm^3 for 3 consecutive days or maximum of 42 days.

ADMINISTRATION

Available as lyophilized powder in 250- and 500-mcg, preservative-free, single-dose vials. Don't reuse single-dose vial. Reconstitute with 1 ml sterile water, directing stream against side of vial and swirling contents gently to minimize foaming. Don't use more than 6 hr after reconstitution or dilution; discard unused portion. Dilute in 0.9% NaCl solution to yield more than 10 mcg/ml. For less than 10 mcg/ml, add human albumin at final concentration of 0.1% to the 0.9% NaCl solution before adding sargramostim to prevent adsorption. For a final concentration of 0.1% human albumin, add 1 mg human albumin/1 ml 0.9% NaCl solution.

Incompatibilities: Don't add other drugs without specific compatibility data. Use only 0.9% NaCl solution for reconstitution and dilution.

Intermittent infusion: Infuse over 2 to 4 hr by a central line; don't use an in-line membrane filter.

Continuous infusion: Give dose over 24 hr.

SPECIAL CONSIDERATIONS

- To accelerate myeloid reconstitution, don't give within 24 hr of last chemotherapy dose or within 12 hr after last radiotherapy dose.
- Closely monitor patient's respiratory status during and immediately after infusion.
- Patient may develop transient rash and reactions at injection site.
- Check CBC with differential biweekly, including examination for blast cells.
- If blast cells appear or increase to 10% or more of WBC count, or if underlying disease progresses, stop therapy. If absolute neutrophil count exceeds 20,000 cells/mm^3 or WBC count exceeds 50,000 cells/mm^3, stop temporarily or reduce dose by half.

scopolamine hydrobromide (hyoscine hydrobromide)

Class: ***antimuscarinic*** *• Pregnancy risk category C*

Premedication to reduce secretions; treatment or prophylaxis for nausea. *Adults:* 300 to 600 mcg (0.3 to 0.6 mg) as single dose. *Children:* 6 mcg/kg (0.006 mg/kg) or 200 mcg/m^2 (0.2 mg/m^2) as single dose.
Premedication as anesthesia adjunct for amnesia. *Adults:* 320 to 650 mcg (0.32 to 0.65 mg) as single dose.
Premedication as anesthesia adjunct for sedation. *Adults:* 600 mcg (0.6 mg) given 30 minutes before procedure. May be repeated three or four times.

Available as 1-ml vials at 0.3 mg/ml, 0.4 mg/ml, and 1 mg/ml. Also available as 0.5-ml ampules at 0.4 mg/ml and 0.86 mg/ml. Store at room temperature; protect from light and freezing. For direct injection, dilute with sterile water for injection according to manufacturer's instructions.
Incompatibilities: Alkalies and methohexital sodium.
Direct injection: Inject diluted drug at ordered rate through patent I.V. line.

- Patient may develop confusion, agitation, excitement, and drowsiness even at typical doses. Reorient and reduce dose if needed.
- When given for pain without morphine or meperidine, drug can act as a stimulant, producing delirium.
- To control excitement or delirium, give small doses of short-acting barbiturate or benzodiazepine, or rectally infuse 2% solution of chloral hydrate. Respiratory depression may require mechanical ventilation. Maintain hydration and treat symptoms.
- Elderly patients and children are especially susceptible to adverse antimuscarinic effects.

secobarbital sodium

Class: ***anticonvulsant*** *• Pregnancy risk category D • Controlled substance schedule II*

Acute agitation in psychosis. *Adults:* No more than 250 mg initially, with additional doses given cautiously after 5 minutes if initial dose fails to produce desired response. Usually, 1.1 to 1.7 mg/kg produces moderate to heavy sedation, 2.2 mg/kg produces hypnosis, and 3.3 to 4.4 mg/kg calms extremely agitated patients. Maximum, 500 mg.
Status epilepticus. *Adults:* 250 to 350 mg.
Tetanic seizures. *Adults:* 5.5 mg/kg, repeated q 3 to 4 hr p.r.n. *Children:* 3 to 5 mg/kg or 12.5 mg/m^2.

Available as 1- and 2-ml prefilled syringe cartridges and 20-ml vials at 50 mg/ml. Refrigerate at 36° to 46° F (2° to 8° C). Protect from light. Discard if solution discolors or precipitates. Drug may be administered as supplied or diluted with sterile water for injection, 0.9% NaCl injection, or Ringer's injection.
Incompatibilities: Alkali-labile drugs (such as penicillin), atracurium, benzquinamide, chlorpromazine, cimetidine, clindamycin, codeine, diphenhydramine, droperidol, ephedrine, glycopyrrolate, hydrocortisone sodium succinate, isoproterenol, lactated Ringer's injection, levorphanol, metaraminol, methadone, methyldopate, norepinephrine, pancuronium, pentazocine, phenytoin, procaine, regular insulin, sodium bicarbonate, streptomycin, succinylcholine, and vancomycin.

- Slow administration usually prevents hypotension in hypertensive patients.
- Avoid extravasation. Use large veins to minimize irritation and risk of thrombosis.
- Monitor patient's vital signs and fluid balance. Maintain a patent airway and keep resuscitation and mechanical ventilation equipment available.
- Stop drug if skin eruptions occur; a potentially fatal reaction may follow.
- Elderly patients may have an increased risk of barbiturate-induced hypothermia, especially with high doses or acute overdose.

(continued)

◆ Also available in Canada. ◇ Available in Canada only.

COMMON INDICATIONS AND DOSAGES	ADMINISTRATION	SPECIAL CONSIDERATIONS
secobarbital sodium *(continued)* **Preoperative anesthesia.** *Adults:* 50 to 250 mg in divided doses. **Insomnia.** *Adults:* 100 to 150 mg.	***Direct injection:*** Inject drug slowly (no more than 50 mg/15 seconds) through a primary I.V. line that contains free-flowing, compatible solution.	

sodium bicarbonate

Class: ***alkalinizer*** • *Pregnancy risk category C*

COMMON INDICATIONS AND DOSAGES	ADMINISTRATION	SPECIAL CONSIDERATIONS
Dosage reflects severity of acidosis, test results, and patient's age, weight, and condition. **Cardiac arrest.** *Adults and children age 2 and older:* 200 to 300 mEq, with additional doses based on ABG measurements, if available. *Children under age 2:* 1 mEq/kg. If ABG and pH levels available, give further doses q 10 minutes, calculated in milliequivalents of $NaHCO_3$. Multiply 0.3 by body weight (kg), then multiply result by base deficit (mEq/L). If ABG and pH levels not available, give 1 mEq/kg q 10 minutes during arrest. Maximum, 8 mEq/kg daily. **Metabolic acidosis from chronic renal failure.** *Adults and older children:* 2 to 5 mEq/kg, with further doses determined by response to drug and lab results (total CO_2, blood pH). **Urinary alkalinization.** *Adults and children:* 2 to 5 mEq/kg.	Available as 5-ml (2.4 mEq) flip-top and pin-top vials of 4% solution (0.48 mEq/ml); 10-ml (5 mEq) disposable syringes of 4.2% solution (0.5 mEq/ml); 500-ml (297.5 mEq) containers of 5% solution (0.595 mEq/ml); 10-ml (8.9 mEq) ampules, 50-ml (44.6 mEq) ampules, and disposable syringes of 7.5% solution (0.892 mEq/ml); and 10-ml (10 mEq) disposable syringes, 50-ml (50 mEq) vials, and disposable syringes of 8.4% solution (1 mEq/ml). Store at room temperature, always below 104° F (40° C), and protect from freezing and heat. Discard if cloudy or precipitated. To dilute for infusion, follow manufacturer's instructions and use sterile water for injection or other standard electrolyte solution. In neonates and children under age 2, use 4.2% sodium bicarbonate solution or dilute 7.5% or 8.4% sodium bicarbonate solution 1:1 with D_5W. ***Incompatibilities:*** Alcohol 5% in dextrose 5%; amino acids; ascorbic acid injection; calcium salts; carmustine; cisplatin; codeine; corticotropin; dextrose 5% in lactated Ringer's injection; dobutamine; dopamine; epinephrine hydrochloride; fat emulsion 10%; glycopyrrolate; hydromorphone; regular insulin; Ionosol B, D, or G with invert sugar 10%; isoproterenol; labetalol; levorphanol; magnesium sulfate; meperidine; methadone; methicillin; methylprednisolone sodium succinate; metoclopramide; morphine; norepinephrine; penicillin G potassium; pentazocine; pentobarbital; phe-	• Overly rapid injection (10 ml/minute) can cause hypernatremia, decreased CSF pressure, intracranial hemorrhage, and severe alkalosis accompanied by hyperirritability or tetany. • Administer repeated small doses to avoid overdose and metabolic alkalosis. • In cardiac arrest, deliver manual or mechanical hyperventilation to lower partial pressure of carbon dioxide before giving drug. • Throughout therapy, monitor patient's ABGs, blood pH, serum bicarbonate, renal function (especially in long-term therapy), and urine pH (especially when drug is used for alkalinization). • Don't attempt full correction of bicarbonate deficit during first 24 hr of therapy. Doing so may cause metabolic alkalosis from delayed compensatory mechanisms.

nobarbital; procaine; promazine; Ringer's injection and lactated Ringer's injection; secobarbital; sodium lactate; streptomycin; succinylcholine chloride; thiopental; vancomycin; and vitamin B complex with vitamin C.
Direct injection: For cardiac arrest, flush I.V. line before and after use. For an adult, inject rapidly into patent primary I.V. line. For neonate or child under 2, inject ordered dose into patent primary I.V. line over 1 to 2 minutes.
Continuous infusion: For metabolic acidosis, flush I.V. line, infuse ordered amount of diluted drug over 4 to 8 hr, as ordered, and flush I.V. line when infusion complete.

sodium chloride • 0.45% Sodium Chloride Injection, 0.9% Sodium Chloride Injection, 3% Sodium Chloride Injection, 5% Sodium Chloride Injection

Class: ***sodium and chloride replacement*** • *Pregnancy risk category C*

Dosage depends on the disorder and on patient's age, weight, and fluid, electrolyte, and acid-base balance. For children, concentration and dosage are based on weight or body surface area.
Fluid and electrolyte replacement. *Adults:* Usually 1 L daily of 0.9% NaCl or 1 to 2 L daily of 0.45% NaCl.
Fluid and electrolyte replacement in ketoacidosis. *Children:* 0.225% or 0.3% NaCl.
Severe NaCl depletion requiring rapid replacement. *Adults:* 100 ml of 3% or 5% NaCl over 1 hr, with further doses based on serum electrolytes.
Adjunct to blood transfusions and hemodialysis. *Adults:* 0.9% NaCl.
Hyperosmolar diabetes. *Adults:* 0.45% NaCl.

Available in glass or flexible polyvinyl chloride containers. Solutions of 0.45% NaCl come in 500- and 1,000-ml containers; 0.9% NaCl in 50-, 100-, 150-, 250-, 500-, and 1,000-ml containers; and 3% and 5% NaCl in 500-ml containers. Solutions of 0.9% NaCl also supplied in 25-, 50-, and 100-ml containers as diluents for drug delivery. Store at room temperature.
Incompatibilities: Amphotericin B, benzquinamide, chlordiazepoxide, diazepam, fat emulsion, methylprednisolone sodium succinate, and phenytoin sodium.
Direct injection: Use only as drug diluent.
Intermittent infusion: Use only as drug diluent.
Continuous infusion: Infuse through a peripheral or central vein at ordered rate. Infuse 3% or 5% solutions through a large vein at no more than 100 ml/hr. Avoid extravasation. Watch infusion site carefully for signs of phlebitis.

- If fluid overload occurs, stop infusion and take corrective measures.
- Monitor patient's serum electrolytes, especially sodium and potassium. Also check chloride and bicarbonate levels.
- Tell patient to report immediately pain at I.V. site.

◆ Also available in Canada. ◇ Available in Canada only.

COMMON INDICATIONS AND DOSAGES	ADMINISTRATION	SPECIAL CONSIDERATIONS

sodium lactate (1/6 M sodium lactate)

Class: ***systemic alkalinizer*** • *Pregnancy risk category C*

Mild to moderate metabolic acidosis. *Adults:* To calculate suggested dosage in ml, multiply 0.8 by body weight (lb), then multiply result by 60 minus the plasma CO_2 level. Actual dosage depends on severity of acidosis, test results (plasma glucose, serum electrolyte levels), and patient's age, weight, and underlying disorder.

Available in 500-, and 1,000-ml containers with sodium and lactate ions, each at 167 mEq/L. Also available as 10-ml flip-top vials with 5 mEq/ml. Store at 104° F (40° C) or below. Protect from freezing and extreme heat. Discard any unused portions. For infusion, dilute in ordered volume of solution if desired concentration is not commercially available.
Incompatibilities: Sodium bicarbonate.
Continuous infusion: Infuse diluted solution through primary I.V. line or piggyback at ordered rate. Don't exceed 300 ml/hr in adults.

- One g of sodium lactate provides 8.9 mEq of sodium and 8.9 mEq of lactate.
- When giving sodium lactate, determine needed volume of I.V. fluid by calculating patient's maintenance or replacement requirements.
- Carefully monitor patient's plasma glucose, fluid and electrolyte balance, and acid-base balance throughout therapy.
- Stop infusion if adverse reaction occurs. Evaluate patient, begin symptomatic treatment, and save remaining solution for examination, if necessary.

streptokinase • Kabikinase, Streptase♦

Class: ***thrombolytic*** • *Pregnancy risk category C*

Pulmonary embolism, deep vein thrombosis, arterial embolism or thrombosis. *Adults:* Loading dose 250,000 IU; maintenance dose 100,000 IU/hr.
Acute, obstructing coronary artery thrombi in evolving acute MI. *Adults:* 1.5 million IU over 60 minutes.
Arteriovenous cannula occlusion. *Adults:* 250,000 IU in 2 ml of I.V. solution.

Available in powder form in varying strengths and in 50-ml infusion bottle of 1.5 million IU. Store unopened vials at room temperature. For cannula clearance, reconstitute using 2 ml of 0.9% NaCl injection or dextrose 5% injection for each 250,000 IU of drug. Add diluent slowly, aiming at side of vial. Roll vial gently. Slight flocculation okay, but solutions with many particles should be discarded. For infusion, reconstitute with 0.9% NaCl injection or dextrose 5% injection. Further dilute, usually to 45 ml (loading dose infusion) or a multiple of 45 ml to maximum of 500 ml (continuous infusion), with the same solution used for reconstitution. Infuse through a 0.22- or 0.45-micron filter using a volumetric or syringe pump. Store reconstituted solutions at 36° to 39° F (2° to 4° C); discard after 24 hr.
Incompatibilities: Dextrans. Don't mix with other drugs.

- Before starting therapy, obtain a blood sample to determine patient's thrombin time, APTT, PT, hematocrit, and platelet count.
- Because streptococci (source of streptokinase) are common, a loading dose is used to neutralize the antibodies present in many patients. Loading dose shouldn't exceed 1 million IU.
- Continue maintenance infusion for 24 hr for pulmonary embolism, 24 to 72 hr for arterial embolism or thrombosis, and 72 hr for deep-vein thrombosis.
- Monitor patient's vital signs and clotting status.
- Watch for bleeding, and avoid noncompressible puncture sites.
- In hemorrhage, stop drug immediately. Give whole blood (fresh, preferably), packed RBCs, and cryo-

Direct injection: To clear obstruction from arteriovenous cannulas, use an infusion pump to slowly deliver reconstituted drug into each occluded cannula over 25 to 35 minutes. Then clamp off the cannulas. After 2 hr, aspirate contents of cannulas and flush with 0.9% NaCl. Reconnect cannulas.
Continuous infusion: For loading dose in pulmonary embolism, deep-vein thrombosis, or arterial embolism or thrombosis, give diluted loading dose over 30 minutes through peripheral I.V. line. Set rate at 30 ml/hr (for 750,000 IU vial) or 90 ml/hr (for 250,000 IU vial) with dilution equaling 45 ml. For maintenance dose, set infusion pump as specified. For coronary artery thrombi, give diluted drug through a peripheral I.V. line as specified. No maintenance dose required.

precipitate or fresh frozen plasma if needed. Don't use dextrans. Aminocaproic acid may be administered in an emergency, although effectiveness as antidote hasn't been established.

streptozocin • Zanosar◆

Class: ***antineoplastic*** • *Pregnancy risk category C*

Dosage depends on renal, hematologic, and hepatic response and tolerance to drug.
Metastatic islet cell carcinoma of pancreas. *Adults:* 500 mg/m^2 daily for 5 consecutive days q 6 weeks. Or, 1 g/m^2 in single weekly dose for 2 weeks; then, if necessary, up to 1.5 g/m^2 weekly.

Follow facility protocol for handling chemotherapy drugs. Available as powder in 1-g vials. Store vials at 36° to 46° F (2° to 8° C) and protect from light. Reconstitute with 9.5 ml of dextrose 5% injection or 0.9% NaCl injection to yield 100 mg/ml. If kept at room temperature, use reconstituted drug within 12 hr. Discard if color changes from pale gold to dark brown, indicating decomposition. Dilute reconstituted drug with dextrose 5% injection, 0.9% NaCl, or dextrose 5% in 0.9% NaCl injection. Usual dilution for intermittent infusion is 100 mg/ml of streptozocin solution added to 10 to 200 ml of dextrose 5% or 0.9% NaCl injection.
Incompatibilities: None reported.
Direct injection: Rapidly inject reconstituted drug through port of primary I.V. line that contains free-flowing, compatible solution.
Intermittent infusion: Infuse diluted drug over ordered duration (usually 15 minutes to 6 hr) via I.V. line that contains free-flowing, compatible solution.

- Keep I.V. dextrose available, especially with first dose, because of risk of hypoglycemia.
- If extravasation occurs, stop infusion. Apply cold compresses and elevate limb. Complete administration in another vein.
- Monitor patient's BUN, serum creatinine, serum electrolytes, urine creatinine levels, and urinalysis before and at least weekly during therapy. After each course, check weekly for 4 to 6 weeks. Watch for proteinuria, commonly the first sign of dose-related, cumulative nephrotoxicity.
- Monitor patient's CBC and liver function studies weekly during and after therapy.
- Encourage patient to drink plenty of fluids to help clear active metabolites.

(continued)

◆ Also available in Canada. ◇ Available in Canada only.

COMMON INDICATIONS AND DOSAGES	ADMINISTRATION	SPECIAL CONSIDERATIONS
streptozocin *(continued)*	***Continuous infusion:*** Infuse diluted drug over ordered duration. Continuous 5-day I.V. infusions have been given, but prolonged continuous administration may cause CNS toxicity.	

succinylcholine chloride • Anectine♦, Anectine Flo-Pack♦, Quelicin

Class: ***skeletal muscle relaxant*** • *Pregnancy risk category C*

Skeletal muscle relaxant for short procedures, such as endotracheal intubation, endoscopy, and orthopedic manipulations. *Adults:* 0.6 mg/kg (range, 0.3 to 1.1 mg/kg), with subsequent doses based on response to drug. *Children:* 1 to 2 mg/kg, with subsequent doses based on first dose.

Skeletal muscle relaxant for prolonged surgical procedures. *Adults:* 2.5 to 4.3 mg/minute (range, 0.5 to 10 mg/minute) by continuous infusion (preferred). Or, 0.3 to 1.1 mg/kg by intermittent injection with further doses at 0.04 to 0.07 mg/kg p.r.n. to maintain relaxation.

Electroshock therapy. *Adults:* 10 to 30 mg given about 1 minute before shock administered. Dosage must be individualized to patient size and condition.

Available in 10-ml vials at 20 or 100 mg/ml, 10- and 20-ml ampules at 50 mg/ml, and as powder in 5-ml unit-dose vials of 100 mg, 500 mg, or 1 g . Reconstitute powder with compatible diluent, such as dextrose 5% injection or 0.9% NaCl, according to manufacturer's instructions. Store solutions at 36° to 46° F (2° to 8° C). Multidose vials stable for 14 days at room temperature. Powders do not require refrigeration. For direct injection, use prepared solution, or dilute with compatible solution to yield concentration, volume, and dosage ordered. For continuous infusion, dilute to 1 to 2 mg/ml. Add 1 g of powder, 10 ml of solution (100 mg/ml), or 20 ml of solution (500 mg/ml) to 1 L or 500 ml of compatible diluent, such as dextrose 5% injection, dextrose 5% in 0.9% NaCl, 0.9% NaCl, or 1/6 M sodium lactate. Or add 500 mg of powder, 5 ml of solution (100 mg/ml), or 10 ml of solution (50 mg/ml) to 500 or 250 ml of diluent to yield 1 or 2 mg/ml succinylcholine, respectively. Discard unused solutions within 24 hr.

Incompatibilities: Barbiturates, nafcillin, and sodium bicarbonate. Decomposes in solutions with pH above 4.5.

Direct injection: Inject ordered amount of commercially prepared or diluted drug over 10 to 30 seconds into a primary I.V. line that contains free-flowing, compatible solution.

Continuous infusion: Infuse diluted drug at 2.5 mg/minute through I.V. line that contains free-flowing, compatible solution, then adjust to 0.5 to 10 mg/minute, depending on patient response.

- Give 10 mg test dose I.V. to determine patient's sensitivity and recovery time, as ordered.
- Premedicate with atropine, scopolamine, or thiopental sodium, as ordered.
- Give drug after unconsciousness has been induced.
- To avoid overdose and detect nondepolarizing neuromuscular blockade, monitor neuromuscular function with a peripheral nerve stimulator when giving drug by infusion.
- When administering succinylcholine, keep emergency resuscitation equipment available.

sufentanil citrate • Sufenta

Classes: ***analgesic, anesthetic*** *• Pregnancy risk category C • Controlled substance schedule II*

Dosage depends on concurrent drug administration (especially anesthetics), type and expected length of surgery, and patient variables.

Adjunct in anesthesia. *Adults:* 1 to 2 mcg/kg (low initial dose), with supplemental doses of 10 to 25 mcg p.r.n. to maintain analgesia or anesthesia. Or 2 to 8 mcg/kg (moderate initial dose), with supplemental doses of 10 to 50 mcg p.r.n. If used with nitrous oxide and oxygen for procedures of 8 hr or longer, total dosage is 1 mcg/kg/hr or less.

Primary anesthesia. *Adults:* 8 to 30 mcg/kg with 100% oxygen, followed by 25 to 50 mcg p.r.n. to maintain anesthesia. Loading dose followed by continuous infusion is recommended for prolonged procedures. *Children under age 12 undergoing CV surgery:* 10 to 25 mcg/kg with 100% oxygen, followed by 25 to 50 mcg p.r.n. to maintain anesthesia. Maximum, 1 to 2 mcg/kg.

Available as preservative-free 1-, 2-, and 5-ml ampules with 50 mcg/ml. Store at room temperature, always below 104° F (40° C). Protect from light and freezing. For continuous infusion, dilute with compatible solution.

Incompatibilities: None reported.

Direct injection: Inject slowly, especially large doses, over 1 to 2 minutes. Use a 1-ml syringe for small doses.

Continuous infusion: After loading dose, infuse 1 mcg/kg or less over 1 hr.

- Keep resuscitation equipment available during therapy.
- Monitor patient's breathing for at least 1 hr after dose.
- Closely monitor for signs of withdrawal when stopping drug after prolonged use.
- High doses may produce muscle rigidity, which can be reversed with neuromuscular blockers.
- For overdose, maintain airway and provide respiratory support. Give naloxone as needed to reverse respiratory depression. Give I.V. fluids and vasopressors, as ordered, to maintain blood pressure and neuromuscular blockers to relieve muscle rigidity.

teniposide (VM-26) • Vumon ◆

Class: ***antineoplastic*** *• Pregnancy risk category D*

Malignant lymphoma. *Adults:* As single therapy, 30 $mg/m^2/day$ q 5 days, 30 $mg/m^2/day$ for 10 days, or 50 to 100 $mg/m^2/day$ once weekly. In combination therapy,

Follow facility protocol for handling chemotherapy drugs. Available as 5-ml ampules that contain 50 mg. Refrigerate and protect from light. For infusion, dilute to 0.1 mg/ml, 0.2 mg/ml, 0.4 mg/ml, or 1 mg/ml with D_5W or 0.9% NaCl. In

- Keep emergency equipment available in case of anaphylaxis.
- Monitor patient's blood pressure before, during, and after infusion.

(continued)

◆ Also available in Canada. ◇ Available in Canada only.

COMMON INDICATIONS AND DOSAGES	ADMINISTRATION	SPECIAL CONSIDERATIONS
teniposide *(continued)* 60 to 70 mg/m^2/day once weekly. **Neuroblastoma.** *Adults:* As single therapy, 130 to 180 mg/m^2/day once weekly. In combination therapy, 100 mg/m^2 daily q 21 days. **Acute lymphocytic leukemia.** *Adults:* 165 mg/m^2/day twice weekly in combination therapy. **Acute lymphocytic leukemia induction therapy in children.** *Children:* Optimum dose unknown. Manufacturer reports I.V. protocol using 165 mg/m^2 teniposide and cytarabine 300 mg/m^2 twice weekly for 8 or 9 doses.	glass container, solutions of 100 to 200 mcg/ml stable 24 hr in D_5W or sterile water; solutions of 100 to 400 mcg/ml stable 24 hr in 0.9% NaCl. In plastic container, solution of 100 mcg/ml stable 8 hr in 0.9% NaCl or sterile water. Drug unstable in plastic containers in solutions over 100 mcg/ml; concentrate may soften or crack plastic. Use glass bottles and administration sets that don't contain polyvinyl chloride. Solution may appear slightly opalescent from surfactants. ***Incompatibilities:*** Heparin sodium. ***Continuous infusion:*** Administer over at least 45 minutes to avoid hypotension. Use distal rather than major veins and a new site for each infusion.	• Monitor patient's CBC and liver function tests during and after treatment. • Watch for phlebitis at injection site. • Stop infusion and notify doctor if systolic pressure falls below 90 mm Hg. • If extravasation occurs, apply ice to the area. Injecting a corticosteroid and irrigating with copious amounts of 0.9% NaCl may decrease swelling.

terbutaline sulfate • Brethine, Bricanyl

Class: ***tocolytic*** • *Pregnancy risk category B*

COMMON INDICATIONS AND DOSAGES	ADMINISTRATION	SPECIAL CONSIDERATIONS
Premature labor (after 20 weeks' gestation). *Adults:* 10 mcg/minute, increased by 10 mcg/minute q 20 minutes until contractions stop or you reach maximum rate of 80 mcg/minute. After 30 to 60 minutes with no contractions, reduce dose by 5 mcg/minute and maintain at minimum effective rate for 4 hr. Then switch to oral form.	Available in 2-ml ampules at 1 mg/ml. Store ampules at room temperature and protect from light. For infusion, add 10 mg of drug to 250 ml D_5W, 0.9% NaCl, or 0.45% NaCl to yield 40 mcg/ml. Solution is clear and colorless; discard if discolored. ***Incompatibilities:*** Bleomycin sulfate. ***Continuous infusion:*** Before administration, start a primary I.V. infusion. Hang terbutaline as secondary I.V. line to allow immediate discontinuation if adverse effects occur. Use an infusion pump.	• To reduce risk of pulmonary edema, avoid using NaCl as a diluent when possible. • Monitor patient's serum potassium and glucose levels closely during infusion. • Continuously monitor maternal and fetal cardiac status. • After delivery, observe neonate for hypoglycemia.

theophylline

Class: ***bronchodilator*** • *Pregnancy risk category C*

Acute bronchial asthma and reversible bronchospasm from chronic bronchitis and emphysema in patients not currently receiving theophylline. Loading dose: 4.7 mg/kg. Maintenance dose based on population. *Adult nonsmokers:* 0.55 mg/kg/hr for first 12 hr, then 0.39 mg/kg/hr. *Adult smokers:* 0.79 mg/kg/hr for first 12 hr, then 0.63 mg/kg/hr. *Elderly patients and those with cor pulmonale:* 0.47 mg/kg/hr for first 12 hr, then 0.24 mg/kg/hr. *Patients with heart failure or liver failure:* 0.39 mg/kg/hr for first 12 hr, then 0.08 to 0.16 mg/kg/hr. *Children ages 6 months to 9 years:* 0.95 mg/kg/hr for first 12 hr, then 0.79 mg/kg/hr. *Children ages 9 to 16:* 0.79 mg/kg/hr for first 12 hr, then 0.63 mg/kg/hr.
Note: If patient receiving theophylline, dosage form, amount, time, and administration rate of last dose determine initial dose. Ideally, initial dose deferred until serum theophylline level known.

Available premixed as 0.4 mg/ml in 1,000 ml D_5W, 0.8 mg/ml in 500 ml or 1,000 ml D_5W, 1.6 mg/ml in 250 ml or 500 ml D_5W, 2 mg/ml in 100 ml D_5W, 3.2 mg/ml in 250 ml D_5W, and 4 mg/ml in 50 or 100 ml D_5W. Store at room temperature and protect from freezing and light. Inspect for precipitates before use.
Incompatibilities: Cimetidine, hetastarch, and phenytoin.
Intermittent infusion: Give slowly at no more than 20 mg/minute.
Continuous infusion: Adjust infusion rate to deliver prescribed amount each hr.

- Base dosage on lean body weight and serum theophylline levels. Optimum therapeutic range is 10 to 20 mcg/ml.
- Expect to reduce dosage in neonates, older adults, and patients with influenza, COPD, or cardiac, renal, or hepatic dysfunction because these patients show reduced drug clearance.
- Monitor patient's vital signs during infusion.
- Ask patient about past or present use of tobacco or marijuana because both affect body's response to theophylline.

thiamine hydrochloride (vitamin B_1)

Class: ***nutritional supplement*** • *Pregnancy risk category A (C if greater than RDA)*

Severe thiamine deficiency (beriberi). *Adults:* 5 to 100 mg t.i.d. *Children:* 10 to 25 mg daily.
Wernicke's encephalopathy. *Adults:* 100

Available as 1-ml ampules, vials, and prefilled syringes and as 2-, 10- and 30-ml vials, each containing 100 mg/ml. Dilute, if necessary, in 0.9% NaCl, D_5W, or a combination of these solutions. Refrigerate drug and protect from freezing and light.

- Never give thiamine by direct injection because of risk of anaphylaxis.

(continued)

COMMON INDICATIONS AND DOSAGES	ADMINISTRATION	SPECIAL CONSIDERATIONS
thiamine hydrochloride *(continued)* mg followed by 50 to 100 mg daily. **During total parenteral nutrition.** *Adults:* 3 to 21 mg daily.	***Incompatibilities:*** Alkali carbonates, amobarbital, barbiturates, citrates, erythromycin estolate, kanamycin sulfate, phenobarbital, streptomycin, and sulfites. ***Intermittent infusion:*** Give ordered amount at less than 20 mg/minute. Use infusion pump for high doses. ***Continuous infusion:*** Add ordered dose to maintenance fluids and infuse at less than 20 mg/minute.	• Use I.V. route only if oral or I.M. administration isn't feasible. • Tell patient that adverse effects usually occur after repeated doses of thiamine.

thiopental sodium • Pentothal♦

Class: ***anesthetic*** • *Pregnancy risk category C* • *Controlled substance schedule III*

COMMON INDICATIONS AND DOSAGES	ADMINISTRATION	SPECIAL CONSIDERATIONS
Dosage individualized based on desired depth of anesthesia, other drugs in use, and patient variables. **Sole anesthesia for brief (15-minute) procedures.** *Adults:* 50 to 75 mg q 20 to 40 seconds until anesthesia established, then 25 to 50 mg p.r.n. *Children age 15 and under:* 3 to 5 mg/kg, then 1 mg/kg p.r.n. **Induction of general anesthesia before administration of other agents.** *Adults:* 3 to 4 mg/kg. **Supplement to regional anesthesia.** *Adults:* 25 to 50 mg p.r.n. **Hypnosis during balanced anesthesia with other agents for analgesia or muscle relaxation.** *Adults:* 50 to 100 mg p.r.n. **Seizure control during or after inhalation or local anesthesia.** *Adults:* 75 to 125 mg as soon as possible after seizure starts.	Available as 250-, 400-, and 500-mg syringes; 500- and 1,000-mg vials; and 500-mg, 1-g, 2.5-g, 5-g, and 10-g containers in kits. Store at room temperature before reconstituting. Reconstitute with 20 to 500 ml sterile water for injection, 0.9% NaCl, or D_5W to yield 0.2% to 5% (usually 2.5%). Compatible solutions include dextrose 2.5% in water, D_5W, 0.45% NaCl, Dextran 6% in D_5W or 0.9% NaCl, and 1/6 M sodium lactate. Refrigerate reconstituted solutions and discard after 24 hr. Drug contains no bacteriostatic agents. ***Incompatibilities:*** Amikacin, benzquinamide, cephapirin, chlorpromazine, codeine, dextrose 10% in water or 0.9% NaCl, dimenhydrinate, diphenhydramine, ephedrine, fructose 10%, glycopyrrolate, human fibrinolysin, hydromorphone, insulin (regular), invert sugar 5% and 10% in 0.9% NaCl, levorphanol, meperidine, metaraminol, methadone, morphine, norepinephrine, Normosol solutions (except Normosol-R), penicillin G potassium, prochlorperazine, promazine, promethazine, Ringer's injection, lactated Ringer's solution, sodium bicarbonate, and succinylcholine. ***Direct injection:*** Inject ordered dose through tubing of I.V. line that contains free-flowing, compatible solution. Repeat as	• Only staff specially trained to give anesthetics and manage their adverse effects should administer. • Monitor patient's serum drug levels and signs and symptoms. Prolonged continuous infusion may cause respiratory and circulatory depression. • Patients tolerant to other barbiturates or alcohol may require higher doses. • Tell patient that psychomotor skills may be impaired for 24 hr, to use caution when operating machinery, and to avoid CNS depressants.

Increased intracranial pressure in neurosurgery (with adequate ventilation). *Adults:* 1.5 to 3.5 mg/kg, repeated p.r.n. **Narcoanalysis and narcosynthesis in psychiatric patients.** *Adults:* 100 mg/minute (2.5% solution) until patient is drowsy but can still speak and respond.

needed to maintain anesthesia.
Continuous infusion: Infuse 0.2% to 0.4% solution (200 to 400 mg/100 ml) at less than 50 ml/hr.

thiotepa (TESPA, TSPA) • Thioplex

Class: ***neoplastic*** • *Pregnancy risk category D*

Dosage reflects response to drug and appearance or degree of toxicity. Maintenance doses reflect hematologic studies. **Adenocarcinoma of breast and ovary, lymphoma, bronchogenic carcinoma (palliative treatment).** *Adults and children age 12 and over:* 0.3 to 0.4 mg/kg q 1 to 4 weeks.

Follow facility protocol for handling chemotherapy drugs. Available as powder in 15-mg vials. Reconstitute with 1.5 ml sterile water for injection to yield 10 mg/ml. Refrigerate powder and reconstituted solution at 36° to 46° F (2° to 8° C) and protect from light. Reconstituted solution stable 5 days if refrigerated (0.5 mg/ml solution in Ringer's injection stable 15 days refrigerated or at room temperature). For infusion, dilute in NaCl injection, dextrose injection, dextrose and NaCl injection, Ringer's injection, or lactated Ringer's injection. Discard if solution becomes grossly opaque or contains precipitates.
Incompatibilities: None reported.
Direct injection: Inject rapidly using a 21G or 23G needle.
Intermittent infusion: Start a primary I.V. line or use infusion port of existing primary line to give diluted drug over ordered duration.

- Drug is highly toxic with a low therapeutic index; many adverse effects are unavoidable.
- Before and during therapy, monitor patient's WBC count, platelet count, BUN, hematocrit, AST, ALT, bilirubin, creatinine, lactic dehydrogenase, and uric acid levels.
- Provide adequate oral hydration to help prevent or delay uric acid nephropathy. Give allopurinol as ordered.
- At first sign of sudden, large drop in WBC (particularly granulocyte) or platelet counts, stop drug or reduce dosage, as ordered, to prevent irreversible myelosuppression.

ticarcillin disodium • Ticar◆

Class: ***antibiotic*** • *Pregnancy risk category B*

Septicemia; infections of respiratory tract, skin, soft tissue, abdomen, pelvis (female), and genital tract. *Adults and children:* 200 to 300 mg/kg/day in divid-

Available as 1-, 3-, and 6-g vials and as 3-g piggyback bottles of white to pale yellow powder or lyophilized cake. Store at room temperature. To reconstitute, add 4 ml 0.9% NaCl, D_5W, or lactated Ringer's solution for each gram of drug.

- Obtain specimens for culture and sensitivity tests before giving first dose.
- Give drug at least 1 hr before bacteriostatic antibiotics.

(continued)

◆ Also available in Canada. ◇ Available in Canada only.

COMMON INDICATIONS AND DOSAGES	ADMINISTRATION	SPECIAL CONSIDERATIONS
ticarcillin disodium *(continued)* ed doses q 4 to 6 hr. *Neonates who weigh 4.5 lb (2 kg) and over:* 75 mg/kg q 8 hr for first week after birth; then 100 mg/kg q 8 hr. **UTI (complicated).** *Adults and children:* 150 to 200 mg/kg/day in divided doses q 4 to 6 hr. **UTI (uncomplicated).** *Adults and children who weigh more than 88 lb (40 kg):* 1 g q 6 hr. *Children who weigh up to 88 lb:* 50 to 100 mg/kg/day in divided doses q 6 to 8 hr. **Dosage adjustment.** Adjust dosage if patient has renal impairment.	Solution should be clear and colorless or pale yellow. Refrigerate or use within 30 minutes. For continuous infusion, dilute further with 10 to 100 ml of compatible I.V. solution. Solutions diluted with sterile water for injection, D_5W, 0.9% NaCl, dextrose 5% in 0.225% or 0.45% NaCl, or 5% alcohol (10 to 50 mg/ml) are stable 72 hr at room temperature. Stable 48 hr at room temperature if diluted with Ringer's injection or lactated Ringer's solution (10 to 100 mg/ml). All solutions stable 14 days when refrigerated at 39° F (4° C), but don't use for multiple doses if stored longer than 72 hr. ***Incompatibilities:*** Aminoglycosides. ***Intermittent infusion:*** To minimize vein irritation, use solutions of 50 mg/ml or less and infuse slowly: 30 minutes to 2 hr for adult or 10 to 20 minutes for neonate. ***Continuous infusion:*** Add total daily dosage of reconstituted drug to ordered volume of compatible solution. Adjust rate to deliver required 24-hr volume.	• Monitor patient's electrolyte levels (especially potassium) and cardiac status frequently, because high sodium content of drug may cause electrolyte imbalance and arrhythmias. • Monitor patient's neurologic status. • If diarrhea persists during treatment, obtain stool culture to rule out pseudomembranous colitis.

ticarcillin disodium and clavulanate potassium • Timentin

Class: ***antibiotic*** • *Pregnancy risk category B*

COMMON INDICATIONS AND DOSAGES	ADMINISTRATION	SPECIAL CONSIDERATIONS
Systemic infection and UTI, especially caused by beta-lactamase-producing organisms. *Adults who weigh more than 132 lb (60 kg):* 3.1 g ticarcillin (as 3 g ticarcillin and 100 mg clavulanic acid) q 4 to 6 hr. *Adults who weigh less than 132 lb and children age 12 and over:* 200 to 300 mg/kg/day in divided doses q 4 to 6 hr. **Dosage adjustment.** If patient has renal impairment, dosage reflects creatinine clearance.	Available as vials that contain 3.1 g (3 g ticarcillin and 100 mg clavulanic acid) of white to pale yellow powder. Also available in pharmacy-mixed reconstituted piggyback infusion bottles. Store powder at 70° to 75° F (21° to 24° C). To reconstitute, add 13 ml sterile water or 0.9% NaCl to yield 200 mg/ml ticarcillin and 6.7 mg/ml clavulanate. Solution potent 6 hr at room temperature, up to 72 hr if refrigerated. Before infusion, dilute in 50 to 100 ml 0.9% NaCl, D_5W, or lactated Ringer's solution. Solutions of 10 to 100 mg ticarcillin/ml using lactated Ringer's or 0.9% NaCl stay potent 24 hr at room temperature, 7 days if refrigerated. Those using D_5W stay potent 24 hr at room temperature, 3 days if refrigerated.	• Obtain specimens for culture and sensitivity tests before giving first dose. • Before giving drug, ask if patient has had allergic reactions to penicillin. • Monitor patient's serum sodium and potassium levels closely. Drug has a high sodium content, and clavulanic acid contributes about 0.15 mEq (6 mg) of potassium per 100 mg. • Monitor patient's CBC, PT, and bleeding times. Watch for bleeding tendencies and discontinue drug if bleeding occurs. • If patient undergoes dialysis, give drug after dialysis

Incompatibilities: Aminoglycosides and sodium bicarbonate. Don't use with other anti-infective drugs.
Intermittent infusion: Give diluted dose over 30 minutes by infusion through Y-tubing or piggyback. Temporarily stop primary solutions during administration.

session complete.
- If diarrhea persists during therapy, obtain stool culture to rule out pseudomembranous colitis.

tirofiban hydrochloride • Aggrastat

Class: ***platelet aggregation inhibitor*** • *Pregnancy risk category B*

Acute coronary syndrome. *Adults:* 0.4 mcg/kg/minute loading dose, then continuous infusion of 0.1 mcg/kg/minute. Continue infusion through angiography and for 12 to 24 hr after angioplasty or atherectomy.
Dosage adjustment. Adjust dosage if patient's creatinine clearance is below 30 ml/minute.

Available as 50-ml vials (250 mcg/ml) or 500-ml premixed vials (50 mcg/ml). Dilute 50-ml injection vials to same strength as 500-ml premixed vial by withdrawing and discarding 100 ml from 500-ml bag of sterile 0.9% NaCl or D_5W and replacing it with 100 ml of tirofiban injection (from two 50-ml vials) or withdraw 50 ml from 250-ml bag of sterile 0.9% NaCl or D_5W and replace it with 50 ml of tirofiban injection. If particles visible or leaks occur, discard solution. Discard unused solution 24 hr after infusion starts. Store drug at room temperature and protect from light.
Incompatibilities: Don't give drug with other medications except heparin. Heparin and tirofiban can be given through the same I.V. catheter.
Continuous infusion: Give I.V. loading dose over 30 minutes, followed by continuous infusion at ordered rate.

- Use cautiously in patients with increased risk of bleeding, including those with hemorrhagic retinopathy or platelet count below 150,000/mm^3.
- Check patient's hemoglobin, hematocrit, and platelet counts before therapy, 6 hr after loading dose, and at least daily during therapy.
- Monitor patient for bleeding. Minimize injections and avoid noncompressible I.V. sites.
- Give drug with concomitant aspirin and heparin.

tobramycin sulfate • Nebcin◆

Class: ***antibiotic*** • *Pregnancy risk category D*

Serious bacterial infection (dosage based on actual pretreatment body weight). *Adults:* 3 mg/kg daily in equal doses q 8 hr. If infection life-threatening, may increase to 5 mg/kg daily in 3 or 4 equal doses. *Children:* 6 to 7.5 mg/kg daily in 3 or 4 equal doses. *Neonates un-*

Available as clear, colorless solution in rubber-stopped vials containing 80 mg/2 ml or 20 mg/2 ml and as pediatric injection in 2-ml vials containing 10 mg/ml. Also available as dry powder (1.2 g) to be reconstituted with 30 ml sterile water for injection to yield 40 mg/ml. For adults, dilute calculated dose in 50 to 100 ml 0.9% NaCl or dextrose 5% injection. For children, dilution depends on patient needs. Diluted solution sta-

- Treatment usually lasts 7 to 10 days.
- Obtain specimens for culture and sensitivity tests before giving first dose.
- Check serum drug levels, especially in neonates, elderly patients, and those with renal impairment. Therapeutic concentration is 4 to 10 mcg/ml.

(continued)

◆ Also available in Canada. ◇ Available in Canada only.

COMMON INDICATIONS AND DOSAGES	ADMINISTRATION	SPECIAL CONSIDERATIONS
tobramycin sulfate *(continued)* *der 1 week old:* 4 mg/kg daily or less in equal doses q 12 hr. **Acute pelvic inflammatory disease.** *Adults:* 2 mg/kg, then 1.5 mg/kg q 8 hr. **Dosage adjustment.** Adjust dosage if patient has renal impairment.	ble 24 hr at room temperature. ***Incompatibilities:*** Beta-lactam antibiotics; cefamandole; cefoperazone; cefotaxime sodium; dextrose 5% in Isolyte E, M, or P; heparin sodium; and I.V. solutions that contain alcohol. Manufacturer recommends against mixing with other drugs. ***Intermittent infusion:*** Infuse diluted solution over 20 to 60 minutes.	• Monitor patient's renal function by obtaining periodic BUN and serum creatinine levels.

tolazoline hydrochloride • Priscoline

Class: ***pulmonary antihypertensive*** • *Pregnancy risk category C*

COMMON INDICATIONS AND DOSAGES	ADMINISTRATION	SPECIAL CONSIDERATIONS
Persistent pulmonary hypertension in newborn. *Neonates:* 1 to 2 mg/kg via scalp vein, followed by 1 to 2 mg/kg/hr.	Available as 4-ml ampules at 25 mg/ml. Store at room temperature of 59° to 86° F (15° to 30° C) and protect from light. For direct injection or continuous infusion, dilute with compatible I.V. solution according to manufacturer's instructions. ***Incompatibilities:*** None reported. ***Direct injection:*** Inject diluted drug into scalp vein over 10 minutes. ***Continuous infusion:*** Infuse diluted drug at 1 to 2 mg/kg/hr.	• Drug stimulates gastric secretion and may activate stress ulcers. Pretreatment with antacids may prevent GI bleeding. • Response, if it occurs, can be expected within 30 minutes of initial dose. • Monitor patient's blood pH for acidosis, which may decrease drug's effect. • Monitor patient's vital signs, oxygenation, and fluid and electrolyte status.

topotecan hydrochloride • Hycamtin

Class: ***antineoplastic*** • *Pregnancy risk category D*

COMMON INDICATIONS AND DOSAGES	ADMINISTRATION	SPECIAL CONSIDERATIONS
Metastatic carcinoma of the ovary after failure of initial or subsequent chemotherapy. *Adults:* 1.5 mg/m^2 daily for 5 consecutive days, starting on day 1 of a 21-day cycle. At least four cycles should be given.	Follow facility protocol for handling chemotherapy drugs. Available in 4-mg single-dose vials. Store at controlled room temperature of 68° to 77° F (20° to 25° C) and protect from light. Reconstitute each 4-mg vial with 4 ml of sterile water for injection and use immediately. Further dilute appropriate volume of reconstituted solution with either 0.9% NaCl intravenous infusion or 5% dextrose I.V. infusion before administration. Diluted solution stable 24 hr at room temperature and	• Check patient's CBC often. • Make sure baseline neutrophil count is above 1,500 cells/mm^3 and platelet count is above 100,000 cells/mm^3 before giving first dose. • Give granulocyte colony-stimulating factor as ordered. • Extravasation causes mild local reactions, such as erythema and bruising.

Dosage adjustment. Reduce dosage if patient has renal impairment or severe neutropenia.

ambient lighting.
Incompatibilities: None reported.
Intermittent infusion: Infuse ordered amount over 30 minutes.

- Bone marrow suppression is drug's dose-limiting toxic effect. Nadir occurs in about 11 days.

torsemide • Demadex

Class: ***diuretic, antihypertensive*** • *Pregnancy risk category B*

Edema from heart failure. *Adults:* 10 or 20 mg once daily. If response inadequate, double dose until desired response obtained. Single doses above 200 mg haven't been fully studied.
Chronic renal failure. *Adults:* 20 mg once daily. Titrate upward by doubling previous dose until desired diuretic response occurs. Single doses above 200 mg haven't been fully studied.
Hepatic cirrhosis. *Adults:* 5 or 10 mg once daily with aldosterone antagonist or potassium-sparing diuretic. Titrate upward by doubling previous dose until desired diuretic response occurs. Single doses above 40 mg haven't been fully studied.

Available as 2-ml (20 mg) or 5-ml (50 mg) ampules at 10 mg/ml. Store at room temperature. Don't freeze.
Incompatibilities: None reported.
Direct injection: Give slowly over 2 minutes.

- In diuretic potency, 10 to 20 mg torsemide is about equivalent to 40 mg furosemide or 1 mg bumetanide. A longer duration of action than furosemide allows once-daily dosing.
- Flush I.V. line with NaCl injection USP before and after administration.
- Watch for evidence of electrolyte imbalance, hypovolemia, or prerenal azotemia.

trace elements (chromium, copper, manganese, selenium, zinc) • MTE-5, Multiple Trace Element with Selenium

Class: ***nutritional supplements*** • *Pregnancy risk category C*

Prevention of trace element deficiencies (combination product) in long-term total parenteral nutrition. *Adults:* 5 ml/day.
Prevention of chromium deficiency. *Adults:* 10 to 15 mcg daily (20 mcg daily with intestinal fluid loss). *Children:* 0.14

Multiple formula available as 10-ml unit dose vials that contain 4 mcg chromium, 0.4 mg copper, 0.1 mg manganese, 20 mcg selenium, 1 mg zinc. Dilute for infusion in the appropriate total parenteral nutrition solution to a minimum dilution of 1:200. Chromium available alone in 5-, 10-, and 30-ml vials. Selenium copper, and manganese available alone in 10- and

- Do not give by direct I.V. injection because solution's acidic pH (approximately 2) may irritate tissues.
- Use serum levels of trace elements to guide further administration, especially when using high mainte-

(continued)

◆ Also available in Canada. ◇ Available in Canada only.

COMMON INDICATIONS AND DOSAGES	ADMINISTRATION	SPECIAL CONSIDERATIONS
trace elements (chromium, copper, manganese, selenium, zinc) *(continued)* to 0.2 mcg/kg daily. **Prevention of copper deficiency.** *Adults:* 0.5 to 1.5 mg daily. *Children:* 20 mcg/kg daily. **Prevention of manganese deficiency.** *Adults:* 0.15 to 0.8 mg daily. *Children:* 2 to 10 mcg/kg daily. **Prevention of selenium deficiency.** *Adults:* 20 to 40 mcg daily (100 mcg daily for 24 to 31 days with selenium deficiency resulting from long-term total parenteral nutrition). *Children:* 3 mcg/kg daily. **Prevention of zinc deficiency.** *Adults:* 2.5 to 4 mg daily (additional 2 mg daily in acute catabolic states; additional 12.2 mg/L in fluid loss from the small bowel; or additional 17.1 mg/kg stool in stool or ileostomy output). *Children up to age 5:* 100 mcg/kg daily. *Premature infants who weigh up to 6.6 lb (3 kg):* 300 mcg/kg daily.	30-ml vials. Zinc available alone in 5-, 10-, 30-, and 50-ml vials. As ordered, dilute for infusion in the appropriate total parenteral nutrition solution. Store at room temperature and avoid excessive heat. Discard if solution isn't clear or seal is broken. Discard unused portion within 24 hr after opening vial. ***Incompatibilities:*** None reported. ***Continuous infusion:*** Give diluted solution through patent I.V. line over ordered duration.	nance doses. • Watch for signs of toxicity. Zinc toxicity produces fever, nausea, vomiting, and diarrhea. Calcium supplements may protect against it. Copper toxicity causes nausea, vomiting, intestinal cramps, diarrhea, intravascular hemolysis, and renal impairment. d-Penicillamine is the antidote.

trastuzumab • Herceptin

Class: ***antineoplastic*** • *Pregnancy risk category B*

Single treatment of metastatic breast cancer in patients whose tumors overexpress the HER2 protein and who have received one or more chemotherapy regimens for metastatic disease, or	Follow facility protocol for handling chemotherapy drugs. Available as vials containing 440 mg lyophilized sterile powder. Vials stable at 36° to 46° F (2° to 8° C) before reconstitution. Reconstitute each vial with 20 ml bacteriostatic water for injection, 1.1% benzyl alcohol preserved, as supplied, to yield	• Use cautiously in elderly patients or those with cardiac dysfunction or known hypersensitivity to drug or its components. • Watch for first-infusion symptom complex, which usually includes chills or fever. Give acetamino-

combined with paclitaxel in patients whose tumors overexpress HER2 but who haven't received chemotherapy for their metastatic disease. *Adults:* 4 mg/kg as loading dose, then 2 mg/kg weekly as maintenance.

a multidose solution of 21 mg/ml. Immediately label vial with expiration date 28 days from date of reconstitution. Reconstituted solution is colorless to pale yellow, transparent solution. Don't freeze. If patient is hypersensitive to benzyl alcohol, reconstitute with sterile water for injection, use immediately, and discard unused portion. For infusion, determine dose based on loading dose of 4 mg/kg or maintenance dose of 2 mg/kg. Calculate volume of 21 mg/ml solution, withdraw this amount from vial, and add it to infusion bag containing 250 ml 0.9% NaCl. Don't use D_5W. Gently invert bag to mix. Store at 36° to 46° F (2° to 8° C) before use. Solution stable up to 24 hr.

Incompatibilities: Don't mix or dilute with other drugs or with dextrose solutions.

Intermittent infusion: Infuse loading dose over 90 minutes, maintenance dose over 30 minutes if patient tolerates loading dose well.

phen, diphenhydramine, and meperidine (with or without reducing infusion rate), as ordered. Other effects may include nausea, vomiting, pain, rigors, headache, dizziness, dyspnea, hypotension, rash, and asthenia. They occur infrequently during later infusions.

- Monitor patient's cardiac status. Treatment may stop if patient develops clinically significant decrease in left ventricular function.

trimetrexate glucuronate • Neutrexin

Class: ***antimicrobial, antineoplastic*** • *Pregnancy risk category D*

Alternative treatment of moderate to severe *Pneumocystis carinii* pneumonia in immunocompromised patient intolerant of or refractory to trimethoprim or in whom trimethoprim is contraindicated, administered concurrently with leucovorin for 72 hr after last trimetrexate dose. Recommended therapy includes trimetrexate for 21 days and leucovorin for 24 days. *Adults:* 45 mg/m² trimetrexate once daily with 20 mg/m² leucovorin I.V. (over 5 or 10 minutes) or P.O. q 6 hr.
Dosage adjustment. Modify doses in response to hematologic toxicity.

Available as single-dose, 5-ml vial with 25 mg of lyophilized powder. Also available as kit with leucovorin 50 mg. Store at 59° to 66° F (15° to 19° C), and protect from light. Reconstitute with 2 ml sterile water or D_5W to yield 12.5 mg/ml trimetrexate. Filter with 0.22-micron filter, then dilute with D_5W to yield 0.25 to 2 mg trimetrexate/ml. Solution should be colorless to pale greenish yellow. Stable up to 24 hr at room temperature or refrigerated; don't freeze. Discard unused portions 2 hr after initial reconstitution.

Incompatibilities: Don't mix with solutions that contain chloride ions or leucovorin because trimetrexate will precipitate on contact.

Intermittent infusion: Infuse over 60 minutes using an infusion pump. Flush line with at least 10 ml D_5W before and

- If drug contacts skin or mucosa, immediately wash thoroughly with soap and water.
- If extravasation occurs, apply warm compresses to site, insert new catheter at another site, and restart infusion. Trimetrexate isn't a vesicant.
- Monitor patient's absolute neutrophil count, platelets, serum creatinine, BUN, ALT, AST, and alkaline phosphatase at least twice weekly during therapy.
- Check and record patient's temperature at least daily. If it exceeds 101° F (38° C), give an antipyretic as ordered.

(continued)

◆ Also available in Canada. ◇ Available in Canada only.

COMMON INDICATIONS AND DOSAGES	ADMINISTRATION	SPECIAL CONSIDERATIONS
trimetrexate glucuronate *(continued)*	after infusion. Leucovorin may be administered before or after trimetrexate; flush I.V. line thoroughly with at least 10 ml of D_5W before and after leucovorin administration. Dilute leucovorin as directed in package insert and administer over 5 to 10 minutes.	

tromethamine • Tham

Class: ***systemic alkalinizer*** • *Pregnancy risk category C*

COMMON INDICATIONS AND DOSAGES	ADMINISTRATION	SPECIAL CONSIDERATIONS
Correction of metabolic acidosis from cardiac arrest or cardiopulmonary bypass surgery. *Adults:* Dosage depends on bicarbonate deficit. When using Tham, required volume (ml) of 0.3 M tromethamine solution is equivalent to weight (kg) multiplied by bicarbonate deficit (mEq/L). Total dose for Tham shouldn't exceed 500 mg/kg. Average dose is 9 ml/kg or a single dose of 500 ml (150 mEq). For severe acidosis, up to 1,000 ml of solution may be given. *Children:* Dosage calculated as for adults. Don't exceed 40 ml/kg. **Reduction of excess acidity in acid citrate-dextrose stored blood before transfusion.** *Adults:* Up to 70 ml solution added to each 500-ml unit of blood. *Children:* About 5 ml solution added to each 50 ml of blood. Usually, 55 ml added to 500 ml of blood is adequate.	Available as 500-ml (150 mEq) single-dose containers. Use undiluted (after cardiac arrest) or dilute in required volume of blood (during bypass surgery or transfusion). Solution concentration shouldn't exceed 0.3 M. Protect from heat and freezing, and discard unused solution within 24 hr. ***Incompatibilities:*** None reported. ***Intermittent infusion:*** Administer over at least 1 hr through 18G needle into central line or antecubital vein. Use infusion pump if possible. In a child, infuse over 6 hr. When infusing peripherally, use largest possible vein to avoid extravasation. If it occurs, infiltrate area with 1% procaine and 150 units of hyaluronidase to reduce venospasm and dilute drug.	• American Heart Association doesn't recommend this drug for cardiac arrest. • Monitor patient's arterial blood gases, serum glucose level, and electrolyte levels before, during, and after therapy. • Assess patient's respiratory function during and after therapy, and keep a mechanical ventilator nearby. • If patient has renal disease, monitor his serum potassium closely and use cardiac telemetry.

tubocurarine chloride (curare, d-tubocurarine chloride)

Class: ***skeletal muscle relaxant*** • *Pregnancy risk category C*

Adjunct to general anesthesia. *Adults:* 6 to 9 mg, then 3 to 4.5 mg over 3 to 5 minutes if needed. Additional doses may be given during long procedures. *Infants and children:* 0.6 mg/kg. *Neonates up to 4 weeks old:* 0.3 mg/kg.
Aid to mechanical ventilation. *Adults:* 0.0165 mg/kg; subsequent dosage determined by response.
Diagnosis of myasthenia gravis. *Adults:* 0.004 to 0.033 mg/kg as a single dose.

Available as 10-ml multidose vials containing 3 mg (20 U/ml. Store at room temperature; avoid excessive heat and freezing. Discard if discolored.
Incompatibilities: Alkaline solutions (including barbiturates, sodium bicarbonate, and other drugs with high pH) and trimethaphan camsylate.
Direct injection: Give ordered dose over 60 to 90 seconds. Give subsequent doses, usually 20% to 25% of initial dose, at 40- to 60-minute intervals. Lengthen intervals, as ordered, in elderly or debilitated patients.

- Only staff trained to give anesthetics and manage their adverse effects should give drug.
- Drug may contain sulfites.
- Maintain patent airway and check vital signs every 15 minutes during therapy.
- Drug doesn't affect consciousness or relieve pain; assess patient's need for analgesic or sedative.
- Monitor patient's baseline electrolyte levels because electrolyte imbalance can potentiate neuromuscular effects. Also measure intake and output because renal dysfunction prolongs duration of action.
- A nerve stimulator and train-of-four monitoring are recommended to assess recovery of muscle strength. Before attempting reversal with neostigmine, some evidence of spontaneous recovery should be apparent.

urea (carbamide) • Ureaphil

Class: ***osmotic diuretic*** • *Pregnancy risk category C*

Reduction of intracranial or intraocular pressure. *Adults:* 1 to 1.5 g/kg infused over 1 to 2.5 hr. *Children age 2 and over:* 0.5 to 1.5 g/kg infused over 30 minutes to 2 hr. *Children under age 2:* 0.1 g/kg infused over 30 minutes to 2 hr.
Rapid correction of hyponatremia in SIADH. *Adults:* 80 g infused over 6 hr.

Available as powder in 40-g vials. Store at room temperature, and protect from heat and freezing. Make sure seal and container are intact. To reconstitute, add 105 ml of D_5W, dextrose 10% in water, or 10% invert sugar injection (unless patient is fructose intolerant) to 40-g vial to yield 30% (300 mg/ml) solution. Warm diluent to 122° F (50° C) to dissolve urea; then cool to body temperature before administration. Each dose should be freshly prepared. Discard if discolored of precipitated.
Incompatibilities: Blood.
Intermittent infusion: Infuse at prescribed rate for adults

- Use in SIADH is unlabeled.
- Infuse diluted dose into large vein but in leg (especially in older patient) because of risk of phlebitis and thrombosis. Avoid extravasation.
- Monitor patient's blood pressure, intake and output, serum electrolytes, and BUN levels before and after administration. Watch for signs of hyponatremia or hypokalemia, such as muscle weakness or lethargy.
- Watch for rebound intraocular and intracranial pres-

(continued)

◆ Also available in Canada. ◇ Available in Canada only.

COMMON INDICATIONS AND DOSAGES	ADMINISTRATION	SPECIAL CONSIDERATIONS
urea *(continued)*	and children. Don't exceed 1.5 g/kg, 120 g in 24 hr, or 4 to 6 ml (30% solution)/minute. Avoid rapid infusion, which can cause hemolysis and cerebral vasomotor symptoms. When used preoperatively, start infusion 60 minutes before ocular surgery or when scalp incision made for intracranial surgery.	sure elevation, which may occur 12 hr after administration. • If BUN levels are 75 to 100 mg, or if diuresis doesn't occur within 2 hr, reduce dosage or withhold drug, as ordered, until patient can be reevaluated and renal function reassessed.

urokinase • Abbokinase, Abbokinase Open-Cath

Class: ***thrombolytic*** • *Pregnancy risk category B*

COMMON INDICATIONS AND DOSAGES	ADMINISTRATION	SPECIAL CONSIDERATIONS
Pulmonary embolism. *Adults:* 4,400 IU/kg initially by infusion, then continuous infusion of 4,400 IU/kg/hr for 12 hr. **Venous catheter occlusion.** *Adults:* 1 ml of 5,000 IU/ml solution for each clearing procedure.	Available as lyophilized white powder in vials containing 250,000 U. Refrigerate vials at 35° to 47° F (2° to 8° C). Reconstitute immediately before use with 5 ml sterile water for injection (preservative-free) to yield 50,000 IU/ml. Don't use bacteriostatic water; it contains preservatives. To avoid filament formation, roll and tilt vial during reconstitution; avoid shaking. Solution may be filtered through a 0.45-micron or smaller cellulose filter. Dilute solution further with 0.9% NaCl or D_5W. Total volume administered shouldn't exceed 200 ml. Reconstituted solution should be clear, practically colorless, and without precipitates. Discard unused portion. Don't use highly colored solutions. ***Incompatibilities:*** None reported, but manufacturer recommends against mixing with other drugs. ***Direct injection:*** To clear venous catheter occlusion, slowly inject solution into occluded line, wait 5 minutes, then aspirate. Repeat aspiration attempts q 5 minutes for 30 minutes. If line isn't patent after 30 minutes, cap it and let urokinase work for 30 to 60 minutes before aspirating. Second injection may be required. ***Continuous infusion:*** Administer initial dose of diluted solution over 10 minutes using an infusion pump. Infuse subsequent doses, as ordered, over 12 hr.	• Have typed and crossmatched RBCs and whole blood available to treat hemorrhage. • Monitor patient's vital signs and condition of limbs (pulses, color, and sensitivity) every hr. • Watch closely for bleeding; avoid noncompressible puncture sites. • Monitor patient's hematocrit, plasma fibrinogen, and plasminogen levels because they may decrease for 12 to 24 hr after therapy stops. Fibrin split products may increase.

vancomycin hydrochloride • Lyphocin, Vancocin, Vancoled

Class: ***antibiotic*** • *Pregnancy risk category C*

Severe systemic infection by susceptible organisms when less toxic drugs are ineffective. *Adults:* 500 mg q 6 hr or 1 g q 12 hr. *Children over 1 month old:* 40 mg/kg daily in divided doses. *Neonates over 8 days old:* 15 mg/kg, then 10 mg/kg q 8 hr. *Neonates 8 days old or younger:* 15 mg/kg, then10 mg/kg q 12 hr.

Prevention of bacterial endocarditis in penicillin-allergic patients undergoing dental or respiratory procedures. *Adults:* 1 g 30 to 60 minutes before procedure, followed by oral erythromycin. *Children:* 20 mg/kg 30 to 60 minutes before procedure, followed by oral erythromycin.

Prevention of bacterial endocarditis in penicillin-allergic patients undergoing GI or GU procedures. *Adults:* 1 g 30 to 60 minutes before procedure together with gentamicin. *Children:* 20 mg/kg 30 to 60 minutes before procedure together with gentamicin.

Dosage adjustment. Adjust dosage if patient has renal impairment.

Available as 500-mg and 1-g vials. Store vials at room temperature. Reconstitute 500-mg vial with 10 ml and 1-g vial with 20 ml sterile water for injection to yield 50 mg/ml. Reconstituted solution is clear and light yellow to light brown. Can be refrigerated 14 days. Before administration, dilute in 100 to 200 ml (500 mg in at least 100 ml, 1 g in at least 200 ml) of D_5W or 0.9% NaCl. For continuous infusion, dilute 1 to 2 g in the ordered volume for 24 hr. Inspect before administration for precipitates or discoloration. Diluted solutions stable 24 hr at room temperature.

Incompatibilities: Alkaline solutions, aminophylline, amobarbital, chloramphenicol, chlorothiazide, corticosteroids, heavy metals, heparin, methicillin, pentobarbital, phenobarbital, secobarbital, and sodium bicarbonate.

Intermittent infusion: Infuse diluted dose over at least 60 minutes to reduce risk of reactions and "red-neck" syndrome.

Continuous infusion: Use only when intermittent infusion isn't feasible. Add ordered dose to compatible solution and give by I.V. drip over 24 hr.

- When used preoperatively, give 60-minute infusion before anesthetic induction to reduce risk of infusion-related reactions.
- If "red-neck" syndrome occurs, stop infusion and notify doctor.
- When treating staphylococcal endocarditis, maintain therapy at least 4 weeks.
- Monitor patient's vital signs, renal function, WBC counts, and auditory function.
- Check serum vancomycin levels for efficacy and toxicity.

COMMON INDICATIONS AND DOSAGES	ADMINISTRATION	SPECIAL CONSIDERATIONS

vasopressin (antidiuretic hormone [ADH]) • Pitressin Synthetic

Classes: ***hemostatic, antidiuretic hormone*** • *Pregnancy risk category C*

COMMON INDICATIONS AND DOSAGES	ADMINISTRATION	SPECIAL CONSIDERATIONS
GI hemorrhage. *Adults:* 0.2 to 0.4 U/minute, increased to 0.9 U/minute if needed. Dosage individualized to patient's response and tolerance.	Available in 0.5-ml and 1-ml ampules with 20 U/ml. For I.V. infusion, dilute to 0.1 to 1 U/ml with 0.9% NaCl or 5% dextrose injection. Store at 59° to 86° F (15° to 30° C). Don't freeze. ***Incompatibilities:*** None reported. ***Continuous infusion:*** Infuse diluted solution through peripheral vein using controlled infusion device.	• Establish baseline vital signs and intake:output ratio before starting therapy. • Monitor patient's blood pressure twice daily, intake and output daily, and weight daily. • Monitor patient's electrolytes and ECG periodically. • Use extreme caution to avoid extravasation because of risk of necrosis and gangrene. • Watch for signs of early water intoxication, including drowsiness, listlessness, headache, confusion, and weight gain. If they occur, stop drug and restrict water intake until polyuria occurs. Severe water intoxication may require osmotic diuresis with mannitol, hypertonic dextrose, or urea, alone or with furosemide.

vecuronium bromide • Norcuron

Class: ***skeletal muscle relaxant*** • *Pregnancy risk category C*

COMMON INDICATIONS AND DOSAGES	ADMINISTRATION	SPECIAL CONSIDERATIONS
As adjunct to general anesthesia, to facilitate endotracheal intubation; to relax skeletal muscles during surgery or mechanical ventilation. Dose depends on anesthetic used, individual needs, and response. *Adults:* 0.08 to 0.1 mg/kg, followed by 0.01 to 0.015 mg/kg 20 to 40 minutes after initial dose, q 12 to 15 minutes, p.r.n. Or, continuous infusion started at 1 mcg/kg/minute (0.001 mg/kg/minute). *Children:* Dosage individualized.	Available as sterile, nonpyrogenic, freeze-dried, buffered cake of fine crystalline particles. Available as 10- and 20-ml vials containing 10 mg drug with or without diluent or 20 mg drug without diluent. Before reconstitution, store at room temperature and protect from light. After reconstitution with bacteriostatic water, use within 24 hr. If reconstituted with a different solution, use within 8 hr. For infusion, dilute further by adding 10 ml reconstituted drug to 100 ml D_5W, 0.9% NaCl, dextrose 5% in 0.9% or 0.45% NaCl, or dextrose 5% in lactated Ringer's solution. Drug is compatible with all I.V. solutions. ***Incompatibilities:*** None reported.	• Only staff trained to give anesthetics and manage their adverse effects should give drug. • Continuously monitor patient throughout infusion. • A nerve stimulator and train-of-four monitoring are recommended to assess recovery of muscle strength. Before attempting pharmacologic reversal, some evidence of spontaneous recovery should be present. • Infants are especially sensitive to drug effects. Recovery time may be 1.5 times that of an adult.

Dosage adjustment. Reduce dosage if patient has renal or hepatic impairment.

Direct injection: Inject dose directly into tubing of I.V. line that contains free-flowing, compatible solution.
Continuous infusion: Begin infusion 20 to 40 minutes after initial dose given by direct injection. Determine rates by carefully observing neuromuscular blockade with a peripheral nerve stimulator. They range from 0.8 to 1.2 mcg/kg/minute (0.0008 to 0.0012 mg/kg/minute) with a 1:10 dilution.

verapamil hydrochloride • Calan, Isoptin◆

Class: ***antiarrhythmic*** • *Pregnancy risk category C*

Supraventricular arrhythmias. *Adults:* 0.075 to 0.15 mg/kg (5 to 10 mg) as bolus, repeated in 30 minutes if no response. *Children ages 1 to 15:* 0.1 to 0.3 mg/kg as bolus, repeated in 30 minutes if no response. *Children under age 1:* 0.1 to 0.2 mg/kg as bolus, repeated in 30 minutes if no response.

Available as a solution of 2.5 mg/ml. Store at room temperature and protect from light and freezing. Drug stable 24 hr at 77° F (25° C) in most common infusion solutions when protected from light. Compatible with D_5W, 0.9% NaCl, and lactated Ringer's solution.
Incompatibilities: Albumin, aminophylline, amphotericin B, ampicillin sodium, co-trimoxazole, dobutamine, hydralazine, mezlocillin, nafcillin, oxacillin, sodium bicarbonate, and trimethoprim.
Direct injection: Give 5 to 10 mg undiluted over at least 2 minutes; 3 minutes in older patient.

- Continuously monitor patient's ECG and blood pressure during therapy.
- If giving digoxin concomitantly, reduce digoxin dose by half and monitor patient's ECG for possible AV block.
- Tell doctor about signs of heart failure, such as dependent edema or dyspnea.

vinblastine sulfate (VLB) • Velban, Velbe◆

Class: ***antineoplastic*** • *Pregnancy risk category D*

May be used alone or in combination. Dosage reflects response to drug and degree of bone marrow depression.
Hodgkin's disease and malignant lymphomas; breast, testicular, renal cell, or head and neck cancer; Kaposi's sarcoma; advanced mycosis fungoides; choriocarcinoma; Letterer-Siwe dis-

Follow facility protocol for handling chemotherapy drugs. Supplied in 10-mg vials. Reconstitute by adding 10 ml of 0.9% NaCl injection containing phenol or benzyl alcohol as a preservative to yield 1 mg/ml. Also available in 10-ml aqueous solution of 10 mg/ml. Store powder and reconstituted solution at 36° to 46° F (2° to 8° C). Solution stable at these temperatures up to 30 days.
Incompatibilities: Furosemide.

- Provide adequate oral hydration and, as ordered, give allopurinol to alkalinize urine.
- Before and during therapy, monitor patient's hematocrit, platelet count, total and differential WBC count, AST, ALT, and serum bilirubin, creatinine, lactic dehydrogenase, BUN, and uric acid levels.

(continued)

◆ Also available in Canada. ◇ Available in Canada only.

COMMON INDICATIONS AND DOSAGES	ADMINISTRATION	SPECIAL CONSIDERATIONS
vinblastine sulfate *(continued)* **ease; germ-cell ovarian tumors; chronic leukemias; neuroblastoma.** *Adults:* 0.1 mg/kg or 3.7 mg/m^2, with successive weekly doses increased by 0.05 mg/kg (or 1.8 to 1.9 mg/m^2) until WBC count falls to 3,000/mm^3, tumor shrinks, or maximum dose of 0.5 mg/kg (or 18.5 mg/m^2) is reached (usual range, 0.15 to 0.2 mg/kg or 5.5 to 7.4 mg/m^2). Maintenance doses are one increment smaller than final initial dose q 7 to 14 days (or 10 mg once or twice monthly) and shouldn't start until WBC count returns to 4,000/mm^3 after preceding dose. *Children:* 2.5 mg/m^2, with successive weekly doses increased by 1.25 mg/m^2 until WBC count falls to 3,000/mm^3, tumor shrinks, or maximum dose of 7.5 mg/m^2 is reached. Maintenance doses are one increment smaller than final initial dose q 7 to 14 days and shouldn't start until WBC count returns to 4,000/mm^3 after preceding dose.	***Direct injection:*** Inject dose rapidly into side port of free-flowing patent I.V. line or inject directly into vein over 1 minute. (Avoid injecting into veins with compromised circulation because of enhanced risk of thrombosis.) If extravasation occurs, stop immediately, inject remaining dose into another vein, and treat affected area.	• Watch for life-threatening acute bronchospasm and notify doctor immediately if it occurs. • Tell patient to report fever, sore throat, chills, sore mouth, or unusual bleeding or bruising, especially if receiving myelosuppressant drugs. • Don't confuse drug with vincristine or vinorelbine.

vincristine sulfate • Oncovin ◆

Class: ***antineoplastic*** • *Pregnancy risk category D*

Leukemias; Hodgkin's disease and malignant lymphomas; osteogenic and other sarcomas; Wilms' tumor; rhabdomyosarcoma; multiple myeloma;	Follow facility protocol for handling chemotherapy drugs. Available as 1-, 2-, and 5-ml vials at 1 mg/ml. Undiluted drug best stored at 36° to 46° F (2° to 8° C) but is stable at room temperature at least 1 month. Protect from light. For infusion,	• Hematologic toxicity is less than with other antineoplastic agents, and mild leukopenia, anemia, and thrombocytopenia are rare at usual doses. However, drug is highly toxic with a low therapeutic index.

medulloblastoma, neuroblastoma, mycosis fungoides; lung, breast, and ovarian carcinoma. *Adults:* Depending on protocol, 0.01 to 0.03 mg/kg or 0.4 to 1.4 mg/m^2 weekly as single dose. *Children who weigh more than 22 lb (10 kg):* 1.5 to 2 mg/m^2 weekly as single dose. *Children who weigh 22 lb or less:* 0.05 mg/kg weekly.
Dosage adjustment. Drug may be used with other drugs to reduce adverse effects; if so, smaller doses may be necessary.

dilute to ordered concentration and volume with compatible solution, such as D_5W or 0.9% NaCl injection.
Incompatibilities: Furosemide.
Direct injection: Inject dose over 1 minute directly into vein or into side port of new I.V. line. Use 23G or 25G winged-tip infusion set. If possible, use distal rather than major vein, which allows repeated venipuncture if necessary.
Intermittent infusion: Not recommended; however, drug has been diluted and given as a slow infusion over 4 to 8 hr.

- Drug is a vesicant, so ensure a patent I.V. line and prepare for possible extravasation. If it occurs, stop injection immediately and inject remaining dose into another vein. Give a local injection of hyaluronidase and apply moderate heat or cold compresses to reduce discomfort and cellulitis.
- Before and during therapy, monitor CBC, ALT, AST, and serum bilirubin, creatinine, lactic dehydrogenase, BUN, and uric acid levels. Leukopenia usually reaches nadir within 4 days.
- Provide adequate oral hydration and give allopurinol, as ordered, to alkalinize urine.
- Don't confuse drug with vinblastine or vinorelbine.

vinorelbine tartrate • Navelbine

Class: ***antineoplastic*** • *Pregnancy risk category D*

Alone or as adjunct therapy with cisplatin for first-line treatment of ambulatory patients with nonresectable advanced non-small-cell lung cancer; alone or with cisplatin in stage IV of non-small-cell lung cancer; with cisplatin in stage III of non-small-cell lung cancer. *Adults:* 30 mg/m^2 weekly. In combination therapy, 30 mg/m^2 with 120 mg/m^2 of cisplatin given on days 1 and 29, then q 6 weeks.
Dosage adjustment. Adjust dosage in response to hematologic toxicity.

Follow facility protocol for handling chemotherapy drugs. Available as 1- and 5-ml single-use vials at 10 mg/ml. Refrigerate vials 36° to 46° F (2° to 8° C), protect from light, and avoid freezing. For direct injection, dilute calculated dose to 1.5 to 3 mg/ml using 5% dextrose injection or 0.9% NaCl injection. For infusion, dilute calculated dose to 0.5 to 2 mg/ml using 5% dextrose injection, 0.9% NaCl injection, 0.45% NaCl injection, 5% dextrose and 0.45% NaCl injection, Ringer's injection, or lactated Ringer's injection. May be used for up to 24 hr in normal room light when stored in polypropylene syringes or polyvinyl chloride bags at 41° to 86° F (5° to 30° C).
Incompatibilities: None reported.
Direct injection: Give over 6 to 10 minutes into side port closest to the I.V. bag in free-flowing I.V. line. Then flush with 75 to 125 ml of one of the solutions; flush with more, if necessary.
Intermittent infusion: Give diluted solution over 6 to 10 minutes as above.

- Extravasation can cause severe tissue irritation, necrosis, and thrombophlebitis. If it occurs, stop drug immediately and use different vein for remaining infusion.
- Watch for evidence of hypersensitivity.
- Monitor patient's peripheral blood count throughout therapy.
- Check patient's deep tendon reflexes because loss may indicate toxicity.
- Tell patient to report fever, sore throat, chills, bleeding, or bruising immediately.
- Don't confuse drug with vinblastine or vincristine.

◆ Also available in Canada. ◇ Available in Canada only.

COMMON INDICATIONS AND DOSAGES	ADMINISTRATION	SPECIAL CONSIDERATIONS
warfarin sodium • Coumadin		
Class: ***anticoagulant*** • *Pregnancy risk category X*		
Dosage must be individualized because requirements vary greatly. **Venous thrombosis, pulmonary embolism, thromboembolism, recurrent MI.** *Adults:* 2 to 5 mg daily with dose adjustments based on INR and PT. Maintenance doses range from 2 to 10 mg daily based on INR and PT.	Available as 5-mg, single-use vials. Store at controlled room temperature and protect from light. For infusion, reconstitute with 2.7 ml of sterile water for injection to yield 2 mg/ml. Store reconstituted solution at controlled room temperature and use within 4 hours. Don't refrigerate. Discard unused portion. ***Incompatibilities:*** None reported. ***Direct injection:*** Inject diluted solution over 1 to 2 minutes in a peripheral vein.	• Monitor patient's PT, PTT, and INR. Dosage adjustments should be based on findings. • Watch for signs of bleeding. • Antidote is vitamin K. • Stay aware of many possible drug interactions and carefully observe for changes in prescribed drug regimens that may cause significant interactions.
zidovudine • Retrovir		
Class: ***antiviral*** • *Pregnancy risk category C*		
Symptomatic HIV infection in patients with history of cytologically confirmed *Pneumocystis carinii* pneumonia or an absolute CD4+ lymphocyte count below 200/mm³. *Adults:* 1 to 2 mg/kg q 4 hr around the clock until oral therapy can start. **To reduce risk of HIV transmission from infected mother to fetus during labor.** *Adults:* 2 mg/kg followed by continuous infusion of 1 mg/kg/hr until umbilical cord clamped. (100 mg given P.O. between 14 and 34 weeks' gestation and continued throughout pregnancy.)	Available as 20-ml vials containing 200 mg. Store at 59° to 77° F (15° to 25° C) and protect from light. To prepare, dilute to no more than 4 mg/ml using D_5W, 0.9% NaCl, D_5W in 0.9% NaCl, lactated Ringer's solution, or D_5W in lactated Ringer's solution. After dilution, solution stable 24 hr at room temperature, 48 hr if refrigerated at 36° to 46° F (2° to 8° C). Give within 8 hr if stored at room temperature, 24 hr if refrigerated. ***Incompatibilities:*** Biological or colloidal solutions. ***Intermittent infusion:*** Infuse over 1 hr. ***Continuous infusion:*** After loading dose, maintain infusion during labor and delivery and until umbilical cord is clamped.	• Significant anemia usually occurs after 4 to 6 weeks of therapy. It usually improves when drug stops or dose is reduced. Patient may need blood transfusions even with lower doses. • Administer syrup (2 mg/kg P.O. every 6 hr for 6 weeks) to infants of infected mothers who received zidovudine to reduce risk of HIV transmission. • Reinforce the importance of checking blood counts for toxicity.

Appendices

Epinephrine infusion rates

Mix 1 mg in 250 ml (4 mcg/ml).

Dose (mcg/min)	Infusion rate (ml/hr)
1	15
2	30
3	45
4	60
5	75
6	90
7	105
8	120
9	135
10	150
15	225
20	300
25	375
30	450
35	525
40	600

Isoproterenol infusion rates

Mix 1 mg in 250 ml (4 mcg/ml).

Dose (mcg/min)	Infusion rate (ml/hr)
0.5	8
1	15
2	30
3	45
4	60
5	75
6	90
7	105
8	120
9	135
10	150
15	225
20	300
25	375
30	450

Nitroglycerin infusion rates

Determine the infusion rate in ml/hr, using the ordered dose and the concentration of the drug solution.

Dose (mcg/min)	25 mg/250 ml (100 mcg/ml)	50 mg/250 ml (200 mcg/ml)	100 mg/250 ml (400 mcg/ml)
5	3	2	1
10	6	3	2
20	12	6	3
30	18	9	5
40	24	12	6
50	30	15	8
60	36	18	9
70	42	21	10
80	48	24	12
90	54	27	14
100	60	30	15
150	90	45	23
200	120	60	30

Dobutamine infusion rates

Mix 250 mg in 250 ml of D_5W (1,000 mcg/ml). Determine the infusion rate in ml/hr, using the ordered dose and the patient's weight in pounds or kilograms.

Dose	**lb 88**	**99**	**110**	**121**	**132**	**143**	**154**	**165**	**176**	**187**	**198**	**209**	**220**	**231**	**242**
(mcg/kg/min)	**kg 40**	**45**	**50**	**55**	**60**	**65**	**70**	**75**	**80**	**85**	**90**	**95**	**100**	**105**	**110**
2.5	6	7	8	8	9	10	11	11	12	13	14	14	15	16	17
5	12	14	15	17	18	20	21	23	24	26	27	29	30	32	33
7.5	18	20	23	25	27	29	32	34	36	38	41	43	45	47	50
10	24	27	30	33	36	39	42	45	48	51	54	57	60	63	66
12.5	30	34	38	41	45	49	53	56	60	64	68	71	75	79	83
15	36	41	45	50	54	59	63	68	72	77	81	86	90	95	99
20	48	54	60	66	72	78	84	90	96	102	108	114	120	126	132
25	60	68	75	83	90	98	105	113	120	128	135	143	150	158	165
30	72	81	90	99	108	117	126	135	144	153	162	171	180	189	198
35	84	95	105	116	126	137	147	158	168	179	189	200	210	221	231
40	96	108	120	132	144	156	168	180	192	204	216	228	240	252	264

Dopamine infusion rates

Mix 400 mg in 250 ml of D_5W (1,600 mcg/ml). Determine the infusion rate in ml/hr, using the ordered dose and the patient's weight in pounds or kilograms.

Dose	**lb 88**	**99**	**110**	**121**	**132**	**143**	**154**	**165**	**176**	**187**	**198**	**209**	**220**	**231**
(mcg/kg/min)	**kg 40**	**45**	**50**	**55**	**60**	**65**	**70**	**75**	**80**	**85**	**90**	**95**	**100**	**105**
2.5	4	4	5	5	6	6	7	7	8	8	8	9	9	10
5	8	8	9	10	11	12	13	14	15	16	17	18	19	20
7.5	11	13	14	15	17	18	20	21	23	24	25	27	28	30
10	15	17	19	21	23	24	26	28	30	32	34	36	38	39
12.5	19	21	23	26	28	30	33	35	38	40	42	45	47	49
15	23	25	28	31	34	37	39	42	45	48	51	53	56	59
20	30	34	38	41	45	49	53	56	60	64	68	71	75	79
25	38	42	47	52	56	61	66	70	75	80	84	89	94	98
30	45	51	56	62	67	73	79	84	90	96	101	107	113	118
35	53	59	66	72	79	85	92	98	105	112	118	125	131	138
40	60	68	75	83	90	98	105	113	120	128	135	143	150	158
45	68	76	84	93	101	110	118	127	135	143	152	160	169	177
50	75	84	94	103	113	122	131	141	150	159	169	178	188	197

Nitroprusside infusion rates

Mix 50 mg in 250 ml of D_5W (200 mcg/ml). Determine the infusion rate in ml/hr, using the ordered dose and the patient's weight in pounds or kilograms.

Dose	**lb 88**	**99**	**110**	**121**	**132**	**143**	**154**	**165**	**176**	**187**	**198**	**209**	**220**	**231**	**242**
(mcg/kg/min)	**kg 40**	**45**	**50**	**55**	**60**	**65**	**70**	**75**	**80**	**85**	**90**	**95**	**100**	**105**	**110**
0.3	4	4	5	5	5	6	6	7	7	8	8	9	9	9	10
0.5	6	7	8	8	9	10	11	11	12	13	14	14	15	16	17
1	12	14	15	17	18	20	21	23	24	26	27	29	30	32	33
1.5	18	20	23	25	27	29	32	34	36	38	41	43	45	47	50
2	24	27	30	33	36	39	42	45	48	51	54	57	60	63	66
3	36	41	45	50	54	59	63	68	72	77	81	86	90	95	99
4	48	54	60	66	72	78	84	90	96	102	108	114	120	126	132
5	60	68	75	83	90	98	105	113	120	128	135	143	150	158	165
6	72	81	90	99	108	117	126	135	144	153	162	171	180	189	198
7	84	95	105	116	126	137	147	158	168	179	189	200	210	221	231
8	96	108	120	132	144	156	168	180	192	204	216	228	240	252	264
9	108	122	135	149	162	176	189	203	216	230	243	257	270	284	297
10	120	135	150	165	180	195	210	225	240	255	270	285	300	315	330

Antidotes for vesicant extravasation

If you must deliver an antidote to an extravasated vesicant, you'll probably do so through the patient's existing I.V. line to infiltrate the area with the antidote. Or you might use a 1-ml tuberculin syringe to inject small amounts of the antidote subcutaneously in a circle around the infiltrated area. Change the needle before giving each injection. Keep in mind that some of the antidotes listed here are used in combination.

Antidote	Dose	Extravasated Drug
Hyaluronidase 15 units/ml Mix a 150-unit vial with 1 ml 0.9% NaCl for injection. Withdraw 0.1 ml and dilute with 0.9 ml NaCl to get 15 units/ml.	0.2 ml × S.C. injections around site	aminophylline calcium solutions contrast media dextrose solutions (concentrations of 10% or more) etoposide total parenteral nutrition solutions nafcillin potassium solutions teniposide vinblastine vincristine vindesine
Sodium bicarbonate 8.4%	5 ml	daunorubicin doxorubicin vinblastine vincristine
Phentolamine Dilute 5 to 10 mg with 10 ml of sterile saline for injection.	5 to 10 mg	dobutamine dopamine epinephrine metaraminol bitartrate norepinephrine
Sodium thiosulfate 10% Dilute 4 ml with 6 ml sterile water for injection.	10 ml	mechlorethamine
Hydrocortisone sodium succinate 100 mg/ml Usually followed by topical application of hydrocortisone cream 1%.	50 to 200 mg 25 to 50 mg/ml of extravasate	daunorubicin doxorubicin vincristine
Ascorbic acid injection	50 mg	dactinomycin

Major electrolyte components of I.V. solutions

Solution	Sodium (mEq/L)	Potassium (mEq/L)	Osmolarity (mOsm/L)
Aminosyn 3.5% M	47	13	477
Aminosyn 7% with electrolytes	70	66	1,013
Aminosyn 8.5% with electrolytes	70	66	1,160
Ammonium chloride 2.14%	-	-	Additive is hypertonic
Dextrose 2.5% in half-strength lactated Ringer's solution	65	2	265
Dextrose 5% in electrolyte no. 48	25	20	348
Dextrose 5% in electrolyte no. 75	40	35	402
Dextrose 5% in sodium chloride 0.11%	19	-	290
Dextrose 5% in sodium chloride 0.2%	34 or 38.5	-	320-330
Dextrose 5% in sodium chloride 0.33%	51 or 56	-	355-365
Dextrose 50% with electrolyte pattern A	84	40	2,800
Dextrose 50% with electrolyte pattern N	90	80	2,875
Dextrose 50% with electrolytes no. 1	110	80	2,917
50% Travert and electrolyte no. 2	56	25	449
FreAmine III 3% with electrolytes	35	24.5	405
Ionosol B in dextrose 5% in water	57	25	426
Ionosol MB in dextrose 5% in water	25	20	352
Ionosol T in dextrose 5% in water	40	35	432
Isolyte E	140	10	310
Isolyte G with dextrose 5%	65	17	555
Lactated Ringer's solution	130	4	275

***Key:** 1 = hypotonic; 2 = isotonic; 3 = hypertonic.

Tonicity*	Calcium (mEq/L)	Magnesium (mEq/L)	Chloride (mEq/L)	Acetate (mEq/L)	Phosphate (mmol)	Other (mEq/L)
3	-	3	40	58	3.5	amino acids 3.5%
3	-	10	96	124	30	amino acids 7%
3	-	10	98	142	30	amino acids 8.5%
3	-	-	400	-	-	ammonium 400
2	1.4-1.5	-	54-55	-	-	lactate 14
2	-	3	24	-	3	lactate 23
3	-	-	48	-	15	lactate 20
2	-	-	19	-	-	-
2	-	-	34 or 38.5	-	-	-
2	-	-	51 or 56	-	-	-
3	10	16	115	-	-	gluconate 13 sulfate 16
3	-	16	150	-	28	sulfate 16
3	-	16	140	36	24	-
3	-	6	56	-	12.5	lactate 25
3	-	5	41	44	3.5	amino acids 3%
3	-	5	49	-	7	lactate 25
2	-	3	22	-	3	lactate 23
3	-	-	40	-	15	lactate 20
2	5	3	103	49	-	citrate 8
3	-	-	149	-	-	ammonium 70
2	2.7-3	-	109 or 110	-	-	lactate 28

(continued)

Major electrolyte components of I.V. solutions *(continued)*

Solution	Sodium (mEq/L)	Potassium (mEq/L)	Osmolarity (mOsm/L)
Normosol-M in dextrose 5% in water	40	13	363
Plasma-Lyte A	140	5	294
Plasma-Lyte R	140	10	312
ProcalAmine	35	24	735
Ringer's solution	147 or 147.5	4	310
Sodium bicarbonate	598	-	1,190-1,203
Sodium chloride 0.45%	77	-	154
Sodium chloride 0.9%	154	-	308
Sodium chloride 3%	513	-	1,030
Sodium chloride 5%	855	-	1,710
Sodium lactate 1/6 M	167	-	330
Travasol M 3.5% with electrolyte no. 45	25	15	450
Travasol 5.5% with electrolytes	70	60	850
Travasol 8.5% with electrolytes	70	60	1,160
Fat emulsion 10%, 20%, 30%	-	-	258-310

***Key:** 1 = hypotonic; 2 = isotonic; 3 = hypertonic.

Tonicity*	Calcium (mEq/L)	Magnesium (mEq/L)	Chloride (mEq/L)	Acetate (mEq/L)	Phosphate (mmol)	Other (mEq/L)
3	-	3	40	16	-	-
2	-	3	98	27	-	gluconate 23
2	5	3	103	47	-	lactate 8
3	3	5	41	47	3.5	amino acids 3% glycerin 3%
2	4 or 4.5	-	155 or 156	-	-	-
3	-	-	-	-	-	-
1	-	-	77	-	-	-
2	-	-	154	-	-	-
3	-	-	513	-	-	-
3	-	-	855	-	-	-
2	-	-	-	-	-	lactate 167
3	-	5	25	52	7.5	-
3	-	10	70	102	30	-
3	-	10	70	141	30	-
2	-	-	-	-	-	-

Estimating surface area in children

Calculate pediatric drug dosages based on body surface area or body weight. If your pediatric patient is of average size, find his weight and corresponding surface area in the box. Otherwise, to use the nomogram, lay a straightedge on the correct height and weight points for your patient and observe the point where it intersects on the surface area scale. *Note:* Don't use drug dosages based on body surface area in premature or full-term newborns. Instead, use body weight.

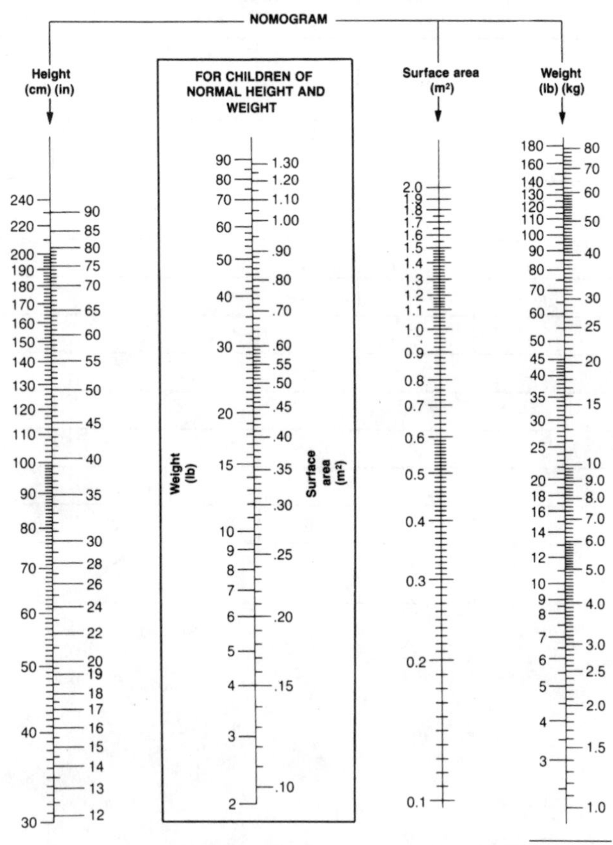

Nelson Textbook of Pediatrics, 15th edition. Courtesy W.B. Saunders Co., Philadelphia, 1996.

Estimating surface area in adults

To estimate an adult patient's body surface area, lay a straightedge from the patient's height in the left-hand column to his weight in the right-hand column. The intersection of this line with the center scale reveals his body surface area. The adult nomogram is especially useful in calculating dosages for chemotherapy.

Height

cm 200, 195, 190, 185, 180, 175, 170, 165, 160, 155, 150, 145, 140, 135, 130, 125, 120, 115, 110, 105, cm 100

79 in, 78, 77, 76, 75, 74, 73, 72, 71, 70, 69, 68, 67, 66, 65, 64, 63, 62, 61, 60, 59, 58, 57, 56, 55, 54, 53, 52, 51, 50, 49, 48, 47, 46, 45, 44, 43, 42, 41, 40, 39 in

Body surface

2.80 m², 2.70, 2.60, 2.50, 2.40, 2.30, 2.20, 2.10, 2.00, 1.95, 1.90, 1.85, 1.80, 1.75, 1.70, 1.65, 1.60, 1.55, 1.50, 1.45, 1.40, 1.35, 1.30, 1.25, 1.20, 1.15, 1.10, 1.05, 1.00, 0.95, 0.90, 0.86 m²

Mass

kg 150, 145, 140, 135, 130, 125, 120, 115, 110, 105, 100, 95, 90, 85, 80, 75, 70, 65, 60, 55, 50, 45, 40, 35, kg 30

330 lb, 320, 310, 300, 290, 280, 270, 260, 250, 240, 230, 220, 210, 200, 190, 180, 170, 160, 150, 140, 130, 120, 110, 105, 100, 95, 90, 85, 80, 75, 70, 66 lb

Geigy Scientific Tables; 1990, 8th ed., Vol 5, p. 105, ©Novartis.

Index

A

t refers to a table.

t refers to a table.

t refers to a table.

t refers to a table.

t refers to a table.

D

t refers to a table.

t refers to a table.

t refers to a table.

G

H

t refers to a table.

t refers to a table.

I

t refers to a table.

JK

t refers to a table.

M

t refers to a table.

t refers to a table.

QR

S

t refers to a table.

t refers to a table.

T

t refers to a table.

XYZ

t refers to a table.